# Pharmacology
# Clear & Simple

## A Guide to Drug Classifications and Dosage Calculations

### SECOND EDITION

# Pharmacology Clear & Simple

## A Guide to Drug Classifications and Dosage Calculations

### SECOND EDITION

Cynthia J. Watkins, RN, MSN

Medical Assisting Program Director
AHA Training Center Coordinator
Lorain County Community College
St. Joseph's Learning Center
Lorain, Ohio

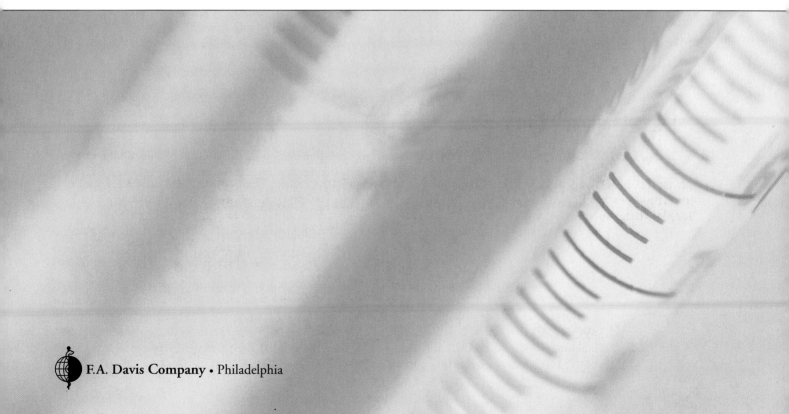

F.A. Davis Company • Philadelphia

F. A. Davis Company
1915 Arch Street
Philadelphia, PA 19103
www.fadavis.com

Copyright © 2013 by F. A. Davis Company

Printed in the United States of America

Last digit indicates print number: 10 9 8 7 6 5 4 3 2

*Acquisitions Editor:* Andy McPhee
*Developmental Editor:* Jennifer Ajello
*Manager of Content Development:* George Lang
*Art and Design Manager:* Carolyn O'Brien

**Library of Congress Cataloging-in-Publication Data**
Watkins, Cynthia J.
  Pharmacology clear & simple : a guide to drug classification and dosage calculations / Cynthia J. Watkins. — 2nd ed.
    p. ; cm.
  Pharmacology clear and simple
  Rev. ed. of: Pharmacology clear & simple / Nina Beaman. c2008.
  Includes index.
  ISBN 978-0-8036-2588-4 (pbk. : alk. paper)
  I. Beaman, Nina. Pharmacology clear & simple. II. Title. III. Title: Pharmacology clear and simple.
  [DNLM: 1. Pharmaceutical Preparations—administration & dosage—Problems and Exercises. 2. Dosage Forms—Problems and Exercises. 3. Drug Administration Routes—Problems and Exercises. 4. Medication Errors—prevention & control—Problems and Exercises. 5. Pharmaceutical Preparations—classification—Problems and Exercises. QV 18.2]

  615'.1—dc23
                                    2012035269

*I would like to dedicate this textbook*
*to the love of my life, Jeffrey Watkins,*
*who has been incredibly supportive of my venture*
*into the realm of being an author.*

# Preface

In my 20 years of pharmacology, I have taught a variety of students in nursing, medical assisting, surgical technology, and respiratory therapy. I have also taught those who may not deliver direct patient care, such as students of psychology and clinical lab science. There is always one constant challenge: to provide students with enough pharmacology knowledge so that they feel confident as they embark on their health profession careers but not so much that they are overwhelmed. For those students who will administer medication, pharmacology is critical; for others, it is a subject that will aid their understanding of the patient care relationship, although they may not be directly involved with the patient.

This edition of the book has been greatly expanded, just as so many of our reviewers asked for. I've tried to build on the solid foundation of the first edition and to expand the coverage of drugs, keeping in mind always the suggestions we received from pharmacology faculty from around the nation. I hope you'll be pleased with the results.

My goal for the second edition of this book is to divide pharmacology into elemental concepts to allow students to understand how medications work and how they are administered as well as health professionals' role in the process. This new edition is divided into four units:

- **Unit 1: Introduction to Pharmacology** discusses the fundamentals of pharmacology, including history, patient safety and regulations, and prescription labels. Each topic lays the foundation for the work ahead.

- **Unit 2: Calculations** begins with Chapter 6, Basic Review of Mathematics, which covers basic mathematical calculations and progresses to more advanced ones. This review provides many testing opportunities for students to assess their knowledge through the Check-Up exercises throughout the chapter. Chapter 7, Measurement Systems, addresses the various measurements systems and shows students how to convert among the metric, household, and apothecary systems. Chapter 8, Dosage Calculations, ends this unit by showing students how to calculate dosages. In this chapter, students have many opportunities to practice dosage calculations using a variety of examples to increase their knowledge and confidence in administering medications.

- **Unit 3: Administration of Medications** includes Chapters 9 and 10, Enteral and Parenteral Medications and Administration, which provide step-by-step instructions through Procedure Boxes with supporting images.

- **Unit 4: Classifications of Drugs** addresses all major drug classifications by body system. Although individual drugs are mentioned, each chapter primarily focuses on key attributes of that particular body system. This focus allows the student to understand how a particular set of drugs works and how individual drugs within that set function the same way.

## FEATURES

New features have been added to the second edition to further facilitate students in their learning and to help them better retain pharmacological content.

- **Check Up** boxes have mathematical calculation exercises in Unit 2. Each Check-Up appears following a math review section to test the student's knowledge and understanding of basic math concepts.

- **Fast Tip** boxes provide brief bits of useful information on various topics within the chapters.

- **Virtual Field Trip** boxes encourage students to use the Internet to research and locate important information on specific drugs, drug safety, and how to educate and instruct patients to use various medications.

- **A Closer Look** boxes examine special topics in each chapter.

- **Drug Spotlight** boxes highlight one or two drugs in each chapter and provide detailed information.
- **Critical Thinking** exercises encourage students to think beyond the chapter and apply their new knowledge to real-life scenarios.
- **Master the Essentials** tables cover indications, side effects, precautions, contraindications, interactions, and examples for each drug classification. They are perfect for study and review because all the drug classifications in the chapters are covered.
- **Chapter Review** questions in multiple formats appear at the end of each chapter to test student comprehension.

## Ancillary Content

- Accompanying the text are resources, both print and online, to help support both students and instructors.

## For the Student...

The student package facilitates easy retention and support for learning. Assets include:

- Dosage Calculation on CD-ROM
- Online Resource—Davis*Plus*:
  - Online review questions
  - Interactive syringe-pull activity in which students can practice pulling on a lifelike syringe plunger to specific marks on the syringe; this is a practice tool for administering parenteral medication
  - Tutorial on how to prevent medication errors
  - Animations showing drug absorption, drug distribution, metabolism, and excretion

## For the Instructor...

An Instructor's Guide accompanies this book with hundreds of multiple-choice, matching, and true-false questions to help prepare students for national certification examinations. PowerPoint slides are also available for every chapter. Instructors also receive the ExamView Pro Test Bank with more than 1,000 review questions. Documentation exercises and Medication Administration/Pharmacology competencies are also available.

I hope this second edition of *Pharmacology Clear & Simple* meets all your teaching and learning needs. And because drug information changes so often, keep track of new developments pertinent to your studies by checking the book's support page on Davis*Plus* (http://davisplus.fadavis.com Keyword: Watkins). Updates will be posted there twice yearly on the Student Resources page.

**Cynthia J. Watkins, RN, MSN**

**Michelle L. Blesi, BA, AA, CMA (AAMA)**
Program Director/Instructor
Medical Assistant Program
Century College
Coon Rapids, Minnesota

**Candy Dailey, RN, MSN, CMA (AAMA)**
Director, MA Program Director
Nicolet Area Technical College
Crandon, Wisconsin

**Alexandra Dell'Amore, RN**
Nursing Program
Santa Fe Community College
Santa Fe, New Mexico

**Gladys S. Gibbons, RN, BSN**
Instructor
Allied Health/Nursing Programs
Southeastern Technical College
Swainsboro, Georgia

**Kris A. Hardy, CMA, RHE, CDF**
Medical Assistant Program Manager
Brevard Community College
Institute of Nursing
Cocoa, Florida

**Glenda H. Hatcher, CMA (AAMA), BSN, RN**
Medical Assisting Instructor/Program Director
Department of Allied Health and Medical Assisting
Southwest Georgia Technical College
Thomasville, Georgia

**Dianna Johnston, MSN, RN**
Nursing Outreach Coordinator
Nursing Department
Eastern Idaho Technical College
Idaho Falls, Idaho

**Geri Kale-Smith, MS, CMA**
Coordinator, Medical Office Programs
Associate Professor
Department of Health Careers
Harper College
Palatine, Illinois

**Brenda Frerichs Ramstad, CMA, BS, MS**
Regional Director of Regulatory Operations
Career Education Corporation
Sioux Falls, South Dakota

**Jackie Shrock, RN, BSN, MEd**
Practical Nursing Instructor
Wayne Adult School of Practical Nursing
Smithville, Ohio

**Karen Snipe, CPhT, MEd**
Program Director, Pharmacy Technician
Department Head, Diagnostic & Imaging Services
Trident Technical College
Charleston, South Carolina

**Richard L. Witt, BS**
Instructor
Special Health Initiatives Department
Allegany College of Maryland
Cumberland, Maryland

# Acknowledgments

I thank Andy McPhee for recruiting me and having faith in my ability to complete this project. Thank you to Jennifer Ajello for all the assistance required to bring this work to publication. I want to acknowledge all the staff of F.A. Davis as well as the editors who have also had input on this project. Thanks to all!

# Contents in Brief

# Contents

# Introduction to Pharmacology

# History of Pharmacology

*Pharmacology has evolved significantly from the days when primarily plants, minerals, and animal products were used to cure the ill. In this chapter, you will learn about the history of pharmacology and sources used for developing drugs; the acceptance of alternative medicine, once considered "folk remedies" by some, and its place in medicine; and the six main categories of drugs and their uses.*

## LEARNING OUTCOMES

At the end of this chapter, the student will be able to:

1.1 Define all key terms.
1.2 List three societies critical to the development and evolution of pharmacology.
1.3 List four sources of drugs.
1.4 List 10 drugs and record their sources.
1.5 Discuss three examples of alternative medicine.

### KEY TERMS

| | | |
|---|---|---|
| Acupressure | Curative | Pharmacology |
| Acupuncture | Destructive | Pharmakon |
| Al-Hawi | Diagnostic | Porcine |
| Alternative medicine | Drug/*droog* | Prophylactic |
| Antineoplastic | Ebers Papyrus | Replacement drugs |
| Aromatherapy | Palliative | Synthetic drug |
| Bovine | Pharmacodynamics | Therapeutic touch |

## ◼ HISTORY OF PHARMACOLOGY

The term **pharmacology** is of Greek origin from two words: **pharmakon,** meaning "medicine," and *ology,* meaning "the study of." Pharmakon also meant poison *and* remedy, poison because some of the early medicines were toxic enough to kill, and remedy because, at times, early medicines cured the illness. The word **drug** has a Dutch origin in which **droog** meant "dry" as in the use of dry herbs.

Most ancient societies had little knowledge about the human body and how it worked, so treating illness was often based on trial and error. Early records document that treatments consisted of plants, minerals, and animal products because no other sources were available.

## Pharmacology in ancient times and cultures

Early documentation of medicine and various remedies is evident in several cultures. For example, "The Yellow Emperors' Inner Classic," a Chinese document, was a very early discussion of yin-yang and **acupuncture.** The first Chinese manual on pharmacology was written in the first century A.D. and included 365 medicines, 252 of which were herbs. In Egypt, a medical document called the **Ebers Papyrus** was written circa 1550 B.C. and lists about 700 "recipes" for a host of illnesses, from crocodile bites to psychiatric illnesses. Another document, the **Al-Hawi,** is a large, 20-volume medical book written by the ancient Iranian physician, Al-Razi. It was translated into Latin in the 13th century and greatly influenced medicine in medieval Europe.

The contributions from these cultures led to the advancement of pharmacology. Through trial and error, treatments for many conditions were discovered, and findings were recorded on papyrus or paper to pass on to future generations. Documenting this early information was extremely important as belief systems have changed over time. Without these earlier writings, much progress could not have been made.

## Pharmacological advances through the 19th and 20th centuries

"Healers" were known as wise men, shamans, witch doctors, medicine men and women, and so on (Fig. 1-1), depending on the culture, and were chosen based on their knowledge of plants. Early treatment was mainly guesswork, such as which herb or other substance to use, how to prepare it, and how much to give the patient.

During the 1800s, chemists were able to isolate the pure chemicals needed from the plant, and this marked the beginning of modern pharmacology. Unfortunately, by the early 1900s, preparing medicine was still very labor-intensive; the pharmacist still had to distill and prepare each medicine when it was ordered (Fig. 1-2). Not until approximately 40 years later, during World War II (1939–1945), did the mass production of medicine begin (Fig. 1-3). More U.S. soldiers died in World War I from infection and accidents than from actual combat injuries; however, the mass production of penicillin minimized the number of deaths from infection during World War II (Table 1.1). For instance, the death rate from pneumonia in the American Army was 18% during World War I, decreasing to 1%

**FIGURE 1-1:** Eskimo medicine man. *(From the Library of Congress Prints and Photographs Division, Washington, D.C.)*

**FIGURE 1-2:** Pharmacist making up a prescription, 1939. *(From the Library of Congress Prints and Photographs Division, Washington, D.C.)*

**FIGURE 1-3:** Mass production of medication, 1944. *(From the Library of Congress Prints and Photographs Division, Washington, D.C.)*

during World War II. Combat injuries, often complicated by infections leading to death, also decreased.

Pharmacology advanced rapidly in the second half of the 20th century as many new drugs were either discovered or developed. Use of natural sources for medicines led to a new belief that the artificial sources (those developed scientifically in a sterile laboratory setting) were far superior to the old "folk remedies," (although today, the value of natural sources in addition to or instead of artificial sources is gaining wider acceptance). Some of these natural or homeopathic sources are referred to as **alternative medicines** and include such modalities as massage, **aromatherapy,** and acupuncture.

## Pharmacology in the 21st century

The development of new medications is ongoing and endless; new technologies are developed daily. Genetic engineering can alter the source of drugs, thus allowing more drugs to be produced or creating different variations of the source. Plant hybrids may make taking multiple drugs unnecessary because scientists may be able to combine drugs that produce more than a single effect. Stem cell research will continue to have an impact on disease and its treatment. New plant discoveries in the rain forest can provide new medications. Soil samples tested daily will help scientists develop new antibiotics.

During the last few decades, the health-care community has gradually accepted that alternative medicine is a valuable complement to traditional treatment. Alternative therapies now seem to have a place in the healing of patients. For example, aromatherapy involves the use of fragrant oils in baths, as inhalants, or during massage to relieve stress and to treat skin conditions. **Acupressure** originates from an ancient Chinese art in which the application of pressure at certain points of the body is used to promote healing. Along similar lines is acupuncture. This therapeutic modality is also a Chinese art in which thin needles are inserted at certain points of the body to foster healing. **Therapeutic touch** involves the use of hand movements to stimulate circulation and healing.

**TABLE 1.1 U.S. Casualties in Major Wars**

| War | Number Serving | Battle Deaths | Disease and Accidents |
|---|---|---|---|
| Civil War | 2,213,363 | 140,414 | 224,097 |
| Spanish-American War | 306,760 | 385 | 2,061 |
| World War I | 4,743,826 | 53,513 | 63,195 |
| World War II | 16,353,659 | 292,131 | 115,185 |

Source: U.S. Department of Justice. From http://pbs.org/greatwar/resources/casdeath_pop.html

Alternative therapies are often used with traditional medication to help patients manage stress, pain, and hypertension. Initially, medication may be prescribed to deal with an acute issue, and alternative therapies may work toward a more long-term goal. As these alternative therapies are used, the medication may be changed, the dosage may be decreased, or the medication may be discontinued altogether.

### Virtual Field Trip

1. Use your search engine to locate a time line of pharmacology. Find information on other societies that contributed to the evolution of pharmacology in addition to the ones discussed in this chapter.
2. Use your search engine to find information on how pharmacology may evolve in the future.

# ■ SOURCES OF DRUGS

Although drugs are now manufactured in laboratories, many agents are still derived from natural substances such as plants, animals, minerals, and toxins. The original or natural source serves as a template for creating a synthetic equivalent. For this reason, scientists are constantly researching natural sources of medication. Some drugs are made by combining chemicals with natural products, such as epinephrine (adrenaline), whereas other drugs are artificially created in a laboratory (synthetic). Barbiturates are an example of synthetic drugs (Fig. 1-4).

## Plants

Many medications are derived from plants. Digoxin (Lanoxin), a drug used to treat heart failure, is made from the foxglove plant and has been used for healing since the 1500s. Epinephrine comes from the ephedra shrub. It is used, as it was in ancient China, as a bronchodilator. Most estrogen hormone replacements come from yams. Procaine (Novocain), used as an anesthetic, is derived from the coca plant. Rose hips are a rich source of vitamin C and are sold as an ingredient in vitamin C supplements. Aspirin comes from the bark of a white willow tree and is used to relieve pain and to treat inflammation.

Unfortunately, as less land becomes available for growing plants, fewer plants will exist for making medications. As the rain forest diminishes, the rare plants that are located only in this environment may become extinct.

#### ✳? CRITICAL THINKING

If people rely on plants for medication, what effect does the increasing human population have on the potential supply of medications?

## Animals

Domesticated animals are also a source of drugs. To ensure the purity of the drugs, donor animals are generally well cared for. Some examples include sheep, which provide lanolin, a topical skin medication that comes from the wool. Cows (**bovine**) and pigs (**porcine**) are good sources of hormone replacements. If a patient's body cannot manufacture a hormone, animal hormones can serve as a substitute. Horses provide humans with the replacement hormone conjugated estrogen (Premarin), which comes from a pregnant mare's urine.

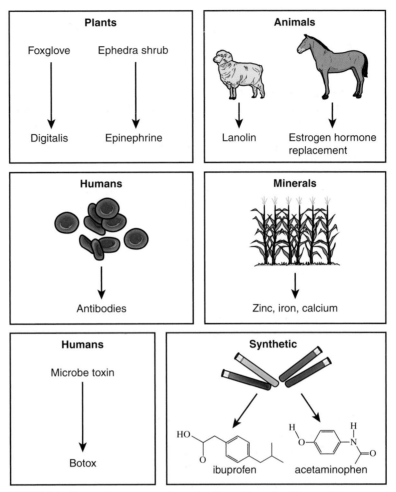

**FIGURE 1-4:** Current sources of medication. *(From the Library of Congress Prints and Photographs Division, Washington, D.C.)*

### CRITICAL THINKING

Cows and pigs are good sources of hormones. Do you think animals may be a better hormone source than humans? Why or why not?

## Minerals

When foods grown from rich soil are unavailable, calcium, iron, zinc, magnesium, copper, and selenium are some of the minerals that are offered as necessary supplements.

For patients taking certain medications, mineral replacement is critical. Diuretic drugs such as furosemide (Lasix) cause the body to lose excess water through the kidneys, and potassium, a vital mineral, is also excreted with the water. Potassium is needed for the heart to function normally, so supplemental potassium chloride is frequently prescribed in addition to the medication. Potassium is also contained in sweet potatoes, bananas, and oranges.

## Toxins

Toxins, by definition, are poisons. Despite this fact, chemical and biological toxins are commonly used in medicine. The key is in the dosage. For instance, certain radioactive chemicals are used to diagnose and treat illnesses. Radioactive iodine, for example, in small doses can help pinpoint problems in a patient's thyroid, a small gland in the neck. In higher doses, radioactive iodine is used to shrink thyroid tumors.

Biological toxins can also be used in medicine. Botulinum toxin (Botox), which comes from a bacterium called *Clostridium botulinum,* is used to reduce skin wrinkling. It is used in tiny doses.

### CRITICAL THINKING

What are some of the dangers of using toxins as medicine?

### Synthetic medications

**Synthetic drugs** can be created by genetic engineering or by altering animal cells. Often, drugs that are obtained from another source can be synthesized in the laboratory, thus preserving natural resources. For example, paclitaxel (Taxol), a drug for patients with cancer, was first made from the bark of the Pacific yew tree and then developed as a synthetic drug. Insulin can be obtained from pigs or cows, but a synthetic source is most commonly used. This change occurred because of concern over the possible transmission of disease from animals to humans. In addition, there is a risk of immune reactions because of impurities found in the animal products. One additional advantage is that synthetic medications are usually more inexpensive because they are mass-produced.

Because scientists have been able to map the human genome, it may be possible to make drugs specifically tailored to a patient. The scientist can manipulate the DNA material by changing it or combining it with DNA from another organism. Therefore, prescribers can choose drugs that work better for one population than for another. Research is also being conducted on the use of existing drugs in targeted populations. For example, BiDil is a combination of two generic drugs—hydralazine hydrochloride and isosorbide dinitrate—and is used to treat African American patients with heart failure.

### CRITICAL THINKING

What are some of the ethical issues with the synthesis of drugs?

### Virtual Field Trip

1. Use your search engine to discover sources of drugs used now and possibly in the future.
2. Use your search engine to locate information on recombinant DNA. How is it used to make medications?

## CATEGORIZING MEDICATIONS

The term **pharmacodynamics** refers to the effect of a drug on the body; or more scientifically, the negative and positive biochemical or physiological changes that a drug creates.. Drugs fall into six categories of desired effects (Table 1.2)

- **Curative.** Some drugs cure problems, as in diuretics, which help the body rid itself of excess fluid.
- **Prophylactic.** These drugs prevent problems, as in antibiotics given before surgery to prevent infection.
- **Diagnostic.** Some drugs help diagnose a disease, such as barium that patients swallow to help highlight digestive problems on a radiograph.
- **Palliative.** Other drugs, such as pain relievers, do not cure disease, but they make patients more comfortable.

### TABLE 1.2    Drug Categories

| Category | Main Action | Examples |
|---|---|---|
| Curative | Cure or treat problem | • Penicillin to treat strep throat |
| Prophylactic | Prevent a problem | • Cefazolin (Ancef, Kefzol) to prevent infections from surgery<br>• Vaccine to prevent measles, mumps, and rubella |
| Diagnostic | Help diagnose a disease or condition | • Diatrizoate meglumine and diatrizoate sodium (Gastrografin)<br>• Barium sulfate (both used for computed tomography scans) |
| Palliative | Treat symptoms to make patient more comfortable | • Morphine to relieve the pain of cancer<br>• Oxygen to make breathing more comfortable |
| Replacement | Replaces a missing substance | • Levothyroxine<br>• Natural thyroid to treat hypothyroidism |
| Destructive | To destroy tumors and/or microbes | • Carbimazole to inhibit the production of thyroid hormone to treat hyperthyroidism |

■ **Replacement drugs.** These drugs "replace" missing substances. Levothyroxine sodium (Synthroid), for example, is a drug that replaces a missing thyroid hormone.

■ **Destructive** medications destroy tumors and microbes. **Antineoplastic** (anticancer) drugs are an example of destructive, toxic drugs.

Medications are used for various reasons during a patient's life span. From infancy through late adulthood, people receive immunizations to prevent disease, antibiotics to treat infections, and pain medications to relieve the pain of an injury or illness. X-ray procedures may be needed to diagnose the presence or absence of cancer, medications are given to destroy that cancer, and women may need hormone replacement therapy of some type once they enter menopause.

CRITICAL THINKING

Identify the following drugs as curative, prophylactic, diagnostic, palliative, destructive, or replacement.

• Synthroid
• Diuretic ("water pill")
• Flu vaccine
• Radiopaque dye
• Fever reducer
• Anticancer drug

## ●●● SUMMARY

Medications, their sources, and their use are older than the written records we have. Many ancient cultures have contributed to the knowledge base and evolution of pharmacology, including Greek, Chinese, Egyptian, and Arabic. Some ancient remedies are still valuable medicines today, whereas others have been discarded as worthless or hazardous. The healers were called by many names, but all shared an extensive knowledge of plants. With the advent of the ability to isolate pure substances and to mass-produce drugs, companies are able to manufacture needed medicines in a timely manner.

Modern medicines are acquired from a variety of sources, from the plants and animals used thousands of years ago, to complete formulation of a drug in a laboratory. Society is again seeing the value in natural healing with plants, herbs, and other alternative medicines, as well as turning to science to create new and better medications.

# Activities

To make sure that you have learned the key points covered in this chapter, complete the following activities.

**Multiple Choice**

Choose the best answer for each question.

1. **Which of the following is the source of lanolin?**
   A. Animal
   B. Plant
   C. Mineral
   D. Human
   E. Synthesis

2. **Which of the following is the source of potassium chloride?**
   A. Animal
   B. Plant
   C. Mineral
   D. Human
   E. Synthesis

3. **Which of the following is the source of digoxin (Lanoxin)?**
   A. Animal
   B. Plant
   C. Mineral
   D. Human
   E. Synthesis

4. **Which of the following is the source of barbiturates?**
   A. Animal
   B. Plant
   C. Mineral
   D. Human
   E. Synthesis

5. **Which of the following is the source of leukocytes?**
   A. Animal
   B. Plant
   C. Mineral
   D. Human
   E. Synthesis

**6. During which war did mass production of penicillin begin?**

A. Civil War

B. World War I

C. World War II

D. Korean War

E. Vietnam War

## Short Answer Questions

Answer the following questions on a separate sheet.

1. Are animals good sources for drugs? Explain your answer.

2. What source of drugs is in danger of disappearing?

## Application Exercises

Respond to the following scenarios on a separate sheet.

1. Muhammed Al-Doost is a devout Muslim. He does not eat pork. Can he have porcine insulin?

2. Mary Littleton is adamantly against stem cell research and is refusing to use Humulin insulin. What do you think? Can you tell her that she can have this because it does not use stem cell research, or is she correct in her thinking?

# Basics of Pharmacology

*Chapter 1 discusses the history and evolution of pharmacology. In this chapter, we look at the science of pharmacology, how medications affect the body, how they interact with each other to produce either a positive or negative effect on the body, and why it is important as a prescriber to understand these effects and interactions. We begin by looking at **pharmacokinetics**, which is the study of metabolism and action of drugs with particular emphasis on the drug cycle and learn what happens once medications are ingested, injected, or applied.*

## LEARNING OUTCOMES

At the end of this chapter, the student will be able to:

2.1   Define key terms.
2.2   List the four steps in the drug cycle and their effects on the body.
2.3   Compare and contrast the usefulness of different drug resources.
2.4   Differentiate between a side effect and an adverse reaction.

### KEY TERMS

| | | |
|---|---|---|
| Absorption | Distribution | Receptors |
| Adverse reaction | Excretion | Side effects |
| Agonist | Half-life | Synergism |
| Antagonist | Idiosyncratic | Teratogenic |
| Biotransformation/Metabolism | Pharmacokinetics | Toxic |

## ■ WHAT IS PHARMACOLOGY?

What is pharmacology, and why is it studied? Pharmacology is the exploration of substances that are used to heal and comfort the sick and in other ways help us to live longer and healthier lives. Do you ever wonder who first felt a spider's web and thought: "This would make a good bandage"? Or who thought to taste a patient's urine to discover whether the patient had "sugar"? These pioneering individuals were extremely brave because they would likely have been banished or killed if they had guessed wrong. They were the first pharmacologists. These courageous men and women and their followers began the journey that led to the wonderful discoveries of the modern era. These advances have enabled us to increase life expectancy by eradicating most childhood illnesses and by producing antibiotics to cure many infections. The science of pharmacology has allowed us to research and produce potential medications without endangering the patient in the process.

# ■ THE DRUG CYCLE

When a medication is ingested, applied, or injected, it enters the bloodstream and begins the drug cycle. This cycle has four main phases: absorption (how the medication enters our bloodstream), distribution (how the medication travels to the appropriate site), metabolism or biotransformation (how our body breaks the medication down into usable components and waste products), and excretion (how our body eliminates the extra medication and waste products) (Fig. 2-1).

Factors influencing the time it takes to complete the drug cycle include the drug itself, the route of administration, and the health of the patient's organs. For example, medication given by mouth takes much longer to enter the bloodstream and to reach the site where it is needed than does medication given directly into the circulatory system. Some medications take longer to break down than others, and the effects of these drugs are prolonged. The estimated time for the cycle to be completed ranges from 15 minutes to days.

## Absorption

**Absorption** is the process by which a substance moves into the bloodstream from the site where it was administered. For example, a medication the patient takes by mouth must be transferred through the stomach or intestinal mucosa into the circulating blood. How quickly a medication is absorbed depends on how it is administered and whether it is topical or systemic. A drug can be administered in one of three ways: (1) enterally, which means the drug is given directly into the gastrointestinal (GI) system orally, rectally, or through a tube entering this system; (2) parenterally, by intramuscular, intravenous, subcutaneous, or intradermal injection; and (3) percutaneously, by inhalation, sublingually (under the tongue), topically, or transdermally.

A topical medication is applied directly to the site of concern. Examples include Desitin and Balmex to treat diaper rash. These creams work quickly in the local area of the rash. Systemic medications are taken by mouth or are administered intravenously or intramuscularly, to circulate throughout the body.

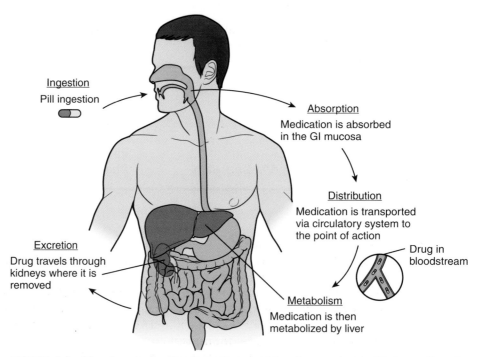

**FIGURE 2-1:** The drug cycle. The four phases of the drug cycle are (1) absorption via the gastrointestinal mucosa, (2) distribution via the circulatory system, (3) metabolism via the liver, and finally (4) excretion via the kidneys.

Liquid medications act faster than pills because pills must first be broken down to be absorbed. Intramuscular injections provide fairly quick absorption because muscles have a rich supply of blood to provide rapid entry into the circulation. Intravenous injection is the fastest way to the blood supply because the drug is injected directly into a vein.

As an allied health professional, you can take steps to facilitate drug absorption. For instance, when administering an ointment for a rash, you can make sure that the skin is clean and dry. If a prescriber orders an intramuscular injection, you will choose which muscle to use for best absorption. A tattooed arm could possibly hinder absorption because of decreased blood flow caused by scar tissue and tattoo paint. You would choose a muscle that is free of any lesions. Conversely, you must be careful when giving intravenous medications so that they are not absorbed too rapidly. For example, if morphine is given too rapidly, a patient may become severely hypotensive and stop breathing.

Other factors that may vary the absorption rate and bioavailability (how much of the drug is absorbed for use) of medications include fat and lipid solubility (ability to dissolve), the pH of the medication, the concentration of the medication, the length of contact, the patient's age, amount of food in the patient's stomach, and the patient's depth of breathing.

- *Fat or lipid solubility:* The more soluble a medication is in fat or lipids, the more easily it is absorbed through the stomach into the bloodstream.

- *pH:* Medications with a low pH (acidic) are easily absorbed in the stomach, whereas those with a higher pH (alkalotic) are less likely to be absorbed effectively.

- *Concentration of the medication:* The higher the medication concentration is, the more easily the medication is absorbed.

- *Length of contact:* The longer a topical medication remains on the skin or mucosa, the greater the absorption will be. If a patient sucks on a lozenge until it dissolves, more medication is released in the mouth than if the patient chews and swallows the lozenge.

- *Age:* Both children and older patients absorb more medication through the skin than do healthy adults, so topical medication is usually applied in a very thin layer.

- *Food:* A large amount of food slows the absorption of systemic medications. Stomach acid facilitates absorption of systemic medications; therefore, medication is absorbed faster when acid in the stomach is increased.

- *Depth of breathing:* For inhalants, the more deeply patients breathe, the more medication they inhale. For example, ask patients to inhale deeply to receive maximum benefit during treatment for asthma.

## CRITICAL THINKING

How does each of the following affect absorption?

Acidity of a drug

Tattoo on the skin

Drug concentration

## Distribution

The second phase in the drug cycle is **distribution,** which is the delivery of a drug to the appropriate site after the drug has been absorbed into the bloodstream. Sometimes the target area is close to the site of administration, but not always. For example, if a patient inhales a medication needed to alleviate the symptoms of asthma, the drug will reach the bronchi fairly quickly. However, an injection of the same drug would take longer to reach the lungs because it would first need to move through the circulatory system. Understanding which area or site the drug is intended to treat is important to help predict how quickly to expect a response to the medication.

Sometimes it is difficult for a drug to travel from the blood to an organ because of physiological "barriers," such as densely packed cells that allow nutrients and certain chemicals, but not other substances, including medications, to pass through them. These densely packed cells include the blood-placental barrier, the blood-brain barrier, and the blood-testicular barrier.

The blood-placental barrier helps to filter drugs and other substances passing from mother to fetus and thereby protects the fetus. However, alcohol, cocaine, and even some over-the-counter drugs can cross this barrier easily and cause harm. Most lipid-soluble and fat-soluble drugs readily cross this barrier, but water-soluble drugs do not. Many drugs, such as psychotropic (mind-altering) drugs, can cross the blood-brain barrier, although antibiotics and other drugs that are easily absorbed in the stomach cannot. The blood-testicular barrier protects the male reproductive organs from toxins that could damage sperm. This barrier also makes certain male reproductive diseases difficult to treat because very little is allowed through it except for substances directly involved in functioning of the testes. Many psychotropic drugs have negative sexual effects, such as decreased libido, because they cross both the blood-brain barrier and the blood-testicular barrier.

 *CRITICAL THINKING*

Why do drugs that cross the blood-brain barrier tend to have strong negative effects?

 *CRITICAL THINKING*

Why should a woman actively trying to become pregnant consult her physician before taking an over-the-counter medication?

## Metabolism

In the phase following distribution, the drug is metabolized by the liver, kidneys, and intestines. **Metabolism** or **biotransformation** means that the medication is gradually "transformed" to a less active or, in some instances, inactive form. A medication is a foreign substance that the body does not normally require. Metabolism is necessary to break this foreign substance down into particles that can be effectively removed from the body. This process could also be considered a way of detoxifying the body by removing substances that should not be there. The liver, kidneys, and intestines metabolize drugs. The liver does most of the work of drug metabolism by means of its enzymes. In some instances, a drug is administered in its inactive form to become activated through metabolism because the metabolite is the desired treatment. This category of drugs is known as prodrugs. An example of a prodrug is fosamprenavir (Lexiva) used in the fight against HIV. Sometimes this process may actually determine the route of administration because metabolism may transform the medication into a useless form too quickly. For example, insulin given by mouth is virtually useless; stomach acid breaks down insulin to an inactive form before it can be absorbed into the bloodstream.

 *CRITICAL THINKING*

David Marchefka has liver damage. How could that damage affect the way his body metabolizes drugs?

## Excretion

Once a medication has acted in the body, it is excreted. This process occurs mainly through the kidneys, although some medications are released as a gas by the lungs, and a few are excreted through bile. Saliva and sweat glands excrete a small amount of drugs, and some medications are excreted through breast milk.

**Excretion** is important because it ensures that waste products are removed and do not build up in the body (called cumulation). If buildup occurs, the patient may become very ill. For example, morphine buildup in a patient with decreased kidney or liver function may cause diminished or absent respiration.

Excretion is necessary also because of the specific time frame needed for exposure to a drug. A medication may not produce the desired effect if it is left in the system too long. Conversely, once a medication is metabolized, it may no longer be able to affect the body, and therefore its metabolites are removed. Scientists work very hard to discover and develop medications in the correct format and strength to provide precise treatment before these drugs are metabolized and excreted.

# ISSUES AFFECTING THE DRUG CYCLE

Therapeutic level, potency, and interactions with other medications affect the drug cycle. The therapeutic level of a medication refers to the point at which the drug has the maximum desired effect. Too little medication renders it less than effective; too much can be **toxic,** or poisonous, to the patient. To be sure the drug level is in the therapeutic range, blood levels may need to be monitored. In addition, if a prescriber orders a drug with known toxic effects, the patient must be monitored for toxicity. An example is gentamicin, which is known to be both nephrotoxic (toxic to the kidneys) and ototoxic (toxic to the ears). Thus, kidney function and hearing would be monitored closely in a patient taking this drug.

### Virtual Field Trip

Use your search engine to research *lithium*. Why is it important to obtain frequent blood specimens from patients who take lithium?

A drug's power or strength is called its potency, which typically increases and then decreases over time (Fast Tip 2.1). Taking more than one drug can affect potency. A drug is called an **agonist** when it is taken with another drug so the two can work together. The drug combination is more powerful than when each drug is taken separately **(synergism).** Common examples of synergistic combinations are

---

**Fast Tip 2.1   The Correct Anesthesia**

A medication's **half-life** is the length of time required for its concentration of a drug to decrease by one-half in the blood plasma and therefore affects the duration of potency for a medication. Drugs with a long half-life may need to be taken less frequently than those with a short half-life. The effects of drugs with shorter half-lives tend to wear off faster. For example, an anesthetic with a short half-life may be chosen if the patient plans to drive home from the facility soon after treatment.

Tylenol with codeine, used for pain relief, and codeine with a cough syrup to diminish the cough reflex and promote rest. **Antagonist** drugs do the opposite by rendering another drug less powerful. For example, birth control pills can become less effective when they are taken with certain antibiotics or minor tranquilizers. Another example is the antibiotic tetracycline, which becomes ineffective when it is taken with penicillin. The therapeutic level of a drug can be affected by other drugs, nutritional factors, body size, environmental factors, gender, and culture.

If a patient is taking several drugs, dosage adjustments may need to be made for each drug. Some drugs potentiate (strengthen) the effects of other drugs, and some weaken them. Natural and herbal remedies can also interact with drugs and affect dosing. Always ask the patient whether he or she is taking natural or herbal remedies. Whenever a combination of drugs is ordered, you must check your drug handbook to verify whether the drugs can be given together.

## ■ THE IMPORTANCE OF SIDE EFFECTS

Every medication carries a risk of side effects. The allied health professional must understand these effects and help the patient to prevent, minimize, or manage them. In addition, it is important to educate the patient about the distinction between symptoms that the patient should try to manage and symptoms that should be reported to the health-care provider immediately.

**Side effects** are usually mild, such as nausea, constipation, or sensitivity to light. Often, the patient can continue to take the medication and manage its side effects by taking the drug with food or by some other intervention such as taking care when rising from a sitting or lying position. An **adverse reaction** is a severe side effect such as shock or death. Adverse reactions may cause the prescriber to change a medication.

A topical drug has fewer side effects than a systemic one. For example, applying an anti-inflammatory drug such as diphenhydramine (Benadryl) directly to itchy skin reduces the chance of systemic side effects. However, when this drug is taken by mouth to treat the inflammation systemically, it can cause side effects such as drowsiness.

Side effects are usually classified by body system or organ. As an allied health professional, you should always check a drug resource guide for the side effects of the medications your patient is taking so you can be aware of them and counsel the patient accordingly. Even though a side effect may not be listed, a patient can have a unique, or **idiosyncratic,** reaction to any drug. The effect may not have occurred in clinical trials because it is so rare, but it must be managed. If the reaction is serious, report it through the MedWatch program. Through this program, run by the Food and Drug Administration (FDA), you can post reports on the Internet or by telephone. Guidelines for what and how to report are available at the FDA MedWatch Web site.

### Virtual Field Trip

1. Visit this Web site: http://fda.gov/safety/medwatch/default.htm
2. Under the spotlight section (right side of the page), find the drug safety communications link.
3. List and discuss at least two current drug safety issues.

### Side effects and the body systems

Any medication given is intended to have a single therapeutic effect, but because of the **receptors** (sites where medication binds to create a physiological effect) throughout every system of the body, many unwanted effects are felt. Side effects of the central nervous system include agitation, hallucinations, confusion, delirium, disorientation, depression, drowsiness, sedation, decreased respiration and circulation, dizziness, and coma. Muscle relaxants such as Flexeril (cyclobenzaprine) cause dizziness and drowsiness along with their intended actions.

As mentioned earlier, the liver is one of the main organs to metabolize medications, and it can be permanently damaged if drugs accumulate in it. Alcohol, acetaminophen, isoniazid, and aspirin can cause liver damage. Early side effects are detected by the presence of high liver enzyme levels in the blood. Jaundice (yellowing of the skin and eye) can occur if liver damage is undetected.

The GI system may suffer the most from medications because the most common side effects occur here. Examples of GI side effects include anorexia, nausea, vomiting, constipation, and diarrhea. With prolonged use of some drugs, stomach ulcers and colitis (inflammation of the intestines) can occur. The side effects are managed on an individual basis, depending on the medication. Some medications require ingestion with milk or food. For certain drugs, adding yogurt to the diet is suggested to prevent diarrhea, and others drugs may require the addition of a high-fiber laxative to the diet to prevent constipation.

Patients who take medications such as nonsteroidal anti-inflammatory drugs on a long-term basis run the risk of developing ulcers. The smallest effective dose is given to try to avoid this adverse effect. In addition, the synthetic prostaglandin misoprostol (Cytotec) may be given because it appears to prevent the development of ulcers. These patients are also urged to stop smoking to reduce the risk of ulcers.

As mentioned previously, the kidneys excrete most medications. Certain kinds of drugs (e.g., ibuprofen and other nonsteroidal anti-inflammatory medications) can damage kidney function because these drugs are primarily metabolized through the kidneys instead of by the liver. This is especially true for patients with preexisting kidney disease. Patients may experience symptoms ranging from fluid and electrolyte imbalance and abnormally high potassium levels. If kidney damage or impairment is suspected, blood urea nitrogen (BUN) levels may be monitored to evaluate kidney functioning. Impaired kidneys cannot effectively metabolize medications processed in the kidneys or excrete most metabolites from all medications. The result is toxic buildup of medications in the body.

Some medications, such as certain types of antibiotics and anticancer drugs, can cause ototoxicity, with resulting loss of hearing or balance. A previous example given is gentamicin, which is ototoxic. If gentamicin levels are not monitored closely, toxicity can cause permanent hearing loss and tinnitus. Another serious problem is the use of oxygen in premature infants. At high doses, oxygen is very damaging to the eyes. For this reason, oxygen is now used at the lowest therapeutic dose possible for all age groups.

Certain drugs can cause problems such as poor coagulation of the blood, bleeding, clotting, and immunosuppression. Anticancer drugs are especially toxic to bone marrow. Bone marrow produces all the blood supply, including the cells responsible for the immune system. Patients who lose large numbers of white blood cells have a high risk of infection. If their red blood cells are decreased, these patients will become anemic, leading to weakness, fatigue, and more difficulty in fighting off illness. Finally, when the platelets are depleted, control of bleeding becomes very challenging. Thus, any patient receiving chemotherapy requires close supervision of the hematological system to prevent serious complications. Any patient taking an anticoagulant such as Coumadin to decrease clotting should be carefully monitored for signs of bleeding, including dark, tarry stool. Coumadin levels should be monitored to ensure that the drug level is therapeutic but not toxic.

## Virtual Field Trip

Go to the following Web sites to find the information. If a Web site is not available, try to find the information through another source.

1. Go to http://mdadvice.com/. List the adverse effects of too much vitamin A (beta carotene, retinol).
2. Visit http://nlm.nih.gov/medlineplus/ and find the side effects of:
   Coumadin
   Ritalin
   Valproic acid
   Lithium
   OxyContin
3. Look at http://nlm.nih.gov/medlineplus/ Methotrexate kills cancer cells. What are its side effects?

# ■ DRUG RESOURCE FOR INFORMATION

Several medication resources are available to health professionals to help with safe administration of drugs to patients. These resources are divided into two categories: comprehensive and clinical. Both types are available in print and online.

### Comprehensive resources

Comprehensive resources cover medications in depth and are usually available only in print. The government produces two major comprehensive resources:

■ *United States Pharmacopoeia/National Formulary (USP/NF)*

■ *United States Pharmacopoeia/Dispensing Information (USP/DI)*

The *USP/NF* is the official source of medication information for drugs approved by the FDA. It is updated every 5 years, with frequent supplements. This publication provides standards for identification, quality, strength, and purity of substances. The *USP/DI* has two volumes; the first is written primarily for the prescriber, and the second is written in lay terms to make it easy for patients to understand.

A more widely used comprehensive resource is the *Physicians' Desk Reference (PDR)*, which is available in most health-care settings. This text contains information about thousands of drugs and is indexed by trade name, generic name, classification, and manufacturer. Color photographs of most common drugs are included to help identify medications when patients are unsure about what they are taking.

---

### A CLOSER LOOK: Organization of the *Physicians' Desk Reference (PDR)*

The *PDR* is organized as follows:

- Section 1 (white): Manufacturer's Index. This is an alphabetical listing of manufacturers with their addresses and phone numbers.
- Section 2 (pink): Brand and Generic Name Index. This is an alphabetical listing of medications by generic and trade names.
- Section 3 (blue): Classification Index. This section lists drugs by classification (e.g., antibiotics, analgesics).
- Section 4 (gray): Product Identification Guide. Manufacturers display photographs of medications. The drugs are listed by manufacturer.
- Section 5 (white): Product Information Section. This section contains the detailed information you would find on package inserts, alphabetized by manufacturer and then product.
- Section 6 (white): This is a catch-all section that includes the following: controlled substances categories; FDA use-in-pregnancy ratings; FDA telephone directory; poison control centers; drug information centers; and look-alike/sound-alike drug names

---

### Virtual Field Trip

Use your search engine and research *fetal alcohol syndrome*. What are the **teratogenic** (interferes with normal fetal development) effects of alcohol ingestion during pregnancy?

---

**Fast Tip 2.2**   Drug Handbook Features

Be sure you can easily find all these features when looking up a drug:

- Classifications of drugs
- Pregnancy categories
- Available forms
- Uses of drugs
- Action and therapeutic effects
- Contraindications and cautious use
- Route and dosage
- Administration
- Adverse effects
- Diagnostic test interference
- Interactions
- Pharmacokinetics
- Clinical implications

---

*CRITICAL THINKING*

**What are the advantages and disadvantages of comprehensive books such as the *PDR*?**

## Clinically based resources

In the daily clinical setting, the allied health professional turns to more user-friendly resources than the comprehensive sources discussed earlier. A pocket guide, or drug handbook, is optimal for easy access and often includes information in terms a patient can understand. Ideally, that handbook will indicate routes of drug administration, list appropriate doses, identify indications and contraindications, and explain how best to educate the patient regarding the medication. Sometimes a book is supplemented with a CD-ROM or digital downloads for your cell phone or other hand-held device (Fast Tip 2.2).

Another clinically based resource is the manufacturer's package insert, which accompanies all drugs. The patient receives the same information from the pharmacy. It is good to have this information on hand in case the patient has any questions.

Another valuable resource is the pharmacist, whether hospital or community based. Pharmacists often can answer questions for both health-care professionals and patients when the answers cannot be found elsewhere.

## SUMMARY

We study pharmacology to discover the most effective medications that cause the least amount of problems for patients. The drug cycle consists of four phases: absorption, distribution, metabolism, and excretion. Each phase has implications for the health-care worker. Health professionals must know how best to administer medications for optimal absorption into the bloodstream. For effective care and education of the patient, health-care professionals must also know where the medications will be distributed and any possible negative side effects. Health-care professionals must be vigilant about knowing how a drug is metabolized and what symptoms or laboratory test results to watch for that may indicate a potential issue. Finally, understanding how drugs are excreted and being aware of potential issues related to drug cumulation are critical. Health-care professionals are the patient's best advocate.

Several drug resources are available to help health professionals administer medication and educate patients. These comprehensive and clinical resources are available in book, digital, and Internet formats.

# Activities

To make sure that you have learned the key points covered in this chapter, complete the following activities.

## True or False

Write true if the statement is true. Beside the false statements, write false and correct the statement to make it true.

Cumulation means a drug causes disease. _____

An antagonist blocks a drug from being effective. _____

A drug's half-life is the time needed to decrease the drug's plasma concentration by 50%. _____

Psychotropic drugs can cross the blood-brain barrier. _____

Anticancer drugs do not cross the blood-placenta barrier. _____

Ototoxicity can damage the eyes. _____

Idiosyncratic means safe for children. _____

The primary organ of metabolism is the kidneys. _____

A package insert is a valuable source of information about medications. _____

BUN is a blood test looking at the function of the kidneys. _____

## Multiple Choice

**1. Which means leaving the body?**

  A. Absorption

  B. Biotransformation

  C. Distribution

  D. Excretion

  E. Metabolism

**2. Which means moving through membranes?**

  A. Absorption

  B. Biotransformation

  C. Distribution

  D. Excretion

  E. Metabolism

**3. Which means chemical alteration to another substance in the body?**

  A. Absorption

  B. Biotransformation

  C. Distribution

  D. Excretion

4. **Which means moving of the medication from site of administration to the target organ?**
   A. Absorption
   B. Biotransformation
   C. Distribution
   D. Excretion

5. **Ototoxicity occurs in the _____?**
   A. Eyes
   B. Ears
   C. Liver
   D. Kidneys
   E. Brain

6. **Nephrotoxicity occurs in the _____?**
   A. Eyes
   B. Ears
   C. Liver
   D. Kidneys
   E. Brain

7. **Which of the following are sources of information about medications?**
   A. *PDR (Physicians' Desk Reference)*
   B. *USP/DI*
   C. *USP/NF*
   D. Package insert
   E. All of the above

8. **What term means the point at which a medication has the maximum desired effect?**
   A. Therapeutic level
   B. Therapeutic range
   C. Toxic level
   D. None of the above

9. **Agonists are taken together to:**
   A. Interact with or counteract each other
   B. Work together
   C. Cause great pain
   D. Relieve great pain

10. **The section of the *PDR* that is a product identification guide is the _____?**
    A. White section
    B. Pink section
    C. Blue section
    D. Gray section

### Short Answer Questions
Answer these questions on a separate sheet.

1. Why would the physician order you to give an antagonist?

2. Why can a drug be toxic to a fetus without hurting the mother?

3. Why should a person abstain from operating heavy equipment if he or she is given a narcotic for nausea and vomiting?

4. Why would a physician give two different drugs at subtherapeutic levels?

5. The cabinet with all the drug resources is locked, and the key cannot be found. Where can you find out about an ordered medication before administering it?

### Application Exercises
Respond to the following situations on a separate sheet.

1. Mary is taking a blood thinner. She does not understand why she needs to have blood drawn monthly. How would you educate her?

2. Daniel has cirrhosis of the liver. How may this affect his metabolism of drugs?

3. Butler is coming in for a flu shot into the muscle. He insists that he wants the injection in his arm, not his buttocks. Both his arms are covered in tattoos. What would you do?

4. Rose has diabetes. Because of her diabetes, she has increased blood pressure and kidney problems. How does this affect the distribution and elimination of drugs from her body?

5. Jerry, an older patient, comes in with a paper bag containing assorted pills. He is not sure which he is supposed to be taking. What would you do?

6. You draw blood from Gary, to check compliance with drug therapy, but the laboratory results show none of that drug in his blood. What could be happening? What would you do?

7. Vera complains that she hears ringing in her ears ever since starting a new drug. What is this called, and what could be causing this?

# Patient Safety in Medication Administration

*This chapter discusses the basics of safe medication administration by identifying the right patient, using the right medication, measuring the right dose, administering the medication at the right time, using the right route, and documenting the right procedure in the right manner. Ethical issues pertaining to the administration of medication are discussed. In addition, this chapter introduces abbreviations used in prescribers' orders and recounts how to respond to allergic reactions and poisoning incidents. Finally, special considerations of which the health professional must be aware in practice are addressed.*

## LEARNING OUTCOMES

At the end of this chapter, the student will be able to:

3.1 Define all key terms.

3.2 List the seven rights of medication administration.

3.3 Explain the various considerations of medication administration.

3.4 Identify common abbreviations used in medicine administration.

3.5 Outline special considerations when administering medications to the elderly and to children.

3.6 Discuss cultural effects on drug use.

3.7 Name the actions taken during an emergency with a patient.

---

### KEY TERMS

Anaphylaxis
Antihypertensive
Geriatric
Health Insurance
    Portability and
    Accountability Act
    (HIPAA)

Lavage
Pediatric
Polypharmacy
Seven rights of
    medication
    administration

Teratogen
Teratogenic
Thrombolytic
Urticaria

---

# ■ PATIENT RIGHTS FOR SAFETY

Allied health professionals play a key role in ensuring that the patient safely receives a medication. When patients come to a medical facility, they may be in pain, grieving, depressed, frightened, or not at their mental or physical best. Therefore, you must take care when explaining and administering medications to patients.

To help you safely administer drugs, follow the **seven rights of medication administration.**

1. Right patient. Know the patient to whom you are administering the medication.
2. Right drug. Know the correct medication to be administered.
3. Right dose. Know the correct dose to give the patient.
4. Right time. Know the correct time the medication should be given, and inform the patient.
5. Right route. Know the correct route of administration by which the drug should be given.
6. Right technique. Know the correct method for administering the medication.
7. Right documentation. Know how to complete a patient's chart accurately, with all pertinent information.

Before you administer any medication, be sure that you have the right patient by asking the patient to verify his or her full name and birth date. Next, verify that you have the correct medication for that patient. In a hospital, the patient's name is on the medicine container, which is then sent to the nursing unit. In an office or a clinic setting, you will likely be the one to select the medication from a medication closet or cabinet, and the patient's name will not appear on the container. In either case, be sure to select the correct drug by using the following steps:

1. Check the label before you take the bottle from the shelf.
2. Check the label before you pour the drug out.
3. Check the label before you put the bottle back on the shelf.

Drug cabinets in medical offices are arranged with both convenience and safety in mind. Arrange medications by classifications or manufacturer. In a hospital, scanning a bar code to double-check a medication with a computer system may help reduce medication errors.

### ✱❓ CRITICAL THINKING

You enter the reception area of a medical office to look for the patient whose name is on the medication container. How can you be certain of giving the medication to the right patient? Because patients are sometimes confused or hard of hearing, how can you be certain that the patient who responds is the right one?

Once you have the right medication, you must ensure that the patient receives the right dose. If you suspect that a prescriber may have ordered an inappropriate dose, do not give the drug until you confirm it. The allied health professional must instruct patients and their caregivers in safe dosing and medication storage (Fast Tips 3.1 and 3.2), as well as emphasize that patients adhere to the exact prescription and avoid self-medication. What works for one patient may not for another. For example, if the patient is elderly or has liver or kidney problems, even a "normal" dose may be too much because the drug may not clear the body well and could accumulate to toxic levels.

Administering the medication at the right time is also critical. When a patient is in the hospital, medications are given according to hospital policy at a time that is convenient to staff members. At home, patients take their medications at a time that suits them. Morning medications, such as allergy pills, are usually taken with breakfast. Evening drugs, such as seizure medications, are taken at dinner. Drugs that help patients sleep at home are taken at the patient's usual bedtime, whereas drugs that help patients sleep in the hospital may be given at a set time. Some medications, such as antibiotics and antiseizure medications, need to be given a standard number of hours apart around the clock to maintain a consistent blood level.

---

### ● *Fast Tip 3.1*   Safe Medication Storage

Most people know that medications should be safely locked away from young children, but they fail to think about others in the household. This negligence can have tragic consequences when individuals lack knowledge about drug safety. For example, teenagers can abuse vitamin pills, cough syrup, cold medications, and inhalable drugs. Older people who are confused may take medications that are left, for example, on the counter. Emphasize to patients the need to store medications safely no matter what the age of others in the household.

---

### ● *Fast Tip 3.2*   Age, Size, and Dosage

Babies and young children require lower dosages because their bodies are small and process drugs faster. A dosage that works on a 150-pound adult is not appropriate for a 75-pound child. Many institutions have a policy requiring you to double-check your calculations with a coworker before administering a dose to a child.

---

Knowing where to administer the medication is also important. Most often, medications are given by mouth (PO). Sometimes drugs are given directly into other areas such as the ears, eyes, nose, vagina, or rectum. At other times, drugs are injected into a vein (intravenous [IV]), a muscle (intramuscular [IM]), skin (intradermal [ID]), or fat (subcutaneous [SC]). The pharmacist dispensing the medication may not know the patient or his or her special needs. For example, a liquid formulation may be necessary if the drug must be given through a feeding tube. In such cases, you need to alert the person dispensing the medication to your patient's individual needs.

Knowing the proper way to administer a medication by these various routes is important. For example, if an oral medication is given improperly, a patient could aspirate the medication into the lungs, thus causing a possible infection or other adverse reaction. If an injection is given at the wrong depth, angle, or site, possible nerve or bone damage could occur. Written procedure manuals are available for every procedure performed in the agency in which the patient is located. These manuals should be consulted whenever the health-care provider is unsure of the technique required.

Finally, be sure to document all pertinent information and know how to document a patient's chart accurately. Although a medical office can be busy, you must take the time for proper documentation whenever you give a medication. Be sure to document not only the medication but also the dose, route, lot number of the drug, and expiration date of the drug.

### Virtual Field Trip

Go to http://drugtopics.com and find the top 50 drugs most frequently associated with medication errors. List the top 10.

### ❋❓ CRITICAL THINKING

What kinds of drugs are usually prescribed to be given at equal intervals throughout the day? Explain why these drugs must be given at exact intervals. What could happen if doses are missed?

# ■ MEDICATION ADMINISTRATION

As an allied health professional, it is your responsibility to be sure that medications are administered safely. This involves learning the many abbreviations used on prescription orders and medicine containers, making sure that the medication schedule is appropriate for the patient's needs while taking into consideration the patient's other medications, and accounting for individual factors such as nutrition, weight, gender, and age.

Many drugs have similar spellings or pronunciations. These drugs, known as "look-alike/sound-alike names," are responsible for some of the most common medication errors. The Institute for Safe Medication Practices (ISMP) publishes the "List of Confused Drug Names." The Joint Commission also publishes a list of commonly confused look-alike/sound-alike drug names and requires that all accredited health-care agencies create a list for use in the institution (Table 3.1).

## Medication abbreviations

Abbreviations abound in medicine, and they are especially important during medication administration (Fast Tip 3.3). Many of these abbreviations are similar but have very different meanings. It is therefore very important to keep a list of abbreviations approved for your agency close at hand for reference. If you are in doubt about an abbreviation, spell out the entire word, look it up, or ask the person who wrote it to explain what was meant.

Sometimes, drugs are taken to coat the stomach before a meal or are taken on a full stomach to reduce the chance of nausea. If a drug is to be given before meals, the prescriber may write a.c. (ante cibum). For after-meal administration, the prescription is written p.c. (post cibum). Some medications can be taken as needed (abbreviated prn). Table 3.2 summarizes common abbreviations related to medication administration. Some of these abbreviations are based on Latin words.

---

### A CLOSER LOOK: Sinister and Dexter

Latin terms can seem daunting unless you can relate them to something familiar or interesting. Here is a story that can help you learn some abbreviations. In many cultures, both hands are washed after urinating or defecation. However, in some countries, running water is not always easily available to wash the hands. In those cultures, people usually designate their left (in Latin, *sinister*) hand as their "evil" hand. They use the left hand for dirty activities and the right (in Latin, *dexter*) hand for courtesies such as shaking hands or eating food from a communal bowl. This is why we customarily extend our right hand when we shake hands. It would be considered rude to extend the left hand because that is considered by many cultures to be the dirty hand. The abbreviation in Latin for ear is a. and for eye is o. Therefore, if a prescriber writes a.s., it means left (sinister) ear; o.s. means left eye.

---

The Joint Commission stated that certain abbreviations are particularly likely to be confused and should not be used (Table 3.3). Any abbreviation not on the official "Do Not Use" list published by the Joint Commission may be used in an institution as long as the abbreviation is included on an official abbreviation list posted in the agency's policy manual and updated annually.

### TABLE 3.1  Sample List of Confused Drug Names

| Drug Name | Confused Drug Name | Drug Name | Confused Drug Name |
|-----------|--------------------|-----------|--------------------|
| Adderall | Inderal | heparin | Hespan |
| Advair | Advicor | Klonopin | clonidine |
| Amicar | Omacor | Leukeran | leucovorin calcium |
| Benadryl | benazepril | OxyContin | Oxycodone |
| Celebrex | Cerebyx | Retrovir | ritonavir |
| Cozaar | Zocor | | |

> ● *Fast Tip 3.3*   Memory Joggers for Frequency of Drug Administration
>
> - *Bi*cycles have two wheels, so *bid* means twice a day.
> - *Tri*cycles have three wheels, so *tid* means three times a day.
> - *Quad*rangles have four sides, so *qid* means four times a day.

## TABLE 3.2   Abbreviations for Drug Administration

| | | | |
|---|---|---|---|
| **a.d.** | Right ear | **o.d.** | Right eye |
| **a.s.** | Left ear | **o.s.** | Left eye |
| **a.u.** | Both ears | **o.u.** | Both eyes |
| **bid** | Two times a day | **PO** | By mouth (orally) |
| **c̄** | With | **qid** | Four times a day |
| **ID** | Intradermally (into skin) | **s̄** | Without |
| **IM** | Intramuscularly (into a muscle) | **SC** | Subcutaneously (into fat) |
| **IV** | Intravenously (into a vein) | **tid** | Three times a day |
| **NPO** | Nothing by mouth | | |

## Medication schedules

The allied health professional may need to help the patient develop a schedule for taking medications at home. Sometimes, it is helpful to write a clear schedule on a chart for the patient to put on a wall at home (Fig. 3.1).

Although most orders are for drugs to be administered, prescribers may order that a drug *not* be given for a period of time or that a drug be discontinued. If a patient is having a test the next day that requires the gastrointestinal system to be clear, either for better diagnostic imaging or to prevent aspiration (inhaling into the lungs) of vomitus, the prescriber may want the patient to take nothing by mouth (abbreviated NPO) after midnight. Patients with diabetes who are NPO usually should not be given insulin because no food is available to interact with the insulin.

The physician may also order a medication to be discontinued. Perhaps the patient does not need it anymore, or the prescriber wants to change the medication. You must tell the patient *not* to take

## TABLE 3.3   Abbreviations to Avoid

| Do Not Use | Potential Problem | Preferred Term |
|---|---|---|
| U (for unit) | Mistaken for zero, four, or cc | Write "unit" |
| IU (for international unit) | Mistaken for IV (intravenous) or 10 (ten) | Write "international unit" |
| q.d. and q.o.d. | Mistaken for each other; the period after the "q" can be mistaken for an "I" and the "o" can be mistaken for "I" | Write "daily" and "every other day" |
| Trailing zero (x.0 mg); lack of leading zero (.x mg) | Decimal point is missed | Never write a zero by itself after a decimal point, and always use a zero before a decimal point (0.5 mg) |
| MS, MSO$_4$, MgSO$_4$ | Confused for one another; can mean morphine sulfate or magnesium sulfate | Write "morphine sulfate" or "magnesium sulfate" |
| **Avoid Using** | | |
| µg (for microgram) | Mistaken for mg (milligrams, resulting in 1,000-fold dosing overdose) | Write "mcg" or "micrograms" |
| > (greater than) | Misinterpreted as the number 7 (seven) or | Write "greater than" |
| < (less than) | the letter L | Write "less than" |
| @ | Mistaken for the number 2 (two) | Write "at" |
| cc | Mistaken for U (units) when poorly written | Write "mL" or "milliliters" |

**Your name**   Chester Earl

| Weekly Medicine Record | | | Week of  August 1, 2012 | | | | | | |
|---|---|---|---|---|---|---|---|---|---|
| **Name of Medicine and Dose** | **Shape, Size, and Color of Pill** | **When to Take** | **Place an X after taking each dose** | | | | | | |
| | | | **Sun** | **Mon** | **Tues** | **Wed** | **Thurs** | **Fri** | **Sat** |
| 1. Digoxin 0.125 mg | Round, 1/4 diameter, white | Daily | X | X | *Need refill* | | | | |
| 2. Coumadin 3–4 mg | Round, 5/16 diameter, blue | Daily | X | X | X | | | | |
| 3. Furosemide 40 mg (Lasix) | Round, 5/16 diameter, white | Daily (morning) | X | X | X | | | | |
| 4. Nitroglycerin 0.4 mg (transdermal system) | Patch | Daily (12-14 hs) | X | X | X | | | | |
| 5. Monopril 20 mg | Elongated, 3/8 diameter, white | Daily | | | | | | | |
| 6. Oyster Shell Calcium 1500 mg | Round, 1/2 diameter, gray | Daily (morning) | X | X | X | | | | |
| 7. Potassium (K-Dur 20 mEq tablet SA Sch) | Large 13/16 x 3/16 x 3/16, white | Daily (morning) | X | X | X | | | | |
| 8. Tylenol 650 mg caplets | Caplet | As needed for headache | | X | | | | | |
| 9. Chlorpheniramine maleate (allergy tablets) 4 mg | Round tablet, 3/16 diameter, yellow | As needed for sleeplessness | X | | X | | | | |

**FIGURE 3-1:** Sample medication schedule for the patient's use at home.

the medication. For example, when a patient is taking a medication to lower blood pressure and the physician decides to change to a different medication with the same effect, the patient's blood pressure may become dangerously low if both medications are taken. Instruct the patient to throw out old prescription medications that have been discontinued, to prevent inadvertent ingestion.

### CRITICAL THINKING

Rachael Smith has been told to be NPO after midnight before an x-ray series of her bowels. She calls to see whether she should take her morning dose of insulin. An office assistant says that she should take it because insulin is not given by mouth. If you had taken her call, what would you have said or done? Explain you answer.

### CRITICAL THINKING

Imagine that you gave Cecile Masse 1 mL of a flu shot in the left deltoid muscle. You took the vaccine from a container that said lot no. 1234567, which expires on 12/01/14. How would you document this procedure?

## Factors affecting medication administration

When administering medications, certain factors must be considered to ensure that, as a health professional, you are following the seven rights. These factors include the following: nutrition and physical activity; age, gender, and culture; environment; pregnancy; and organ dysfunction.

### Nutrition and physical activity factors

Some nutrients are needed for absorption; a poor diet may reduce therapeutic levels. For instance, administering tetracycline (an antibiotic) with calcium prevents the absorption of tetracycline. Most antibiotics work best when taken on an empty stomach. Food high in vitamin $B_6$ can impair the actions of drugs used to treat Parkinson's disease. Grapefruit juice inhibits the effectiveness of some drugs if both are ingested at the same time. A patient who is dehydrated may have a medication blood level that is higher than normal. Consult your drug reference for any food interactions that the patient should be made aware of before a new medication is begun. Additionally, exercise can influence metabolism and cause medications to be absorbed more quickly. Exercise also decreases the need for insulin and is used to control blood glucose concentrations in patients with diabetes. Chewing gum increases saliva, which enhances food breakdown and absorption.

Drug dosing is usually based on total body weight. Normal doses are based on an average adult body weight of 70 kg (about 150 lb). However, size and distribution of fat in the patient can change the way the drug is processed. If a drug that does not penetrate fatty tissues is used in obese patients, the dose may have to be higher than usual.

Similarly, underweight patients may need smaller amounts of drugs because of their lower body weight. Patients with amputated limbs also require lower doses because of lower body weight.

### Age, gender, and culture

A patient's age, gender, and cultural background may influence medication administration. These factors must be taken into consideration.

In terms of age, drug administration guidelines are based on the average weight and height of an adult patient. However, a health-care professional must consider two populations when administering medications: the elderly, or **geriatric,** population and the young, or **pediatric,** population.

#### Geriatric patients

In patients more than 55 years old, decreased absorption results from diminished gastrointestinal function and congestion of abdominal blood vessels. Distribution can also be altered by low plasma protein levels, particularly if the patient is malnourished. When plasma proteins are decreased, a larger amount of unbound drug increases the drug's action. Thus, toxic drug levels can be found in elderly patients, even at normal doses. The aging process also alters liver and kidney function and leads to accumulation of medications. Body composition changes as we age. Elderly patients have increased fatty tissue and decreased skeletal muscle and water. All these age-related changes slow drug absorption and distribution.

Because of these factors, doses may need to be adjusted for elderly patients. Of special concern are sedative-hypnotics (anticoagulants, nonsteroidal anti-inflammatory drugs [NSAIDs]), **antihypertensives** (drugs that lower blood pressure), and **thrombolytics** (drugs that break up blood clots). These medications are most commonly associated with adverse drug events. For example, sedative-hypnotics may be used to calm a patient, but they can worsen agitation and exacerbate dementia.

Another concern for geriatric patients is **polypharmacy,** defined as taking several medications for more than one problem. Multiple medications increase the risk of drug interactions and side effects. The health professional must spend more time on educating the elderly patients because their treatment regimens are often more complex, and it may take these patients more time to understand the specifics of each medication.

#### Pediatric patients

Pediatric patients comprise a unique population. Children have a higher metabolism but lower weight than adults and therefore require less medication. Dose amounts and administration vary, depending on the age of the child.

A neonate or premature baby has special needs. Because the renal system and some endocrine systems of these infants are not mature at birth, drug metabolism and excretion are impaired. Their nervous system and blood-brain barrier of these children are also not mature at birth; thus, the central nervous system is more susceptible to the effects of medications. In addition, because these infants are so small, any dosage miscalculation could be devastating. Medications such as digoxin and certain antibiotics that are used in older infants may therefore be much trickier to use in the newborn. The prescriber must be extremely meticulous in determining the proper dose for infants younger than

1 month. Drugs that are ototoxic and nephrotoxic are not given or are given very cautiously in the newborn. Premature infants have developed both hearing loss and kidney disease from some of these drugs, but the alternative is death from infection. The gastric pH and gastrointestinal motility of neonates and premature infants differ from those of an older child or an adult. Because weight changes rapidly in infants, frequent dose adjustments must be made.

Infants also have poorly developed arm muscles. Therefore, medications that must be given intramuscularly are injected into the infant's thigh because it has more muscle. The blood vessels of infants and children are more fragile than adult blood vessels, and these patients can easily become overhydrated if intravenous therapy is not carefully monitored. Children are frequently afraid of injections and other interventions, so age-appropriate explanations about the procedures to these patients may be necessary.

Most drugs are not tested on pediatric patients, and a drug tested in adults may not act the same way in a child (Table 3.4). Be especially alert to side effects, and fill out a MedWatch form if the child has an adverse reaction.

## CRITICAL THINKING

How do pediatric patients differ from adult patients regarding the following?

Dosage amount

Site of administration

Length of needle for parenteral administration

Fat and muscle body composition

Metabolism of medication

Blood vessel fragility

Blood volume

Cooperation with therapy

Gender must also be considered when administering medication. Men typically have more muscle than fat, as compared with women. Therefore, medications are absorbed and distributed in the body more quickly in men than in women. Other gender differences are body water content, metabolic rate, and gonadal hormone variations. Men tend to respond to different antidepressants than women because of the hormones found in each.

## TABLE 3.4 Pharmacology in Neonates, Infants, and Young Children*

| Developmental Factor | Effect |
| --- | --- |
| Gastric pH is higher in neonates and infants; adult levels at 20–30 months | Decreased absorption in younger patients |
| Irregular emptying time for stomach; adult functioning at 6–8 months | Unpredictable absorption |
| Decreased lipase secretion in infants | Poor absorption of lipid-formulated drugs |
| Thin stratum cornea in infants | Increased absorption of topical medications applied in the eye |
| Rectally administered drugs absorbed more | Increased absorption possibly leading to toxicity quickly in infants |
| Variable blood flow to muscles of neonates | Unpredictable absorption of drugs injected into muscle |
| Larger percentage of extracellular and total water in the body in neonates and infants | Wider distribution of drugs |
| Higher ratio of water to lipid in neonates and young adults in adipose tissue | Lower level of drug in bloodstream |

*Because children's bodies are not fully developed, it is especially important to monitor drug effects in these age groups.

A person's culture can also affect the use of medications.. Some cultural beliefs are grounded in scientific research, and people in these cultures find comfort in knowing that medications have been rigorously tested before approval. These patients are more likely to depend on their primary health-care provider to choose drugs for them.

Conversely, more holistic cultures believe that imbalances in a person's life cause disease. People with a holistic outlook may be less likely to use conventional drugs and more inclined toward herbal remedies.

Other cultures believe that illness comes from evil spirits who hurt people if taboos (rules) are broken. People in these cultures may search for alternative healers and may or may not continue to take medications prescribed by their primary health-care provider.

### CRITICAL THINKING

Seth Eaton comes to the office with a wound that does not seem to be healing. As he is leaving he states: "I am going to see my herbalist. Your drugs can't help me!" What would you do or say?

### Environmental factors

Smoking cigarettes induces liver enzymes to metabolize drugs more rapidly. For this reason, patients who smoke cigarettes may need larger doses of liver-metabolized drugs than do nonsmokers. The effects of active and second-hand smoke may persist for months.

### Pregnancy

Pregnancy is another consideration when administering medications. Drugs affect not only the mother, but also the fetus she is carrying. The blood-placental barrier protects the fetus from the effects of certain medications. Water-soluble medications such as heparin are kept from crossing this barrier, although fat-soluble medications are more like to cross it. Severe malformations or death of the fetus can occur if a **teratogenic** (causing deformities) drug crosses the placenta.

The fetus is especially vulnerable to medications during the first trimester, when vital organs are forming, and the last trimester, when the baby is prone to accumulating drugs before birth. The Food and Drug Administration (FDA) classifies drugs according to their safety during pregnancy (Table 3.5). Always check your drug handbook before giving a drug to a pregnant woman, to ensure that it is not a **teratogen** (substance that impairs normal fetal development).

### CRITICAL THINKING

If an obstetric patient calls and asks what over-the-counter drugs she can take for a cold, where would you find that information? How would you explain your responses?

**TABLE 3.5  Food and Drug Administration Drug Safety Categories for Pregnancy**

| Category | Risk | Description | Examples |
|---|---|---|---|
| A | Lowest | Studies have not shown a risk to mother or fetus | Levothyroxine (Synthroid) |
| B | Slight | Animal studies have not shown a risk to the fetus, or if they have, human studies have not | Insulin (Humulin R) |
| C | Moderate | Animal studies have shown a risk to the fetus, but controlled studies have not been performed on women | Furosemide (Lasix) |
| D | Risky | Studies show these drugs may cause harm to the fetus, so the prescriber must weigh risk against. benefit; may use if another, safer therapy is not available | Warfarin (Coumadin) |
| X | Highest | Studies have shown significant risk to mother and fetus | Castor oil (Purge) |

### Patients with organ dysfunction

As discussed in Chapter 2, great care must be taken when medications are administered to patients with organ dysfunction because drugs can easily build up to undesirable levels. Pay close attention to the kidneys, liver, and heart, the organs most affected by systemic drug accumulation. The liver and kidneys metabolize and excrete medications, and the heart may change how quickly and effectively a medication is distributed throughout the circulatory system.

Because the liver metabolizes drugs, poor functioning of this organ leads to an accumulation of drugs and to toxic effects. Patients who abuse alcohol on a long-term basis may have destroyed much of their liver's ability to function. Decreased serum protein levels can alter the capacity of a drug to bond. More unbound medication is therefore available, and this can lead to side effects. Unfortunately, no laboratory test adequately predicts appropriate doses when the liver is not working properly.

### CRITICAL THINKING

How does liver disease affect the accumulation of drugs in the body?

Most drugs are metabolized in the liver and are excreted through the kidneys. Other drugs are excreted unmetabolized through the kidneys. Not only can this process destroy the kidneys, it also puts patients with kidney disease at risk for accumulating toxic amounts of drugs. To determine proper doses of drugs in patients with kidney disease, blood specimens are drawn for laboratory tests, such as blood urea nitrogen (BUN) and creatinine clearance (CrCl).

In patients with heart failure, the heart fails to pump fluid adequately. This condition can cause congestion of blood vessels in the gastrointestinal tract that decreases drug absorption and drug delivery to the liver. Kidney function is also compromised by the congestion, with resulting delayed excretion and thus drug accumulation in the patient. For these reasons, patients with heart failure usually take lower doses of medications.

## ■ PROTECTING THE PATIENT: ETHICAL AND SAFETY CONSIDERATIONS

As an allied health professional, it is your responsibility to see that medications are administered safely and to ensure that the patient's rights, consent, and privacy are equally protected. You also have the responsibility of responding quickly, safely, and ethically should a patient have a medication emergency such as accidental ingestion of too much medication or an acute allergic reaction.

### Patient information

Patients have a right to participate in planning their treatment. Thus, it is important to teach patients about their medications in terms they can understand. Although you may understand medical terminology, the patient most likely does not. Misunderstandings can lead to injury, overdose, or subtherapeutic treatment. For example, patients may believe that taking more pain medication will relieve pain better or faster. If a patient is told to take a narcotic every 6 hours as needed for pain, he or she may take it more often and may not know that this could cause confusion, respiratory depression, or death. It is your responsibility as a health professional to educate the patient about the risks associated with taking more than the prescribed dose.

One way to ensure that patients receive enough information is to teach them to ask the questions in box 3.1 whenever they start a new medication.

### Virtual Field Trip

Go to http://ismp.org (Institute for Safe Medication Practices), and list the topic of this month's alert.

---

**BOX 3.1 What You Need to Know About Prescription Medicines**

As an allied health professional, you should encourage patients to discuss their medication regimens with their health-care providers. When a new medicine is prescribed, patients can refer to the following list of questions to ask the prescriber or pharmacist.

- What are alternative names for this medication?
- What is it supposed to do?
- Is there a less expensive alternative?
- Why am I taking it?
- How and when do I take the medicine and for how long?
- Should I store it in the refrigerator or the cabinet?
- Should I take it with water, food, or with another medication?
- Can it be taken with over-the-counter medicines? Alcohol?
- What do I do if I miss or forget a dose?
- How long should I wait between doses?
- If taken "as needed," how will I know I need it?
- What food, drinks, other medicines, dietary supplements, or activities should I avoid while taking this medication?
- Will any tests or monitoring be required while I am taking this medicine? Do I need to come to the office with a certain frequency?
- What are the possible side effects, and what should I do if they happen?
- When should I expect the medication to start working, and how will I know if it is working?

---

## Patient consent

Patients have the right to refuse treatment, including medications. If patients do not understand why they are required to take a medication, you should first give them the appropriate information. If they are still reluctant to take a medication, inform the prescriber. Giving a medication to someone who refuses to take it can be considered assault and battery.

A disoriented patient may not understand the treatment plan. Therefore, you may need to advocate for the patient. If the patient is frightened or confused, he or she may refuse an injection or to swallow a medication; educating the patient may facilitate understanding.

A patient who is taking an experimental drug has the right to informed consent, which means understanding the treatment, its effects, alternative treatments, and the possible outcome if the treatment is declined. It is essential to document informed consent. Ensure that the patient is comfortable with the decision and that the informed consent is documented correctly. If the patient seems reluctant to sign the consent form, notify the physician of your observation.

## Patient privacy

Patients have rights to privacy. Medication records, like many items in the patient's medical record, are to be kept confidential, except for release to pharmacists and other professionals involved in the care of the patient.

Patients also have a right to receive medications in a quiet, private place. The **Health Insurance Portability and Accountability Act (HIPAA)** holds allied health professionals accountable to the government to protect the privacy of the patient. Health professionals should take the steps necessary to ensure that all communications are confidential. For instance, to call a colleague across a waiting room to announce that a drug is ready for a patient whose name has been called out loud is illegal as well as unprofessional.

HIPAA standards also allow patients access to their own medical records and offer them more control over how the information in their records is shared. All health-care providers must supply patients with a notice alerting them to their rights and that medical information cannot be revealed to other people without the patient's consent. For more information on HIPAA, visit http://dhhs.gov/.

## CRITICAL THINKING

While entering a crowded reception room, a medical assistant calls back to a colleague that she has to tell a patient the results of her test for a sexually transmitted disease. Immediately afterward, the medical assistant calls the patient's name aloud. Is this appropriate? How could she have better handled patient confidentiality?

## Patient emergencies

If a patient comes to your office or facility and presents with signs of accidental or deliberate medication overdose, you must respond quickly. Refer to office or facility protocols, but usually the first step is to notify the physician immediately and begin the ordered treatment.

If you receive a call from a patient who has ingested a toxic substance, call 911 or ask the patient to do so immediately. Usually, when you activate the emergency response system, the dispatcher will connect you to a poison control center. Experts at poison control hotlines are trained to manage toxic substance emergencies and have access to the latest research and recommended treatments. If possible, identify the substance so the staff can better diagnose and treat the problem.

The staff members at a poison control center may ask you to do any of the following, depending on the type of toxin:

■ Administer activated charcoal, which will bind with the poison. Activated charcoal is usually administered by emergency medical personnel in the field or in emergency departments. This treatment is usually administered after **lavage** (pumping) of the patient's stomach to remove the toxin. If the toxin is caustic, lavage is not done because of the damage caused on ingestion: removing the substance may cause further harm.

■ Have the patient drink a large amount of water to dilute the poison.

■ Have the patient drink milk to reduce acidity.

■ Monitor the patient for symptoms such as changes in vital signs (heart rate, respiratory rate, blood pressure, and temperature), seizures, and altered level of consciousness.

Follow the directions of the experts carefully. Immediate treatment of a toxin overdose can save the patient considerable discomfort and harm. Most poison control centers no longer suggest that vomiting be induced with syrup of ipecac because it is not completely effective and can cause complications. There has been some discussion of taking syrup of ipecac off the market.

### Virtual Field Trip

Visit http://aapcc.org (American Association of Poison Control Centers) and find which drug most commonly poisons patients.

In an emergency situation, ask the patient whether he or she has any allergies to medications *before* giving another medication. An allergic reaction may include **urticaria** (hives), in which the skin becomes red and itchy. Notify the physician immediately if this occurs.

A severe allergic reaction is called **anaphylaxis.** It is especially dangerous if swelling occurs in the neck because the swelling can constrict the trachea and cause death from suffocation. Patients experiencing anaphylaxis have difficulty breathing and may have other symptoms, such as itching, wheezing, anxiety, and light-headedness. The physician may order you to give a medication to reverse the anaphylaxis, such as epinephrine or diphenhydramine (Benadryl). It is safe and best practice to observe a patient for 15 minutes following an injection, an antibiotic, or an allergy shot to be sure that an allergic reaction is not missed. Document your observation period, such as in the following example: "Patient observed for 15 minutes after allergy shot. No signs of anaphylaxis noted."

● ● ● S U M M A R Y

Medication administration is regulated for the public's safety. As an allied health professional, you are responsible for the safe administration of medications. This includes always administering the right drug, in the right dose, at the right time, by the right route, to the right patient, using the right technique, and then documenting the administration correctly.

To administer medications safely, you need to know the acceptable abbreviations used to understand the medication order. Medication administration is affected by many variables, such as the patient's nutrition status and physical activity, as well as his or her size, age, and gender. In addition, patients' cultural beliefs, their home environment, and their pregnancy status affect the medication they may use.

Always remember that as an allied health professional, you must respect patients' rights to receive accurate information, obtain informed consent, and protect patients' privacy. In addition, remember that patients have the right to refuse treatment. Be alert to signs of poisoning or anaphylaxis and act appropriately to correct any problems. Documenting your observation of the patient and your response to symptoms is vital.

# Activities

## True or False

Write true if the statement is true. Beside the false statements, write false and correct the statement to make it true.

In patients more than 55 years old, decreased absorption occurs because of diminished gastrointestinal function and congestion of abdominal blood vessels. _____

If a patient is NPO, he or she takes the medication only as needed. _____

Drugs that are given a.d. are given in the right eye. _____

There are five rights to medication administration. _____

You should compare the order with the bottle at least three times. _____

In case of anaphylaxis, administer syrup of ipecac. _____

Patients have the right to refuse treatment. _____

HIPAA refers to standards holding health professionals accountable to protect the privacy of patients. _____

Patients should be discouraged from discussing their prescriptions with the physician. _____

Lavage refers to the use of a large tube place through a patient's nose to the stomach to remove remnants of poisons. _____

## Multiple Choice

**1. Which of the following is a sign of anaphylaxis?**

A. Hallucinations

B. Bleeding nose

C. Fixed pupils

D. Wheezing

**2. Which abbreviation means "before meals" ?**

A. a.c.

B. a.d.

C. a.m.

D. a.s.

E. a.u.

**3. In an examination room in a medical office, which of the following is the best way to identify a patient?**

A. Check the patient's wrist identification band.

B. Call the patient by name.

C. Ask the patient his or her name.

D. Compare the photograph in the patient's chart with the patient.

E. Ask one of your coworkers who the patient is.

**4. What does teratogenic refer to?**

    A. Causing birth defects in the unborn fetus

    B. Endangering the health of the mother

    C. Endangering the elderly

    D. None of the above

**5. Which of the following is NOT one of the seven rights of medication administration?**

    A. Right patient

    B. Right route

    C. Right time

    D. Right place

    E. Right documentation

**6. Why should you have a patient remain seated in the examination room for 15 minutes after receiving an injection, antibiotic, or allergy shot?**

    A. This gives you time to chart and clean up.

    B. The purpose is to watch for allergic reaction symptoms.

    C. Your next patient does not need to be seen for at least 15 minutes.

    D. The patient does not have to wait and can leave immediately.

**7. If a patient presents in your office and states that he has ingested a poisonous substance, what should you monitor while awaiting arrival of the emergency medical service?**

    A. Changes in vital signs (heart rate, blood pressure, respiratory rate, temperature)

    B. Seizures

    C. Level of consciousness

    D. All of the above

**8. What are some of the possible instructions that poison control may give you for the patient who has overdosed or ingested poison?**

    A. Administer activated charcoal.

    B. Have the patient drink large amounts of water to dilute the poison or medication.

    C. Have the patient drink milk to decrease the acidity of the poison.

    D. Any of the above

**9. Which of the following means to administer three times a day?**

    A. bid

    B. tid

    C. qid

    D. None of the above

**10. Documenting items correctly would include documenting which of the following?**

    A. Medication

    B. Dose

    C. Route

    D. Signature

    E. All of the above

## Short Answer Questions

Answer these questions on a separate sheet.

1. What are the three steps to confirm you have the right drug?

2. What precautions should be taken in a medical office to ensure the safe dispensing of medications? What precautions are taken in a hospital setting?

3. What should you do if a patient begins itching after you gave an immunization?

4. What are some possible instructions that a poison control center may give you?

5. What information should you have ready when you call a poison control center?

## Application Exercises

Respond to the following situations on a separate sheet.

1. In a closet, the office stores drug samples from drug company representatives. What would be the most efficient way to store these samples: by classification, company, or expiration date? Defend your answer.

2. You inject measles, mumps, and rubella vaccine into Brian's left leg. The drug was from lot no. 2468, expiration date 03/1/14. After you give the injection, he begins to cry. How would you document this medication administration in baby Dale's chart?

3. You pull the chart for Walter Roberts, and you notice that five patients named Walter Roberts are seen at this practice. What information would you need to find the correct chart?

4. Inger frequently forgets to take her medications. She is 77 years old and claims that she cannot remember well. What would you do to help her learn her medication schedule?

5. Derrick is a diabetic patient who lives with his daughter, who also has diabetes and wonders why they do not take the same dose of insulin. What would be your response?

6. Mrs. Valenzuela does not understand English well, but her son, who does understand English, is with her. How can you be sure that she understands how and when to take her medications?

7. Elaine is receiving an experimental drug. Write how you would document her informed consent.

8. Beth is pregnant. She calls the office to see what drugs she can use for cold symptoms. Where would you look to find out which drugs are safe for her?

9. Mickie is a diabetic patient with impaired vision. How should an allied health professional make sure he can take his medication safely?

10. Valentina wants to know why she needs less of a medication as she ages. Because her liver is becoming more impaired, she insists that she should be taking more medication, not less. What would you say to her?

## Abbreviation Study

Take a few minutes to study the abbreviations you have learned in this chapter. Then, test yourself. How did you do? If you missed any, you may want to make flash cards to help you learn. Put the abbreviation on one side of a 3 × 5 inch index card, and write its definition on the other side. Take these cards with you, and study whenever you get a chance. You will be able to learn the abbreviations quickly.

a.u. _____          a.d. _____          IM _____

IV _____          SC _____          tid _____

bid _____          p.c. _____          a.s. _____

prn _____          o.d. _____          o.u. _____

NPO _____          ID _____          o.s. _____

## Matching

1. bid          _____after meals

2. o.s.          _____as needed

3. tid          _____both ears

4. prn          _____left eye

5. a.u.          _____right eye

6. a.c.          _____three times a day

7. p.c.          _____twice a day

8. o.d.          _____before meals

# Regulations

*To ensure public safety, the United States government enacts and enforces laws and regulations related to drugs. The Occupational Safety and Health Administration (OSHA), the Food and Drug Administration (FDA), the Drug Enforcement Agency (DEA), and other government agencies safeguard the public by protecting workers, approving drugs, and enforcing drug laws. This chapter reviews the roles of these agencies, the process for developing new drugs to be sold in the United States, the way in which drugs are classified, and the illegal use of drugs.*

## LEARNING OUTCOMES

At the end of this chapter, the student will be able to:

4.1  Define key terms.

4.2  Describe the roles of OSHA, FDA, and DEA in patient safety.

4.3  Discuss how drugs are developed.

4.4  Distinguish among brand, generic, and trade names.

4.5  Know the slang names for illegal street drugs.

4.6  Discuss why some drugs are controlled more strictly than others.

4.7  Give an example of a drug from each controlled substances schedule and explain its classification.

4.8  Discuss the role of allied health professionals in recognizing and reporting impaired patients and professionals.

## KEY TERMS

Addiction

Chemical name

Clinical trials

Compassionate use

Control group

Controlled Substances Act

Double-blind

Drug Enforcement Agency (DEA)

Food and Drug Administration (FDA)

Generic name

Investigational New Drug (IND)

New drug application (NDA)

Occupational Safety and Health Administration (OSHA)

Patent medicine

Placebo

Substance abuse

# ■ HISTORY OF DRUG REGULATIONS

Drug regulations were created both in response to the sale of toxic substances to unsuspecting people who were promised a cure for their ailments and out of concern over food safety. These toxic substances were often referred to as "tonics," "elixirs," or "therapeutic agents." More addictive than curative, these substances contained alcohol, morphine, heroin, or opium, which caused temporary euphoria and therefore relief from pain. Additionally, in the late 1800s, Coca-Cola was developed. It was rumored to use coca leaves, from which cocaine is produced. By the early 1900s, approximately 1 in every 200 people was addicted to some form of **patent medicine.** The early definition of patent medicine referred to remedies of questionable value that had the potential to cause intentional or accidental harm.

In addition to these addictive substances falsely advertised as cure-alls, serious concerns arose regarding public food consumption and its safety. During the Spanish-American War, it was rumored that the soldiers were fed "embalmed beef," which caused serious illness. As a result of these concerns and the patent medicine problems, Congress passed the first federal drug law: the Pure Food and Drug Act of 1906 (Table 4.1). This bill required accurate labeling of drugs to prevent substitution or mislabeled ingredients.

The Food, Drug, and Cosmetic Act of 1938 (Table 4.2) replaced the previous law with more specific regulations including holding the drug developer responsible for drug safety. This change helped form the **Food and Drug Administration (FDA),** which oversees the safe development of new drugs. The roots of this organization can be traced back to the mid-1800s, when the office was formed to evaluate agricultural products. With the passage of the Pure Food and Drug Act of 1906, this office took on its familiar role in regulating medications. The Durham-Humphrey Amendment (1951) defined prescription drugs as drugs that must be administered under the supervision of a physician. In 1962, Kefauver-Harris Amendment (Table 4.3) was enacted in response to thalidomide use during pregnancy and the drug's direct link to birth defects. This act requires drug manufacturers to show product effectiveness and safety, to report adverse events to the FDA, and to ensure that any advertisements to physicians disclose a product's risks and benefits.

The **Controlled Substances Act** of 1970 established the **Drug Enforcement Administration (DEA).** This law provided the legal foundation for preventing abuse of drugs and other substances. The DEA regulates the manufacture and distribution of nartcotics, stimulants, depressants,

---

### TABLE 4.1   The Pure Food and Drug Act of 1906

- States are outlawed from buying and selling food, drinks, and drugs that have been mislabeled and/or tainted.
- Ingredients now must be clearly labeled by quantity or percentage.
- Imitation of popular items is banned.
- False or misleading claims are banned, including claims about contents of the labeled item.
- Habit-forming drugs must now have a warning label.

---

### TABLE 4.2   The Food, Drug, and Cosmetic Act of 1938

Responsible for formation of the FDA

- Placed cosmetics and medical devices under government control
- Required preapproval of all new drugs after manufacture proved safety to the FDA
- Prohibited false advertising about medication therapeutic properties
- Required correction of deficiencies in food quality and packaging
- Authorized manufacturing inspections

---

FDA, Food and Drug Administration

## TABLE 4.3 Amendments to the Food, Drug, and Cosmetic Act of 1938

Durham-Humphrey Amendment of 1951

- Defines which types of drugs cannot be used without medical supervision
- Limits sale of these drugs to prescription only by a medical professional
- All other drugs available without prescription

Kefauver-Harris Drug Amendments

- Requires drug makers to prove their drug works before approval for sale
- Advisory Committee on Investigation Drugs to advise FDA on product approval and policy making

FDA, Food and Drug Administration

hallucinogens, and anabolic steroids, as well as the substances used in their production. Although the FDA determines which drugs are available by prescription only, the DEA decides which drugs are controlled and assigns drugs a schedule or category. Of the five categories, which outline the addictive potential and use of the drug, Schedule I drugs are the most addictive and Schedule V the least (Table 4.4).

The Orphan Drug Act of 1983 was established to facilitate the development of drugs for rare diseases (i.e., diseases that affect fewer than 1 in 200,000 people). Pharmaceutical manufacturers had been reluctant to produce these drugs because of poor return on investment. In addition, these drugs were often expensive for patients. The Orphan Drug Act encouraged the development of these "orphan" drugs by guaranteeing marketing exclusivity, tax credits, and waiver of other fees.

### Virtual Field Trip

Visit http://accessdata.fda.gov/scripts/opdlisting/oopd and find two orphan drugs under current research and their orphan designation.

## TABLE 4.4 Controlled Substances Schedules

| Schedule | Examples | Information |
|---|---|---|
| Schedule I | Heroin, LSD, methaqualone | High abuse potential<br>No medically acceptable use |
| Schedule II | Morphine, PCP, cocaine, methadone, methamphetamine, Ritalin | High abuse potential<br>Acceptable medical use<br>Severe dependence risk |
| Schedule III | Anabolic steroids, codeine, hydrocodone, and some barbiturates | Lower abuse potential<br>Acceptable medical use<br>Moderate to low dependence risk |
| Schedule IV | Darvon, Valium, Xanax | Low abuse potential<br>Acceptable medical use<br>Limited dependence risk |
| Schedule V | Cough medicines with codeine | Lower abuse potential than Schedule IV drugs<br>Acceptable medical use<br>Limited physical or psychological dependence compared with Schedule IV drugs |

# ■ MODERN REGULATING AGENCIES

Several governmental authorities regulate and oversee the safe delivery of medications, as well as ensure safe practices among health-care workers (Table 4.5). The **Occupational Safety and Health Administration (OSHA),** the FDA, and the DEA have established laws and regulations to enforce safety for health-care professionals, patients, and the public.

## Occupational Safety and Health Administration

OSHA is a branch of the Department of Labor that helps ensure that all workers not be exposed to unnecessary job-related risks, such as electrical cords placed where workers could fall over them or a lack of portable fire extinguishers. In addition, as a health-care worker, you have the right to be protected from patients' diseases. In turn, you must take steps to protect yourself. The following are some of OSHA's regulations for protecting yourself on the job:

- Hand washing is required before any patient is handled.
- Medications should not be touched unless the health-care worker is wearing gloves.
- Gloves should be worn in case of exposure to blood or other bodily fluids.
- Sharp objects (e.g., needles) should be disposed of in specialized sharps disposal containers.

To ensure that health-care employees practice safe work habits, OSHA requires that all employees who may have access to blood-borne pathogens undergo annual training in workplace safety practices and the use of personal protective equipment (e.g., gloves, face shield). OSHA requires that employers provide safe supplies for workers, such as safety needles to avoid accidental needle sticks while drawing blood. Every practice setting must also have protective supplies, such as sharps disposal containers, gloves, masks, and eyewash solutions, readily available.

### Virtual Field Trip

Explore OSHA's Web site: http://osha.gov/. Find out where your regional office is located. Discover how you can report violations of OSHA regulations.

Occupational injuries, such as being stuck with a dirty needle and falls, must be reported to OSHA. Further training may be required for organizations that report several occupational injuries. Because OSHA is a regulatory agency, its representatives can inspect a medical organization at any time to ensure adherence to regulations. Organizations that are not compliant may be fined.

## Food and Drug Administration

The FDA was created to establish guidelines and regulations for food quality and drug development to maintain public safety. The FDA requires that drugs be scientifically researched before they are approved and regulates drug distribution. Once a drug is approved by the FDA, it is added to the

### TABLE 4.5   Federal Agencies

| Agency | Responsibility | Associated Department |
|---|---|---|
| Occupational Safety and Health Administration (OSHA) | Health-care worker safety | Department of Labor |
| Food and Drug Administration (FDA) | Safety of food and drug supply, approval of new drugs | Department of Health and Human Services |
| Drug Enforcement Administration (DEA) | Enforcement of Controlled Substances Act, public safety | Department of Justice |

*United States Pharmacopoeia/National Formulary,* or *USP/NF,* which is a comprehensive listing of all approved drugs in the United States.

All approved drugs must be proven safe and effective before they can be marketed. This means that the drugs must perform the indicated action without causing unacceptable harm. For example, one medication may work to eliminate lung cancer; however, it may also cause many patients to suffer cardiac arrest. The benefit is therefore not worth the risk. The FDA insists on high standards of scientific research, so it may take 8 years or longer for a company to gain approval of a drug, even if that drug is approved and sold in another country. Since 1997, the FDA has had the authority to accelerate the approval process (to as quickly as 6 months) for drugs needed by patients who are in a critical or life-threatening stage of illness.

All drugs have side effects, which are unintended consequences of a drug. Common side effects include headache, nausea, vomiting, and diarrhea. A side effect that can cause severe harm or death is commonly called an adverse reaction. An example is airway swelling, which can lead to suffocation and death if it is not treated immediately.

It is your responsibility as an allied health professional to report an adverse reaction to a medication to the FDA's MedWatch. The appropriate form is available on the FDA Web site (www.fda.gov/medwatch) (Fig. 4-1). Although the reporting of these problems is voluntary, it helps the FDA track trends. If a drug has multiple reports of adverse reactions or a serious event such as death, the manufacturer may voluntarily recall a drug, or the FDA may order a recall. In a recall, the manufacturer of the drug must stop distributing it and must contact customers to inform them of the product name, size, lot number, code or serial number, reason for recall, and instructions on how to proceed. Recalled drugs are listed in a weekly FDA Enforcement Report, available on the FDA Web site. If the adverse event was caused by a vaccine, the Vaccine Adverse Event Form shown in Figure 4-2 is used.

## Virtual Field Trip

Check out the FDA's Web site at http://fda.gov and download MedWatch Form 3500. Fill it out as though you were reporting adverse effects of a medication.

To monitor public safety continuously, the FDA also holds annual public meetings to hear comments from patients, pharmaceutical manufacturers, and health-care professionals about the safety and effectiveness of drugs.

 *CRITICAL THINKING*

Mr. Dupee is upset that he is unable to obtain a drug in the United States. He knows of a Web site from which he can order the medication from Mexico.
What are the potential dangers of ordering a drug from another country? How would you discuss this with him?

## Drug Enforcement Administration

The DEA enforces the laws on drug use. Although some medications may be obtained without a prescription as over-the-counter (OTC) drugs, many medications require a prescription from a licensed health-care provider.

OTC drugs are generally safe if they are taken as indicated. However, prescription drugs require the control of a prescriber to ensure that the patient does not take dangerous or inappropriate medication. The physician or other prescriber must first evaluate the patient to diagnose the illness or condition requiring medication. For example, although patients may be able to choose an OTC medication to treat mild headaches, they need health-care providers with medical training to evaluate the cause of severe or debilitating headaches and to identify an appropriate medicine. The more serious the illness requiring medication is, the more likely it will be that the medication is available by prescription only.

U.S. Department of Health and Human Services

Form Approved: OMB No. 0910-0291, Expires: 12/31/2011
See OMB statement on reverse.

# MEDWATCH

The FDA Safety Information and
Adverse Event Reporting Program

For VOLUNTARY reporting of
adverse events, product problems and
product use errors

Page 1 of _____

| FDA USE ONLY |
| --- |
| Triage unit sequence # |

### A. PATIENT INFORMATION

| 1. Patient Identifier | 2. Age at Time of Event or Date of Birth: | 3. Sex | 4. Weight |
| --- | --- | --- | --- |
| In confidence | | ☐ Female ☐ Male | _____ lb or _____ kg |

### B. ADVERSE EVENT, PRODUCT PROBLEM OR ERROR

Check all that apply:

1. ☐ **Adverse Event**   ☐ **Product Problem** *(e.g., defects/malfunctions)*
   ☐ **Product Use Error**   ☐ **Problem with Different Manufacturer of Same Medicine**

2. Outcomes Attributed to Adverse Event
   *(Check all that apply)*
   ☐ Death: _____ *(mm/dd/yyyy)*
   ☐ Life-threatening
   ☐ Hospitalization - initial or prolonged
   ☐ Required intervention to Prevent Permanent Impairment/Damage (Devices)
   ☐ Disability or Permanent Damage
   ☐ Congenital Anomaly/Birth Defect
   ☐ Other Serious (Important Medical Events)

| 3. Date of Event *(mm/dd/yyyy)* | 4. Date of this Report *(mm/dd/yyyy)* |
| --- | --- |

5. Describe Event, Problem or Product Use Error

6. Relevant Tests/Laboratory Data, Including Dates

7. Other Relevant History, Including Preexisting Medical Conditions *(e.g., allergies, race, pregnancy, smoking and alcohol use, liver/kidney problems, etc.)*

### C. PRODUCT AVAILABILITY

Product Available for Evaluation? *(Do not send product to FDA)*
☐ Yes   ☐ No   ☐ Returned to Manufacturer on: _____ *(mm/dd/yyyy)*

### D. SUSPECT PRODUCT(S)

1. **Name, Strength, Manufacturer** *(from product label)*
   #1 Name:
      Strength:
      Manufacturer:
   #2 Name:
      Strength:
      Manufacturer:

*PLEASE TYPE OR USE BLACK INK*

| 2. | Dose or Amount | Frequency | Route |
| --- | --- | --- | --- |
| #1 | | | |
| #2 | | | |

3. Date of Use *(if unknown, give duration) from/to (or best estimate)*
   #1
   #2

4. Diagnosis or Reason for Use *(Indication)*
   #1
   #2

| 6. Lot # | 7. Expiration Date |
| --- | --- |
| #1 | #1 |
| #2 | #2 |

5. Event Abated After Use Stopped or Dose Reduced?
   #1 ☐ Yes ☐ No ☐ Doesn't Apply
   #2 ☐ Yes ☐ No ☐ Doesn't Apply

8. Event Reappeared After Reintroduction?
   #1 ☐ Yes ☐ No ☐ Doesn't Apply
   #2 ☐ Yes ☐ No ☐ Doesn't Apply

9. NDC # or Unique ID

### E. SUSPECT MEDICAL DEVICE

1. Brand Name

2. Common Device Name

3. Manufacturer Name, City and State

| 4. Model # | Lot # | 5. Operator of Device |
| --- | --- | --- |
| Catalog # | Expiration Date *(mm/dd/yyyy)* | ☐ Health Professional ☐ Lay User/Patient ☐ Other: |
| Serial # | Other # | _____ |

| 6. If Implanted, Give Date *(mm/dd/yyyy)* | 7. If Expiration, Give Date *(mm/dd/yyyy)* |
| --- | --- |

8. Is this a Single-use Device that was Reprocessed and Reused on a Patient?
   ☐ Yes   ☐ No

9. If Yes to Item No. 8, Enter Name and Address of Reprocessor

### F. OTHER (CONCOMITANT) MEDICAL PRODUCTS

*Product names and therapy dates (exclude treatment of event)*

### G. REPORTER *(See confidentiality section on back)*

1. Name and Address
   Name:
   Address:

   City:            State:            Zip:

| Phone # | E-mail |
| --- | --- |

| 2. Health Professional? | 3. Occupation | 4. Also Reported to: |
| --- | --- | --- |
| ☐ Yes   ☐ No | | ☐ Manufacturer ☐ User Facility ☐ Distributor/Importer |

5. If you do NOT want your identity disclosed to the manufacturer, place an "X" in this box: ☐

**FORM FDA 3500 (1/09)**   Submission of a report does not constitute an admission that medical personnel or the product caused or contributed to the event.

**FIGURE 4-1:** MedWatch form. This form is completed to report serious adverse events that result from drug administration. *(Reprinted from U.S. Department of Health and Human Services, Food and Drug Administration. Retrieved June 22, 2011, from http://fda.gov/downloads/Safety/MedWactch/HowToReport/DownloadForms/ucm084725.pdf)*

WEBSITE: www.vaers.hhs.gov   E-MAIL: info@vaers.org   FAX: 1-877-721-0366

## VACCINE ADVERSE EVENT REPORTING SYSTEM

**VAERS**

24 Hour Toll-Free Information  1-800-822-7967
P.O. Box 1100, Rockville, MD 20849-1100
**PATIENT IDENTITY KEPT CONFIDENTIAL**

| *For CDC/FDA Use Only* |
| --- |
| VAERS Number _____ |
| Date Received _____ |

Patient Name:

Last          First          M.I.

Address

_____

_____

_____

City          State          Zip

Telephone no. (____) _____

Vaccine administered by (Name):

_____

Responsible
Physician _____
Facility Name/Address

_____

_____

_____

City          State          Zip

Telephone no. (____) _____

Form completed by (Name):

_____

Relation      ☐ Vaccine Provider   ☐ Patient/Parent
to Patient    ☐ Manufacturer       ☐ Other
Address *(if different from patient or provider)*

_____

_____

_____

City          State          Zip

Telephone no. (____) _____

| 1. State | 2. County where administered | 3. Date of birth / / mm dd yy | 4. Patient age | 5. Sex ☐ M ☐ F | 6. Date form completed / / mm dd yy |
|---|---|---|---|---|---|

**7.** Describe adverse events(s) (symptoms, signs, time course) and treatment, if any

**8.** Check all appropriate:
☐ Patient died      (date ___/___/___ )
                          mm  dd  yy
☐ Life threatening illness
☐ Required emergency room/doctor visit
☐ Required hospitalization (_____days)
☐ Resulted in prolongation of hospitalization
☐ Resulted in permanent disability
☐ None of the above

9. Patient recovered    ☐ YES   ☐ NO   ☐ UNKNOWN

12. Relevant diagnostic tests/laboratory data

**10.** Date of vaccination
___/___/___  mm dd yy  AM
Time _____ PM

**11** Adverse event onset
___/___/___  mm dd yy  AM
Time _____ PM

**13.** Enter all vaccines given on date listed in no. 10

| | Vaccine (type) | Manufacturer | Lot number | Route/Site | No. Previous Doses |
|---|---|---|---|---|---|
| a. | | | | | |
| b. | | | | | |
| c. | | | | | |
| d. | | | | | |

14. Any other vaccinations within 4 weeks prior to the date listed in no. 10

| | Vaccine (type) | Manufacturer | Lot number | Route/Site | No. Previous doses | Date given |
|---|---|---|---|---|---|---|
| a. | | | | | | |
| b. | | | | | | |

| 15. Vaccinated at: ☐ Private doctor's office/hospital ☐ Public health clinic/hospital ☐ Military clinic/hospital ☐ Other/unknown | 16. Vaccine purchased with: ☐ Private funds ☐ Public funds ☐ Military funds ☐ Other/unknown | 17. Other medications |
|---|---|---|

| 18. Illness at time of vaccination (specify) | 19. Pre-existing physician-diagnosed allergies, birth defects, medical conditions (specify) |
|---|---|

20. Have you reported    ☐ No          ☐ To health department
this adverse event
previously?            ☐ To doctor   ☐ To manufacturer

*Only for children 5 and under*

22. Birth weight _____ lb. _____ oz.

23. No. of brothers and sisters

21. Adverse event following prior vaccination (check all applicable, specify)

| | Adverse Event | Onset Age | Type Vaccine | Dose no. in series |
|---|---|---|---|---|
| ☐ In patient | | | | |
| ☐ In brother or sister | | | | |

*Only for reports submitted by manufacturer/immunization project*

| 24. Mfr./imm. proj. report no. | 25. Date received by mfr./imm.proj. |
|---|---|

| 26. 15 day report? ☐ Yes  ☐ No | 27. Report type ☐ Initial  ☐ Follow-Up |
|---|---|

Health care providers and manufacturers are required by law (42 USC 300aa-25) to report reactions to vaccines listed in the Table of Reportable Events Following Immunization. Reports for reactions to other vaccines are voluntary except when required as a condition of immunization grant awards.

Form VAERS-1(FDA)

**FIGURE 4-2:** Vaccine Adverse Event Reporting System. If an adverse event results from a vaccine, the allied health professional must complete the Vaccine Adverse Event Reporting System form. *(Reprinted from U.S. Department of Health and Human Services, Food and Drug Administration. Retrieved June 22, 2011, from http://fda.gov/BiologicsBloodVaccines/Safety Availability/ReportaProblem/VaccineeAdverseEvents/default.htm)*

Some OTC medications are now found only behind the pharmacy counter because they contain ephedrine, which is an ingredient used in the production of crystal meth, an illegal street drug. Valid identification (ID) and the patient's signature are required to buy these medications. Some discussion has suggested adding these drugs to the controlled substances list; that would make them at least schedule V drugs.

Be sure the person ordering the medication is lawfully allowed to do so. In some states, nurse practitioners and physician assistants are allowed to prescribe medications. Some prescription medications are considered controlled substances and can cause addiction or harm if they are misused. Prescribers must register with the DEA to prescribe these drugs, and in the case of controlled substances, the registry number must be printed on the prescription.

## Drug development

Drug development begins after researchers discover, identify, or create agents that show promising effects against a disease or disorder. These agents must pass through many stages of development and exploration and meet strict regulatory requirements before they can be tested on humans. The FDA evaluates premarket drugs through its Center for Drug Evaluation and Research (CDER). The Center's goals are to ensure that beneficial drug products are safe, available, and labeled with information on risks and benefits. The FDA approves a drug when it deems that the benefits of the drug outweigh the risks for the intended population and use.

After a drug is on the market and available for use, it is continually monitored and evaluated for its benefits and risks, not only by the FDA, but also by health-care providers and patients taking the drugs. Figure 4-3 demonstrates the FDA's role in risk management.

A major part of drug development requires that developers conduct **clinical trials** or studies. After testing in laboratories and/or on animals, a drug must be carefully tested in humans. Researchers use clinical trials with human subjects to test the effects of a drug with the goal of determining effectiveness, side effects, toxicity, and interactions. During the study or trial, the effect of the active drug is compared

**FIGURE 4-3:** Role of the Food and Drug Administration in risk management of approved drugs. *(Reprinted from U.S. Department of Health and Human Services, Food and Drug Administration. Retrieved June 22, 2011, from http://fda.gov/ downloads/Safety/SafetyofSpecificProducts/UCM180522.pdf)*

with a **placebo.** A placebo is an inactive (inert) substance that is sometimes given to participants in clinical trials to compare it with an active substance. The study drug may also be compared with a drug already on the market. For example, ibuprofen was possibly compared with other, well-known pain relievers such as aspirin or acetaminophen (Tylenol).

### Clinical trials

Study participants are randomly assigned to one of at least two groups (Fig. 4-4). One group is the placebo or **control group;** the other group receives the active study drug or drugs. Because the participants do not know whether they are receiving the active or inactive drug, they are prevented from invalidating the study by reporting effects they were not truly experiencing. Similarly, if the clinician conducting the study knew which patients were taking the active drug, the scientist could change the results, consciously or subconsciously. Therefore, to be sure the results of the drug trials are accurate, most studies are **double-blind**, meaning that neither the participants nor the clinicians know who is receiving the active drug. Computers are used to generate random numbers to assign to patients, and the study drug and placebo look alike.

To encourage volunteers, treatment is usually free. Volunteers also may be paid for participating or may receive funds to cover transportation costs to and from the trial facilities. These volunteers must sign a detailed consent form.

Clinical trials are conducted in several phases (Table 4.6). The goal of phase I trials is to determine safety. A few healthy participants take a drug for several months to measure any harmful effects.

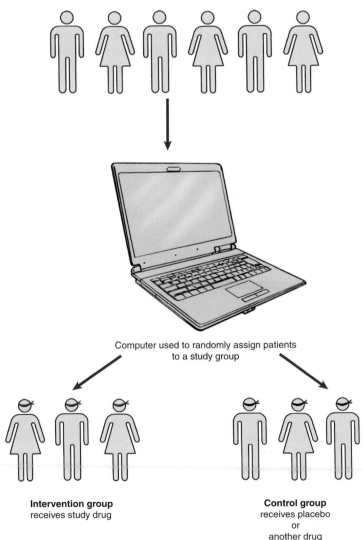

Computer used to randomly assign patients
to a study group

**Intervention group**
receives study drug

**Control group**
receives placebo
or
another drug

**FIGURE 4-4:** Double-blind clinical trial. In a randomized, double-blind clinical trial, neither patients nor clinicians know who is receiving the drug or placebo.

**TABLE 4.6 Clinical Trials**

| Phase | No. of Patients | Length | Purpose |
|---|---|---|---|
| I | 20–100 | Several months | Safety—does the drug do harm? |
| II | Up to several hundred | Several months–2 yr | Efficacy—does the drug help the patient? Also looks at safety |
| III | Several hundred to thousands | 1–4 yr | Dosage—how much should the patient take to be helped without overdosing? Also looks at safety and efficacy |
| IV (postmarketing trials) | Thousands | Ongoing | Continuing evaluation through MedWatch |

For example, a drug may cause diarrhea or may negatively affect vital signs. If the drug causes significant harmful effects, the trial stops. Usually, the participants are men because of concern over giving experimental drugs to women who could become pregnant. One disadvantage of this practice is that researchers may not become aware of any harmful effects that occur only in women until a later research phase.

Phase II clinical trials involve hundreds of patients (all of whom have the disease targeted by the drug) for longer periods of time. Although safety is important, the main goal of these trials is to see whether a drug works as desired (efficacy). For example, if a drug is meant to lower cholesterol, samples of participants' blood are checked to see whether blood cholesterol levels are lower while participants are taking the medication.

Phase III trials are for drugs that have been proven to be safe and effective. These trials involve hundreds to thousands of participants and can last 1 to 4 years. Frequently, phase III trials are conducted in several facilities (e.g., hospitals, physicians' offices, clinics), each of which enrolls hundreds of patients. The manufacturer is testing for safety, effectiveness, and dosage. The therapeutic (best) dose is evaluated during this phase; the goal is to give the least amount of drug possible to gain the necessary effect.

## CRITICAL THINKING

Not all people who volunteer for clinical trials are acceptable for the research. What do you think could eliminate a patient from clinical trials?

During the first three phases of clinical trials (Fig. 4-5), the drug is known as an **investigational new drug (IND),** and its use is limited to persons who meet specific criteria for inclusion in the trial. If the drug is being developed to help critically ill patients, special exceptions can be made. The FDA allows some physicians the **compassionate use** of INDs before approval. If a patient is suffering greatly and may die without the drug, a physician can prescribe it before FDA approval. However, most Health Maintenance Organizations (HMOs) do not cover the costs of experimental drugs because these drugs are expensive to obtain if you are not participating in the research.

If the clinical trials show that the drug is safe and effective, and a therapeutic dose is established, the manufacturer next applies to the FDA for approval. The manufacturer submits a **new drug application (NDA),** with the results of the scientific testing. Depending on the drug, the approval process can take 6 months to several years, and up to 12 years may pass from preclinical trails to approval.

Because the process of drug approval is long and expensive, and only about 1 drug is marketed for every 5,000 to 10,000 compounds tested. The manufacturer usually receives a 17- to 20-year patent to recover the cost and make a profit.

Once approved by the FDA, a drug can be marketed and distributed outside clinical trials groups. However, surveillance for any problems not previously identified continues through the MedWatch

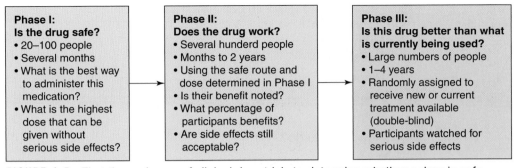

**FIGURE 4-5:** First three phases of clinical drug trials to determine whether a drug is safe, whether it works, and whether it is an improvement over drugs in current use.

program. Additional research may also be conducted. These activities are referred to as postmarketing (or phase IV) trials.

### CRITICAL THINKING

Canadians are protected by the Health Protection Branch (HPB) of the Department of Health and Welfare. Why would it be important for countries to cooperate in drug research?

## Naming drugs

Part of the process of developing drugs and taking them through FDA approval involves assigning names. When a drug is first developed, it is known as a mix of chemicals. The **chemical name** is meaningful to the researchers and to those companies who want to copy a successful drug, but it means little to others. For example, the chemical name of aspirin is acetylsalicylic acid, and morphine's chemical name is (5alpha, 6alpha) 7,8-didehydro-4,5-epoxy-17-methylmorphinan-3,5-diol. Complicated chemical names would be difficult for the allied health professional to memorize.

Once a drug clears phases I to III of clinical trials, it is ready to be put on the market and is given a **brand** or **trade name** (also sometimes called a *proprietary name*), to which the company owns the rights. Because the brand name is used in advertising, the company selects a name that is easy to remember and may indicate the drug's purposes. For example, Restoril® helps patients sleep. Another example is Aleve®, which helps relieve pain. The initial letters of brand names are capitalized. A brand name is usually followed by the letters R or TM with circles around them, to signify that the name is a registered trademark and no other manufacturer can use that name during the patent period.

Once a drug's patent period has ended, the drug's trademark status is not protected, so other companies may produce the drug under its common or **generic name.** No one except the manufacturer holding the trademark status can use the brand name, but other companies can manufacture the drug. Because these other companies did not do the research or spend as much on marketing, they can produce the medication much more cheaply than the original manufacturer.

### CRITICAL THINKING

Drug names can reflect their treatment effect. Try to determine what the drugs listed here could be used for, and then check a drug reference book to see how close you were.

Azmacort

Bronkaid

Elimite

Flexeril

Glucotrol

*Continued*

*CRITICAL THINKING—cont'd*

Lipitor

NasalCrom

Nicoderm

Pepcid

Rythmol

How did you do?

The FDA has specific requirements for manufacturers of generic drugs (Box 4.1). If the company uses the generic name, the drug must have the active ingredient the generic name specifies, but different fillers can be used. In some patients, the drug is more effective in the brand name form than in the generic form, but most adapt well to a generic brand. Because the generic drug is less expensive, HMOs often require that patients and prescribers use it or forfeit reimbursement.

Unlike the brand name, the first letter of the generic name is capitalized only if it begins a sentence. The generic name can also provide a clue to a drug's class (type) (see Fast Tip 4.1). The generic name becomes the official name of the drug.

Sometimes the prescriber uses shortened names. If the chemical is followed by the terms carbonate, citrate, gluconate, hydrochloride, hydroxide, phosphate, sodium, or sulfate, the prescriber assumes that the pharmacist understands the generic name without the second term. For example, potassium chloride is often ordered as potassium, although the drug label should contain the complete name. If you have any doubt about the correct name, check with the pharmacist or prescriber.

The generic drug may have a different shape and/or color from the trade drug. A change in the appearance of medications can confuse patients. Encourage patients to contact the pharmacy if they are

### BOX 4.1 Food and Drug Administration Requirements for Generic Drugs

- An FDA-approved brand name drug must be the reference for the proposed generic. The generic drug must have the same active ingredient or ingredients and the same labeled strength as this reference product. It must have the same dosage form: tablets, patches, and liquids are examples of dosage forms. It must be administered in the same way (e.g., swallowed as a pill or given as an injection).
- The manufacturer must show the generic drug is "bioequivalent" to the brand name drug. This means that the generic version delivers the same amount of active ingredients into a patient's bloodstream in the same amount as the brand name drug.
- The generic drug's labeling must be essentially the same as that of the approved drug.
- The firm must fully document the generic drug's chemistry, manufacturing steps, and quality control measures. Each step of the process must be detailed for FDA review.
- The firm must assure the FDA that the raw materials and the finished product meet USP specifications, if these have been set. The USP is the nonprofit, scientific body chartered by Congress to set standards for drug purity in the United States.
- Before the generic drug can be sold, the manufacturing firm must show that the drug maintains stability as labeled. Once the drug is on the market, the firm must continue to monitor the drug's stability. The firm must show that the container and its closure system will not interact with the drug. Firms making sterile drugs must submit sterility assurance data showing microbiologic integrity of these products.
- The firm must provide a full description of the facilities it uses to manufacture, process, test, package, label, and control the drug. It must certify that it complies with federal regulations about current good manufacturing practices and must undergo FDA inspection of the manufacturing facility to ensure compliance.
- Before the FDA approves a generic drug, it usually conducts an inspection at the proposed manufacturing site to make sure the firm is capable of meeting its application commitments and to ensure the firm can manufacture the product consistently.

FDA, Food and Drug Administration; USP, United States Pharmacopoeia. Source: U.S. Food and Drug Administration.

---

● *Fast Tip 4.1*    Drug Suffixes (Ending of Words)

Sometimes drug suffixes provide clues to the type of drug.

| Drugs With These Endings | Usually Belong to This Class |
|---|---|
| -caine | Local anesthetics |
| -cillin | Antibiotics |
| -dine | Antiulcer agents |
| -done | Opioid analgesics |
| -ide | Oral hypoglycemics |
| -iam | Antianxiety agents |
| -micin | Antibiotics |
| -mide | Diuretics |
| -mycin | Antibiotics |
| -nium | Neuromuscular blocking agents |
| -olol | Beta blockers (cardiovascular) |
| -oxacin | Antibiotics |
| -pam | Antianxiety agents |
| -pril | ACE inhibitors |
| -sone | Steroids |
| -statin | Antilipemics |
| -vir | Antivirals |
| -zide | Diuretics |

ACE, angiotensin-converting enzyme

---

unsure of a change in drugs. The pharmacy may have purchased the drug from a different manufacturer, but the change may also be an error.

Sometimes both legal and illegal drugs are known by *street* or slang names. Although you may not know the names of illegal drugs used on the street, your patients may use these terms; therefore, you should be familiar with them. Box 4.2 provides common street names for drugs that are frequently used.

---

## BOX 4.2 Street Names for Commonly Abuse Drugs

Sometimes both legal and illegal drugs are known by street or slang names. The following are street names for selective addictive drugs.

**Cannabinoids**

Hashish—boom, chronic, gangster, hash, hash oil, hemp

Marijuana—blunt, dope, ganja, grass, herb, joints, Mary Jane, pot, reefer, sinsemilla, skunk, wacky weed, weed, widow

**Depressants**

Barbiturates—barbs, phennies, reds, red birds, tooies, yellows, yellow jackets

Benzodiazepines—candy, downers, sleeping pills, tranks

Flunitrazepam—forget-me pill, Mexican Valium, R2, Roche, roofies, roofinol, rope, rophies

GHB—G, Georgia home boy, grievous bodily harm, liquid ecstasy

Methaqualone—ludes, mandrex, quad, quay

Sleep medications—A-minus, zombie pills

*Continued*

**BOX 4.2 Street Names for Commonly Abuse Drugs—cont'd**

**Dissociative Anesthetics**

Ketamine—cat Valiums, K, special K, vitamin K

PCP and analogs—angel dust, boat, hog, love boat, peace pill

**Hallucinogens**

LSD—acid, blotter, boomers, cubes, microdot, red/green dragon, yellow sunshines

Mescaline—buttons, cactus, mesc, peyote

Psilocybin—magic mushroom, purple passion, shrooms

**Opioids and Morphine Derivatives**

Codeine—Captain Cody, Cody, schoolboy, doors and fours, loads, pancakes and syrup

Fentanyl—Apache, China girl, China white, dance fever, friend, goodfella, jackpot, murder 8, TNT, Tango and cash

Morphine—M, Miss Emma, monkey, white stuff

Opium—big O, black stuff, block, gum, hop

Other opiod pain relievers—Hillbilly heroin, oxy, oc, oxycotton, percs, happy pills, vikes

**Stimulants**

Amphetamines—bennies, black beauties, crosses, hearts, LA turnaround, speed, truck drivers, uppers

Cocaine—blow, bump, C, candy, Charlie, coke, crack, flake, nose candy, rock, snow, toot

Methamphetamine—chalk, crank, crystal, fire, glass, go fast, ice, meth, speed

Methylphenidate—JIF, MPH, R-ball, Skippy, the smart drug, Vitamin R

**Other**

Anabolic steroids—juice, roids

Inhalants—bombers, buzz bomb, laughing gas, poppers, snappers, whippets

Source: National Institute of Drug Abuse (NIDA).

# ■ DRUG CONTROL

The purpose of the DEA is to enforce the controlled substances laws and regulations for the United States. This includes the provisions of the Controlled Substances Act as they pertain to the manufacture, distribution, and dispensing of legally produced controlled substances.

## Drug schedules

Controlled substances are those that must be tracked or "controlled." Most of these drugs are available by prescription only. Some do not require a prescription, but they must be signed for with a valid ID at the pharmacy. This protocol may vary from state to state. Controlled substances are categorized into schedules, designated by Roman numerals. It is not necessary to memorize all these drugs, but knowing the categories is important, to understand the effects of each type of drug on the patient. The most highly controlled drugs are Schedule I drugs, and the least controlled are Schedule V drugs (Table 4.7).

Schedule I drugs are considered to be highly addictive, both physically and psychologically, and they have no medical use. Heroin is considered a Schedule I drug. These drugs are considered so dangerous that they are illegal to process, distribute, and use. Schedule I drugs are not prescribed except in carefully controlled research facilities in which patients are closely monitored, such as the study of the street drug ecstasy in the treatment of post-traumatic stress disorder. Allied health professionals should never possess these drugs because criminal prosecution may result.

Schedule II drugs have a high potential for physical and psychological addiction. The use of these drugs is heavily restricted because they are popular with addicts. These drugs are dispensed through

**TABLE 4.7   Drug Enforcement Agency Controlled Substance Schedules**

| Schedule | Abuse Potential | Medications | Examples |
|---|---|---|---|
| I | High | No accepted medical use in the United States | Heroin, marijuana, LSD, methaqualone |
| II | High; may lead to severe dependence (psychological or physical) | Has a currently accepted medical use; may have severe restrictions | Cocaine, methadone, methamphetamine, morphine, PCP, OxyContin, Ritalin |
| III | Less than drugs and substances in Schedules I and II; may lead to moderate or low physical dependence or high psychological dependence | Has a currently accepted medical use | Anabolic steroids, codeine and hydrocodone with aspirin or Tylenol, some barbiturates |
| IV | Low relative to substances in Schedule III; may lead to limited dependence | Has a currently accepted medical use | Valium, Xanax |
| V | Low, relative to substances in Schedule IV; may lead to limited dependence (psychological or physical) | Has a currently accepted medical use | Cough medicine |

Source: http://usdoj.gov/dea/pubs/abuse/1-csa.htm

written prescription only; an office assistant cannot call in the prescription to the pharmacy. Additionally, no refills are permitted. This does not mean that patients cannot have more of the medication, but they must have a written prescription for each new supply. The office staff may fax the prescription to the pharmacy, but the patient must also give a handwritten prescription to the pharmacist to receive the medicine. In an emergency, the prescriber may phone in an order to a nurse (e.g., if the patient is in the hospital), but a handwritten copy of the prescription must be submitted within 72 hours. This category includes drugs that suppress the central nervous system such as morphine, as well as amphetamines, which stimulate it. Examples include cocaine, PCP, methylphenidate (Ritalin), and oxycodone (OxyContin).

Schedule III drugs are moderately addictive and may lead to limited dependence. Refills are allowed up to five times in 6 months. This category includes combination drugs that contain a small amount of a narcotic with a less-addictive medication, such as acetaminophen or aspirin. The patient absorbs less of the narcotic dose in each tablet, but the drug is still powerful. Examples are anabolic steroids, hydrocodone (Hydrocet), and Tylenol 3. Allied health-care professionals may write the prescription for the drug, but the prescriber must sign it.

Schedule IV drugs have lower abuse potential but are still controlled. As with Schedule III drugs, allied health-care professionals may write the prescription (e.g., name, route, dosage), but the prescriber must sign it. A health-care professional can fax or phone in these orders to the pharmacy or facility. Refills of drugs in this category are allowed up to five times in 6 months. Examples include lorazepam (Ativan), diazepam (Valium), and alprazolam (Xanax).

Schedule V drugs have the lowest potential for abuse. They include OTC cough suppressants to which a small amount of codeine has been added, as well as preparations for diarrhea, such as paregoric and opium tincture. Because the syrup is thick, overdose is difficult. However, small children like the taste of syrup, so advise parents to store the medicine away from children. Examples are diphenoxylate hydrochloride and atropine sulfate preparations (Lomotil), Robitussin A-C, and Children's Tylenol 3.

Drugs may be prescribed in more than one schedule. For example, full-strength codeine is a Schedule II drug because it is a highly addictive narcotic. If a manufacturer adds more acetaminophen or aspirin so that only a small amount of the narcotic is present in the medication, it can be classified as a Schedule III drug. If the manufacturer adds a small amount of narcotic to a large amount of syrup, the medication can be classified as Schedule V (e.g., Children's Tylenol® with Codeine syrup) because the narcotic is less addictive when taken in such a small quantity.

**Virtual Field Trip**

Type the following URL into your browser: http://deadiversion.usdoj.gov. According to the DEA controlled substances schedules list, under which schedule is each of the following classified?
Marinol
Kaolin Pectin PG
Meperidine
Midazolam

## Controlled substances management

If you work in an office that stores controlled substances, you need to keep an inventory log to document when you receive certain controlled medications and to whom you dispensed them. Be sure to sign off regarding which patient received what dosage and sign your name to the documentation. Also sign your name to the drug count only if you have counted the drugs to show that the count is accurate. Be aware of agency policies mandating the timing of a narcotic count. The count may be performed as often as once per day or once per shift, depending on the type of facility. In a narcotic count, two professionals count the controlled substances on hand. One person counts the actual medications, and one compares that count with the narcotics log to verify that the numbers match.

Notify the physician immediately if the controlled drug count is not as recorded. For example, if the log shows eight remaining Demerol tablets but only five tablets are present in the narcotics cabinet, you would immediately notify the physician. These records must be kept for 2 years. See the DEA Web site for complete information. In the hospital setting, nurses usually count and log out the controlled substances. These drugs should be kept double-locked in a safe place whenever they are not in your sight. Patients should not know where these drugs are stored. Be suspicious of a patient who asks you for this information. If controlled substances are stolen or lost, the prescriber who has a DEA number must file DEA Form 106 Report of Theft or Loss of Controlled Substances, which is also available on the DEA Web site. Theft of a significant amount should be reported to the local police department.

If you need to dispose of a controlled medication, you must have someone witness the disposal, and the medication must be destroyed beyond any possible reuse. Many states require that you return unused medications to a pharmacy or state police facility for incineration, to ensure complete disposal. Controlled substances must be clearly marked as controlled. The label on the medication bottle shows a "C" for controlled substances. Do not put controlled substances in unmarked containers.

## ■ SUBSTANCE ABUSE

**Substance abuse** is a maladaptive pattern of behavior marked by the use of chemical agents. The key to substance abuse is that the patient does not adapt well under the influence of the substance.

Each year, numerous deaths in the United States result from substance abuse. Some substances are commonly and legally used, such as nicotine and alcohol (ETOH). Others are illegal drugs. Still others, such as steroids, are seen as a way to enhance athletic performance (Fast Tip 4.2). Any drug can be abused if it is used improperly. For example, a person obsessed with losing weight may choose to use laxatives as aids but may harm himself or herself in the process. Allied health professionals may see patients who show signs of substance abuse, including tremors (shaking), poor judgment, or slurred speech. Because these signs can also reflect disease states, include all the facts when documenting such signs in the medical record.

Some drugs are particularly addictive. **Addiction** means being compulsively driven to take a drug, often to the exclusion of all other activities. Most patients do not start taking a drug with the thought of becoming addicted, but over time they may become dependent on the drug and crave it either psychologically or physically. For example, a patient experiencing pain after an injury may take an increasing amount of pain medication. Soon more of the drug is needed to produce the same effect because the person has developed a tolerance to it.

Other people become **habituated** to drugs. This means they are psychologically tolerant of the drug and need an increased amount to achieve the desired effect. They may not physically need the drug but

> **● Fast Tip 4.2** Steroid Abuse
>
> The National Institute on Drug Abuse (NIDA) reports that anabolic steroids are frequently abused by people who want to build muscles, reduce body fat, and improve sports performance. Abuse is estimated to be high among competitive body builders and athletes. Men usually abuse steroids to become larger and more muscular, whereas women abuse steroids to become lean and muscular. Doses taken by abusers can be up to 100 times greater than doses used for treating medical conditions, such as the muscle wasting seen in AIDS. Anabolic steroids can cause hormonal system disruptions, musculoskeletal system effects, infections, cardiovascular diseases, liver and skin dysfunction, and behavioral effects. (Source: National Institute of Drug Abuse: NIDA Notes 15[3], 2000.)

believe that they cannot live without it. For example, a patient may be prescribed an antianxiety medication to help her cope with stressful work situation, but she begins to enjoy the way the drug makes her feel. She may take more of the medication to cope with perceived anxiety. Soon she takes increasing amounts of the drug because she has developed a **tolerance** to it. Having the drug in her system becomes "normal."

It is vital to keep patients free of pain when they are in the acute stage of a disease or are recovering from surgery. However, prescribers are typically reluctant to increase dosages over the long term. If patients engage in drug-seeking behavior (i.e., requesting more medication out of proportion to physiological needs), the prescriber may reduce the amount of medication allowed and refer the patient for psychological counseling. Patients who stop taking a medication may experience symptoms of **withdrawal,** such as tremors, emotional distress, and hallucinations. Chronic pain is a particular challenge, especially in patients who are terminally ill (dying). These patients may experience increasing, not decreasing, pain as the disease worsens. The health-care provider may prescribe more painkillers as time goes on but must be careful not to overprescribe drugs that can injure the patient by suppressing respiration.

### CRITICAL THINKING

A patient calls frequently and begs for more pain medication. The doctor and staff are frustrated by the repeated requests and attribute them to drug-seeking behavior. How would you handle this situation?

## Preventing substance abuse

One of the best ways to mitigate behavior that may lead to tolerance or habituation is education. Frequently, patients do not understand the purpose of the medication or the reason for adhering to the ordered dose. You can help educate patients by teaching them about side effects and cautionary situations (e.g., do not take during pregnancy).

Perhaps a more difficult situation is learning that a member of your office staff is abusing substances. If a health-care provider is impaired (not fully functional mentally or physically) when caring for patients, the consequences can be deadly. The provider, under the influence of alcohol or other substances, may prescribe a wrong drug or be unable to perform minor surgery safely. An addicted staff member may steal drugs from the health-care provider's stock, a facility's medication cart, or even from patients. Persons suffering from an addiction go to extreme lengths to obtain their drugs of choice and often lie to cover their behavior. This is the major reason that allied health professionals must be vigilant in maintaining the security of controlled substances. These substances should be locked in a cabinet with two locking doors. Only one person should have responsibility for the key, and the controlled substances should be frequently inventoried. Strict security can prevent the use of an agency's drugs for addictive purposes.

**Virtual Field Trip**

The following Web site offers information on drug misuse: http://usdoj.gov/dea. Find out how to obtain information on teaching children not to abuse drugs.

## Signs of substance abuse

Substance abuse is sometimes extremely difficult to detect until the abuse has become chronic. Many individuals have learned to function adequately under the influence of drugs and/or alcohol and appear normal. Not until you notice the physical changes in their appearance and the deterioration of their work do you begin to suspect that something is wrong. If the person is someone you have worked with for a long time, substance abuse may be the farthest thing from your mind as you try to discover the cause of these changes. Abuse of drugs and/or alcohol can affect most organs of the body. In addition to the physical signs caused by damage done to the liver, kidneys, and other organs, certain behaviors can signal substance abuse. These symptoms and behaviors are summarized in Box 4.3. Some of the most common physical symptoms are as follows:

- Changes in sleep habits (either too much or too little energy alters sleep patterns)
- Excessive weight change
- Excessive sweating
- Excessive tremors
- Poor coordination
- Needle marks

Some behaviors signaling substance abuse are as follows:

- Poor work performance (i.e., a health-care provider spends an inappropriate time away from patients and makes strange excuses for the absences)
- Sloppy charting or other written work
- Moodiness, including restlessness, irritability, and violent temper outbursts
- Forgetfulness
- Change in personal hygiene (e.g., clothes, bathing)

These signs may not positively indicate drug or alcohol abuse, but they should trigger an investigation into the cause of these changes to protect patients and coworkers, as well as the employee. Typically, people who are addicted may deny substance abuse or minimize the effects of their habit. If you have noticed that someone is impaired, you must focus on ensuring that the person receives treatment.

## Treating substance abuse

Follow your facility's protocol on referral of impaired employees for substance abuse treatment. Many employers have employee assistance programs or support groups organized through the human resources department. If a patient or family member is suspected of substance abuse, again follow your facility's protocol. Usually, the issue is discussed with the physician before any action is taken.

Be familiar with local resources for treatment, so you can help your colleague or patient by suggesting community resources. Patients and/or families may also come to you for advice about helping a loved one. Having these resources on hand will help them, too.

You must set boundaries and not accommodate the substance abuse by covering up inappropriate behavior. Abusers sometimes lose their families and jobs before they receive help. As a health-care professional, you have the knowledge and ability to help these people obtain the assistance they need.

**Virtual Field Trip**

Visit the Association of Addiction Professionals at http://naadac.org and find a list of clinicians who treat impaired professionals in your area.

| BOX 4.3 Signs of Possible Substance Abuse in a Coworker |
|---|
| Is frequently late or absent from work because of "illness" |
| Documents poorly |
| Is irritable and defensive or withdrawn |
| Makes frequent mistakes |
| Does not keep scheduled appointments |
| Has difficulty working with many staff members |
| Relates to patients unprofessionally |
| Has physical symptoms such as:<br>    Confusion<br>    Sweating<br>    Tremors<br>    Slow reflexes |
| Has changes in appearance such as:<br>    Weight change<br>    Jaundice<br>    Dilated or constricted pupils<br>    Needle tracks<br>    Poor or deteriorated hygiene |

## Substance abuse and legal issues

If any of your colleagues is impaired, report the behavior to your supervisor or office manager immediately. If the impaired colleague has a license, your supervisor should report the behavior to the state Board of Medicine, Board of Nursing, or another board, depending on the license. Most licensing boards will not take away someone's license to practice permanently unless that person has caused serious harm while impaired. The board may limit this colleague's practice for a period of time or indefinitely. For example, a nurse who is having an addiction problem may be barred from working in a facility with controlled substances on the premises. If you fail to report this colleague and he or she harms a patient, coworker, or himself or herself, you could be held responsible because you could have prevented the situation.

If you suspect any other member of the community (e.g., patients, their families, clergy) of being impaired, you need to follow your agency policy regarding the steps to take to handle the situation appropriately. If no one is in danger from the impairment, following your agency policies should protect you legally from any repercussions of your actions.

### Virtual Field Trip

Go to your favorite search engine and search for your state's board of medicine and board of nursing. Write the address and phone number for each.

● ● ● S U M M A R Y

Drug regulations are instituted to protect the public from the use, sale, and consumption of worthless or dangerous medications. OSHA enacts laws geared toward protecting health-care workers from patients' diseases and requires yearly education to ensure the safety of workers. The FDA approves drugs for sale in the United States, and the DEA ensures that addictive drugs are carefully controlled. The allied health-care worker has a professional responsibility to know the main laws and regulations related to medications.

Although drugs can be helpful, they can harm people if they are used inappropriately. The allied health professional must be alert to signs of addiction in both patients and colleagues. If you detect a substance abuser or impaired health-care provider, report the facts to your supervisor or the state professional board and suggest that the addicted person obtain treatment.

## Activities

To make sure that you have learned the key points covered in this chapter, complete the following activities.

### True or False

Write true if the statement is true. Beside the false statements, write false and correct the statement to make it true.

The DEA approves drugs for dispensing in the United States. _____

Schedule II drugs are highly addictive. _____

OHSA is part of the Department of Health and Human Services. _____

MedWatch is a way of reporting adverse reactions. _____

The DEA is a part of the Department of Justice. _____

Clinical trials in drug development have two phases. _____

Phase IV clinical trials happen after the drug is released to the public. _____

In a double-blind clinical trial, neither patients nor clinicians know who is receiving a drug or a placebo. _____

Generic drugs are trademark protected. _____

The drug suffix -cillin is closely associated with antibiotics. _____

### Multiple Choice

Choose the best answer for each question.

**1. The governmental department that enforces the Controlled Substances Act:**
  A. DEA
  B. DOJ
  C. FDA
  D. DHHS
  E. OSHA

**2. During the first three phases of clinical trials, a drugs is known as a/an:**
  A. Experimental new drug
  B. Investigational new drug
  C. Orphan drug
  D. Generic drug
  E. Chemical drug

**3. Once a drug clears the first three phases of clinical trials, it is given a _____ name:**
  A. Generic
  B. Trade
  C. Brand
  D. Chemical
  E. B or C

**4. The most addictive schedule of drugs, with no accepted medical use, is _____ drugs:**

A. Schedule I

B. Schedule II

C. Schedule III

D. Schedule IV

E. Schedule V

**5. An example of a Schedule II drug is:**

A. Heroin

B. Valium

C. Tylenol with codeine

D. Cocaine

**6. A damaged controlled substance should be disposed by:**

A. Flushing it down the toilet

B. Throwing it in the garbage

C. Destroying it beyond any possible use in the presence of a witness

D. None of the above

**7. What schedule includes anabolic steroids?**

A. Schedule I

B. Schedule II

C. Schedule III

D. Schedule IV

E. Schedule V

**8. Symptoms of substance abuse include:**

A. Tremors

B. Poor judgment

C. Slurred speech

D. Change in behavior

E. All of the above

**9. OSHA mandates that employers:**

A. Provide yearly safety training to all employees

B. Provide protective supplies to employees

C. Report all occupational injuries

D. All of the above

**10. The Orphan Drug Act:**

A. Facilitates the development of drugs for rare diseases

B. Facilitates the development of drugs for children

C. Facilitates the development of drugs for almost eradicated diseases

D. None of the above

### Application Exercises

Respond to the following situations on a separate sheet of paper.

1. You just started a new job in Dr. Johnson's office. When you ask about safety needles for injections, you are told that the office is using nonsafety needles. Is this a problem? What would you do?

2. You have a patient diagnosed with a rare form of leukemia. She is thinking of entering clinical trials for a new drug and wants your opinion. What would you say to her?

3. At the end of the day, you are counting the scheduled drugs in the locked cabinet and discover that an entire box of morphine is missing. What do you do?

4. You are administering an antibiotic injection to a patient. Five minutes after the injection, he has a grand mal seizure. The patient has never had a seizure before, and the physician thinks it may be related to the medication. What do you do, and to whom do you report this?

5. You are the office manager in a busy family practice. You have a medical assistant who has incurred a dirty needle stick four times this month. What should you do?

# Prescriptions and Labels

*A key element in keeping the patient safe is ensuring the accuracy of prescriptions for medications. Drugs have a variety of names, are developed from several sources, are administered by different routes, and act in various ways. Therefore, the prescriber must give specific information to avoid mistakes when prescriptions are filled or medications are administered. This chapter discusses the types of prescriber orders, the parts of prescriptions, and medication labels.*

## LEARNING OUTCOMES

At the end of this chapter, the student will be able to:

5.1 Define key terms.

5.2 Discuss precautions to ensure patient safety.

5.3 Identify the parts of a legal prescription.

5.4 Differentiate among three different types of medication orders.

5.5 List which health-care providers are able to write prescriptions.

5.6 Define abbreviations used in prescriptions.

5.7 Interpret labels safely.

5.8 Discuss the impact of e-prescribing on health-care consumers.

### KEY TERMS

| | | | |
|---|---|---|---|
| Automatic stop orders | Medication orders | Standing orders | Superscription |
| Electronic prescription | Rx | STAT orders | Verbal orders |
| Inscription | Signature | Subscription | |

## ■ MEDICATION ORDERS

**Medication orders** are the prescriptions provided by a physician for a patient for a specific medication. Medication orders include written orders, verbal or standing orders, and stop orders. The prescription order itself contains some basic information, such as the preprinted prescriber's name and contact information. Knowing the basic parts of a medication order aids in ensuring the patient's safety because of the many different medications, routes of administration, and times for taking them. This knowledge also helps to prevent errors and to teach patients important facts about their medications. Review the abbreviations presented in Chapter 3 (Tables 3.2 and 3.3); in addition, Box 5.1 lists common abbreviations

## BOX 5.1 Abbreviations Related to Medication Administration

| Abbreviation | Meaning | Abbreviation | Meaning | Abbreviation | Meaning |
|---|---|---|---|---|---|
| cap | Capsule | mcg | microgram | tab | tablet |
| elix | elixir | mEq | milliequivalent | T, Tb | tablespoon |
| g | gram | mL | milliliter | t, tsp | teaspoon |
| gr | grain | mg | milligram | | |
| gtt | drops | oz | ounce | | |

used. Abbreviations can vary from one setting to the next, so be sure to check which are—and are not—accepted at your workplace.

### Written orders

Obtain a written order for a prescription whenever possible, to decrease the chance of misinterpretation of information written on the order and subsequent errors. Legally, every drug that is ordered, administered, or dispensed must also have written documentation by the prescriber. Having this information in writing protects the health-care professional who administers or dispenses the drug from possible later discrepancies between what the prescriber meant to order and what was actually given or administered. The prescriber should write or type the prescription accurately. A health-care facility is a busy workplace, and errors result from haste or sloppy penmanship. As an allied health professional, you help ensure the patient's safety by proofreading a prescription before the patient takes it to the pharmacy. If a prescriber has poor handwriting, offer to write or type the prescription, and then have the prescriber read and sign it. The exception is a prescription for a Schedule II drug, which must be written by the prescriber.

### Verbal orders

When a prescriber has the health-care professional write the prescription, these instructions are **verbal orders.** For example, a physician may not be present, so the order is given over the telephone. Check with your supervisor to see whether you are allowed to take a verbal order. If so, write words and numbers carefully, and be sure to read what you have written back to the prescriber to ensure that the information is correct. Some offices require that the prescriber also repeat the information back to you. In rare instances, a physician may give a verbal order during an emergency situation. This is known as a **STAT** order, meaning to give immediately. This should be the only instance in which you give a patient a medication without a written order when the prescriber is present. If the situation is not an emergency, you should write the order, and have the prescriber sign it before the medication is administered or dispensed. In all instances, the prescriber must sign the order as soon as possible. Again, this procedure legally protects the health-care worker from discrepancies between what the prescriber intended and what was actually administered. Verbal orders are not permitted for Schedule II drugs.

### Electronic prescription orders

A newer type of medication order is the **electronic prescription** (e-prescription). The prescriber creates the prescription electronically and sends it directly to the patient's pharmacy. In many instances, the electronic prescribing network can immediately verify insurance coverage for medications. Some programs manage the patient's medication history, to identify any medication interactions or other problems before the patient receives the ordered medication. E-prescriptions bypass the typical problems of written prescriptions, such as illegible writing, loss of the written document, and missing information on the prescription.

---

### A CLOSER LOOK 5.1: Internet Pharmacies

With the soaring cost of prescription medication in the United States and the high numbers of Americans without medical insurance, many people are turning to Internet pharmacies. Many legitimate Canadian companies take a written prescription and fill it with lower-cost Canadian medications.

### Standing orders

A prescriber may leave a list of **standing orders** to be used in specific routine circumstances. For example, before a diagnostic test, a prescriber may require the patient to have nothing by mouth (NPO) after midnight, have an enema, follow with a clear liquid diet, and take an antibiotic. It is important to verify standing orders with the prescriber. These standing orders need to be reviewed and updated regularly, usually on an annual basis. Like all other orders, standing orders are not exempt from a timely signature and must be signed by the prescriber as soon as possible.

### Stop orders

**Automatic stop orders** are given for a limited time only. A common example is an order for Schedule II and III drugs after an injury or surgical procedure. Most likely, the patient will experience some level of pain for a short time following the injury or surgery, and the physician therefore orders a Schedule II narcotic analgesic to be taken every 4 hours as needed. Because this prescription cannot be refilled unless the prescriber renews it, the patient is less likely to become addicted to the medication. Another example is an antibiotic to be taken twice a day for 10 days. The order stops after 10 days and is not refilled unless the prescriber renews it. To "d/c" an order is to discontinue it.

Regardless of the order, the prescription must be clear. Patients can suffer serious consequences or possibly die if a pharmacist misinterprets a prescription and gives the wrong medication or the wrong dose. Your role is to be the safety check before the prescription is sent to the pharmacist, to make sure the information is accurate and legible.

*CRITICAL THINKING*

**You review a prescription and find that you cannot determine whether the medication is Trileptal (an antiseizure medication) or Tylenol 3 (a narcotic pain reliever). What would the difference mean to the patient if the wrong drug were given? What should you do in this situation?**

## ■ PARTS OF A PRESCRIPTION

The prescription is a written record of the prescriber's order. In addition to physicians, nurse practitioners and physician assistants are allowed to prescribe medications. On every prescription pad, the prescriber is identified by name and Drug Enforcement Administration (DEA) number. Research and learn who can prescribe medications in your state.

Prescriptions are dispensed only by health-care professionals who are licensed to do so, and only the patient whose name is on the prescription should take the medication. Drugs are ordered in facilities such as hospitals, outpatient surgery centers, and prescribers' offices. Because you will probably have the most contact with prescriptions in a prescriber's office, that setting area is the main focus of this discussion.

Every prescription must include the following: name, address, telephone number, the DEA number of the prescriber; name and address of the patient; date of the order; **Rx** or the **superscription,** which means "take thou" and is an abbreviation for prescription or treatment; **inscription** (name of drug, dosage, and quantity to be dispensed); directions for taking the drug **(signature)**; refill numbers **(subscription)**; a notation about whether a generic drug can be used; and the signature of the prescriber (Fig. 5-1). The following list details some of these parts:

■ **Date.** Including the date of the order is important for filing insurance claims and for linking the drug therapy with the office visit. The date of the order should match the date of the office visit, even though patients may not fill the prescription for up to a month after the visit because they may receive free samples at the office or emergency department. Prescriptions should never be postdated.

■ **Physician's name, contact information, and DEA number.** Large medical groups may use one prescription form with all the legal prescribers listed, or they may have separate prescription forms for each prescriber. All prescribers licensed to prescribe scheduled drugs must have their DEA numbers preprinted on the prescription form.

---

## A CLOSER LOOK 5.2: Drug Enforcement Administration Numbers

Pharmacists can verify the legitimacy of the DEA number found on a prescription by the following method: Each number has two letters followed by seven digits. The first letter is always A or B, based on when the number was issued (A is earlier than B). The second letter is the first letter of the prescriber's name. The seven digits have a mathematical relationship that is always followed. Try the formula to see whether BW1342586 is a valid DEA number:

- Add the first, third, and fifth numbers. in this case, $1 + 4 + 5 = 10$
- Now add the second, fourth, and sixth numbers: $3 + 2 + 8 = 13$
- Double the sum just calculated: $13 \times 2 = 26$
- Add this to the first sum: $26 + 10 = 36$
- Take the last digit in that sum (36, the first digit is 3, the last digit is 6).
- The final digit in this DEA number must be 6.
- If the final digit in this number were anything but a 6, the DEA number would be fraudulent.

---

■ **Patient's name, address, and date of birth.** Be sure that the current address of the patient appears on the prescription form; write it on the form if it is not there already, and check with the patient to be sure it is correct. Including the patient's birth date on the prescription helps the pharmacist ensure that the drug and dosage prescribed are appropriate for the age group of this patient.

■ **Inscription (name of drug, dosage, and quantity to be dispensed).** The drug name must be clearly identified. The prescriber may write the generic or brand name on the order. The prescriber also notes whether a generic drug can be substituted for a brand name drug. This information

---

(A) CARL NEWELL, M.D.    DEA# _____
125 Main Street
Hometown, VA 22958
(703) 555-0106

(B) Connie Martin                    (C) Date: _11/14/2012_
789 Beach Tree Drive
Hometown, VA 22958

(D) R<sub>x</sub>

(E) Claritin syrup
Qty: 150 mL

(F) Sig: 1 tsp daily

(G) Refills:    None    1    2    3    4

(H) May substitute generic          ☐

May not substitute generic    ☐    (I) _____
                                         Signature

**FIGURE 5-1:** Sample prescription. A prescription has several parts: (A) name, address, telephone number, and Drug Enforcement Administration (DEA) number of the prescriber; (B) patient's name and address; (C) date; (D) Rx (abbreviation for prescription or treatment); (E) inscription (name of drug, dosage, and quantity to be prescribed); (F) signature (directions to the patient); (G) number of refills; (H) whether a generic drug can be used; and (I) prescriber's signature.

may be indicated with a checked box, or it may be written out as "do not substitute" or "dispense as written" if the prescriber prefers the brand name drug. As noted in Chapter 4, insurance companies and health maintenance organizations (HMOs) usually prefer paying for the less expensive drug. However, some patients are allergic to dyes or fillers found in certain generic drugs. For these patients, the brand name drug is the best choice.

The dosage is a crucial piece of information. Make sure that the strength of the drug is clearly indicated. Missing a decimal point or a zero (e.g., 25 mg instead of 2.5 mg or 0.25 mg instead of 25 mg) can harm a patient. If a dose seems inappropriate, check your drug resources before giving the patient the prescription, and if the dose still does not seem right, check it with the prescriber.

The quantity to be dispensed is indicated by a number after a pound sign (#). In addition, this number should be written out. Adding a 0 at the end or a 1 in front of a number is simple, but a number that is also written out is not so easily changed. For an acute problem, the drug may be given for only a short time. Thus, perhaps only a 1-week or 1-month supply is given. A patient with a chronic condition may require a 90-day supply and three refills to continue the drug treatment for a year.

■ **Signature.** The signature is from *signetur,* a Latin word for "write on the label." It instructs the patient when and how to take the drug. Prescribers use standardized abbreviations when writing prescriptions. For example, a prescriber may write "1 tab q4h prn." This Latin is not understood by most patients, so the pharmacist writes the following on the medication label: "Take one tablet by mouth every 4 hours as needed."

■ **Subscription (refill).** The prescriber may specify how many refills are allowed before the patient must return to the office. Patients with chronic conditions may not return to the office for some time. For these patients, refill orders facilitate the continuity of care.

■ **Physician's signature.** Prescriptions are not valid unless they are signed by the physician. Although the prescription may be completely written by the allied health professional (except for Schedule II drug prescriptions), the prescriber must sign the prescription.

### CRITICAL THINKING

If most patients do not understand Latin, why do you think physicians write the signature in Latin?

If a patient calls for a refill, the prescriber may refill the prescription without asking to see the patient again, especially if the patient has a chronic condition or is taking birth control pills. After the refill has been approved, the allied health professional must document in the patient's medical record that the prescription was telephoned to the pharmacy.

### CRITICAL THINKING

You work in a busy gynecologist's office. Many women run out of birth control pills before you can schedule them to come to the office. Create a protocol for refilling oral contraceptives without seeing the patient.

## ■ DRUG LABELS

Drug labeling is all the printed information that is found with a drug, including the label and the package insert from the manufacturer. This labeling is regulated by the Food and Drug Administration (FDA), which specifies exactly what must appear on the label, such as foods, drugs, and activities to be avoided while taking the drug; clear instructions to health-care practitioners; and drug ingredients.

## Medication labels

A medication label contains important information. It includes the pharmacy's name, address, and telephone number (Fig. 5-2A), which are useful in case the patient needs to contact the pharmacy with problems or questions. The dispensing date is also on the label (Fig. 5-2B). This date may differ from the date when the prescriber wrote the prescription. The pharmacist originates an Rx number that identifies this unique prescription in the computer system and on the label (Fig. 5-2C). The patient can refill the prescription by using this number. The patient's full name and address is included (Fig. 5-2D), as are the name of the medication, the strength, the dosage form, the quantity, and the manufacturer (if the drug is generic) (Fig. 5-2E). Refill information must also be included (Fig. 5-2F). The label contains the name of the prescribing physician (Fig. 5-2G). For accuracy, the prescriber's name and perhaps license classification (e.g., MD or FNP) are included. The pharmacist also adds the date when the medication will expire or lose its potency and should be discarded.

The pharmacist translates the Latin abbreviations into English for the patient (compare Fig. 5-1 with Fig. 5-2). It is important for the patient to understand the order but may be hesitant to ask a pharmacist about it. Therefore, before the patient leaves the medical office, be sure the patient knows how to take the drug. Also instruct the patient to read the label on the medication bottle carefully

---

### 🖉 CHECK UP: ABBREVIATIONS

Before completing the rest of the chapter, test yourself on the following abbreviations. If you do not know some of them, make flashcards to help you memorize them.

| | | |
|---|---|---|
| $\bar{a}$ _____ | gtt _____ | o.u. _____ |
| a.c. _____ | hs _____ | oz _____ |
| a.d. _____ | ID _____ | $\bar{p}$ _____ |
| a.s. _____ | IM _____ | p.c. _____ |
| a.u. _____ | IV _____ | prn _____ |
| bid _____ | mcg _____ | $\bar{s}$ _____ |
| $\bar{c}$ _____ | mEq _____ | SC _____ |
| cap _____ | mg _____ | STAT _____ |
| d/c _____ | mL _____ | Tb _____ |
| elix _____ | NPO _____ | tid _____ |
| g _____ | o.d. _____ | tsp _____ |
| gr _____ | o.s. _____ | |

---

■ **Amount of drug dispensed.** The amount of medication contained in the prescription bottle must be listed. This information is listed as a number and, if the medication is in liquid form, the unit of measure, such as 120 mL or 8 ounces. Labels for liquid medications also give the concentration of the liquid (e.g., 100 mg per 5 mL). Labels for pills, tablets, and capsules usually state simple quantity (e.g., Qty: 60).

(A) R<sub>x</sub> Pharmacy    Rx Pharmacy    (B) Date filled: 11/14/2012
345 Cherry Lane
Hometown, VA 22958

(C) Rx 001234789

(D) Martin, Connie
789 Beach Tree Drive
Hometown, VA 22958

(E) Take 1 teaspoonful every day    (F) 3 refills
Claritin 10 mg/10 mL syrup Qty: 150 mL         Discard after 11/14/2013

Mfg: Scherring Corp

(G) Carl Newell M.D.
125 Main Street
Hometown, VA 22958

**FIGURE 5-2:** Sample medication label. A drug label has several parts: (A) name, address, and telephone number of the pharmacy; (B) date when the prescription was filled; (C) Rx (prescription) number; (D) name and address of the patient; (E) drug name, dosage, frequency, and quantity (Latin terms are translated into English for the patient), as well as the manufacturer for generic drugs; (F) number of refills and expiration date; and (G) name of the prescriber.

■ **Warning labels.** The pharmacist places appropriate warning labels on the prescription container to make sure that patients understand the best way to take the medication and become aware of possible situations to avoid. These warning labels are usually a bright color, to preclude their being overlooked (Fast Tip 5.1).

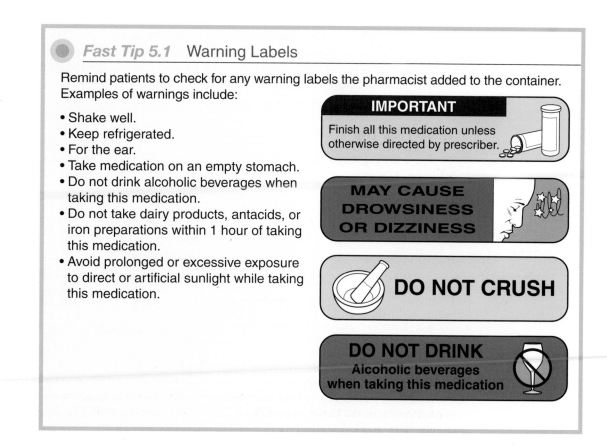

*Fast Tip 5.1*   Warning Labels

Remind patients to check for any warning labels the pharmacist added to the container. Examples of warnings include:

• Shake well.
• Keep refrigerated.
• For the ear.
• Take medication on an empty stomach.
• Do not drink alcoholic beverages when taking this medication.
• Do not take dairy products, antacids, or iron preparations within 1 hour of taking this medication.
• Avoid prolonged or excessive exposure to direct or artificial sunlight while taking this medication.

**IMPORTANT**
Finish all this medication unless otherwise directed by prescriber.

**MAY CAUSE DROWSINESS OR DIZZINESS**

**DO NOT CRUSH**

**DO NOT DRINK**
Alcoholic beverages when taking this medication

## Manufacturer labels and names

Stock medications stored the office must contain necessary information to ensure safe administration. This information should include the brand (trade) name, generic name, drug strength and drug form, route of administration, total amount of medication in the container, directions for reconstitution if necessary, manufacturer, National Drug Code (NDC), expiration date, and lot number (Fig. 5-3).

The manufacturer's name is listed, as are the city and state in which the manufacturer is located. More contact information is available on the drug insert (detailed drug information included with the medication container), which also contains the following information:

- **Trade name.** This is the brand name given to the drug by the manufacturer with the patent rights to this drug. The trade name is always capitalized to differentiate it from the generic name.

- **Generic name.** This is the official name given to the drug by the U.S. Pharmacopeia. Because it is capitalized only if it begins a sentence, the generic name is almost always lower case.

- **Dosage strength and form.** The amount of active drug (e.g., milligrams, micrograms, grains) is listed on the label, as is the form or unit of measure in which the active drug is contained (e.g., tablets, capsules, teaspoons, milliliters).

- **Route of administration.** This instruction explains how the patient is to take the medication. Most medication labels on drugs for parenteral use list the acceptable administration routes. For oral drugs, the common assumption is that a tablet will be given by mouth, and the oral route therefore is not listed.

- **Total quantity.** The quantity indicates the total amount of medication in the container in tablets, capsules, caplets, or milliliters. If the drug is in powder form, the quantity designation will identify the total medication weight in the package, as well as the total concentration and total number of milliliters in the package if reconstituted according to label instructions.

- **NDC number and lot number.** The NDC number assigned to each medication identifies the manufacturer, product, and size of the container. This information is listed on the label as NDC followed by a 10-digit number. The lot number links this package to a specific batch of drugs manufactured in a particular place over a given period of time. This information is important when a problem is found with a drug, such as contamination by a pesticide or other substance. The FDA can usually pinpoint the problem to a specific lot and can issue a recall for that lot number alone.

### Virtual Field Trip

Visit www.walgreens.com and list five different languages (besides English) in which labels can be printed for patients.

NDC 1562-1578-48

**ITCHASIN**
**(diphenhydramine capsules)**
**25 mg**
(100 capsules)

**Dist. By: CICA, INC.**
**589 N. Ruston Dr.**
**Ormond Beach, FL**
**32179, USA**

EXP: 0/30/14
LOT: 15676131

**FIGURE 5-3:** Sample manufacturer label. The manufacturer's label should include the brand (trade) name, generic name, drug strength and drug form, route of administration if other than oral, total amount of medication in the container, directions for reconstitution if necessary, manufacturer, National Drug Code (NDC), expiration date, and lot number.

Prescription drugs are not the only medications that include medication labels. Over-the-counter (OTC) drugs, purchased without a prescription, also contain labels or instructions on drug use based on age and weight. The FDA has determined that, if the consumer takes an OTC medication as directed on the label, the drug is safe for the general population, although the medication may cause side effects, which are also listed on the label. As with prescription drugs, it is important for patients taking OTC drugs to read the label, including the dosage and any possible side effects. OTC drugs can interact negatively with prescription drugs. For example, some cold medicines increase the action of sedatives, so a person taking both medications would be sleepier than expected.

## Virtual Field Trip

Visit the Web site http://bemedwise.org and:
  Print out a brochure in English and Spanish.
  Print out a drug facts label.
  Take the MedWise quiz and report your score.

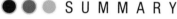 S U M M A R Y

To prescribe drugs safely, the prescriber must write legibly and accurately. As an allied health professional, you must ensure the safe transfer of information from the prescriber through the patient to the pharmacist. To do so, you must memorize abbreviations and understand the parts of the prescription. You also need to be able to read labels and prescriptions to educate patients about taking their medication safely.

## Activities

To make sure that you have learned the key points covered in this chapter, complete the following activities.

### True or False

Write true if the statement is true. Beside the false statements, write false and correct the statement to make it true.

Physicians are the only health-care professionals allowed to write prescriptions. _____

The DEA issues a specific number to those prescribers who write prescriptions for scheduled drugs. _____

There is only one type of medication order. _____

The abbreviation gtt stands for drops. _____

NDC code stands for National Drug Code. _____

OTC medications are never dangerous. _____

A pharmacist can decide whether a generic drug can be used for a brand name drug. _____

A STAT order is a standing order. _____

An automatic stop order means to discontinue the medication after a specified period of time. _____

Rx is the abbreviation for prescription or treatment. _____

### Multiple Choice

Choose the best answer for each question.

**1. Which of the following explains how to take a medication?**
  A. Inscription
  B. Superscription
  C. Subscription
  D. Signature

**2. The abbreviation for three times per day is:**
  A. bid
  B. o.d.
  C. hs
  D. tid

**3. Which abbreviation means without?**
  A. $\bar{p}$
  B. x
  C. $\bar{s}$
  D. $\bar{c}$
  E. w

4. **Which means drops?**
   A. g
   B. gr
   C. gtt
   D. mg

5. **Which means to give the drug immediately?**
   A. prn
   B. STAT
   C. NPO
   D. d/c

6. **The abbreviation for two times per day is:**
   A. bid
   B. o.d.
   C. hs
   D. tid

7. **Which abbreviation means with?**
   A. w
   B. x
   C. $\bar{c}$
   D. $\bar{s}$

8. **Which of the following means to take as needed?**
   A. STAT
   B. prn
   C. NPO
   D. tid

9. **Which abbreviation means that the patient should take nothing by mouth?**
   A. prn
   B. STAT
   C. NPO
   D. d/c

10. **The following are examples of warning labels:**
    A. Shake well.
    B. Keep refrigerated.
    C. Do not take with dairy products.
    D. Avoid prolonged exposure to the sun.
    E. All of the above.

Respond to the following situations on a separate sheet of paper.

1. What standing orders may be necessary for Henry Krause to have a barium enema diagnostic test?

2. Write a prescription for Brittany for the following: Feldene 20-mg capsules. Quantity of 30. Take one every day with food or milk. Before breakfast.

3. The physician frequently misplaces prescription pads. How should these pads be stored to ensure that they are not misused?

4. Prednisone is ordered: four pills today, three tomorrow, two the day after tomorrow, one the day after that, then stop. How many pills are dispensed?

5. How does the label read for the following prescription? Warren Short. Nitroglycerin tablets. 0.4 mg sublingually every 5 minutes, up to three tablets for chest pain. Dr. Clark Castillo wants him to have 60 tablets. The prescription may be refilled as needed, but once the bottle is opened, the tablets should be used for only 6 months.

6. Donna is prescribed doxycycline 100-mg tablets. This prescription is for 20 tablets, with two taken as an initial dose, then one tablet every 12 hours until the supply is exhausted. How would you document this prescription in Donna's chart?

7. Create a prescription for the following: Dr. Campbell wants Peter to have Tylenol 3 (a controlled substance) for pain: one to two tablets every 4 to 6 hours as he needs the medication. Dr. Campbell wants the patient to have 30 tablets. No refills.

8. Theresa, a nurse practitioner, wants Sharon to take potassium tablets daily. Write the prescription for K-Dur, 20 mEq once daily in the morning for 90 days. The prescription can be refilled three times.

# Calculations

6

# Basic Review of Mathematics

*The next three chapters cover dosage calculations. This chapter includes a basic review of mathematics. If you fear mathematics and do not master the problems included in the chapters, you will continue to struggle with mathematical concepts. The more you read these chapters and the more problems you solve, the easier it will be to understand how to calculate dosages safely.*

## LEARNING OUTCOMES

At the end of this chapter, the student will be able to:

6.1 Define all key terms.
6.2 Discuss numerical relationships.
6.3 Perform calculations involving whole numbers.
6.4 Calculate problems using fractions.
6.5 Find the least common denominator.
6.6 Perform calculations involving decimals.
6.7 Calculate percents, ratios, and proportions.
6.8 Solve problems for an unknown quantity.

### KEY TERMS

| | | |
|---|---|---|
| Decimal | Improper fraction | Proper fraction |
| Denominator | Invert | Proportion |
| Dividend | Least common denominator | Ratios |
| Divisor | Means | Scored |
| Extremes | Mixed number | Whole numbers |
| Factors | Numerator | |
| Fraction | Percents | |

## ■ BASIC MATH CONCEPTS

This section covers basic addition, subtraction, multiplication, and division, first with whole numbers, then with fractions and decimals. **Whole numbers** have no subdivisions and are simply a whole amount (1, 2, 3...).

### Addition calculations

Frank has a fluid restriction of 30 oz. To calculate what he consumes, simply add amounts.

He drinks:

| | |
|---|---|
| A 12-oz soda | 12 oz |
| An 8-oz glass of water | 8 oz |
| 6 oz of apple juice    + | 6 oz |
| | 26 oz |

Did he exceed his fluid restriction? His total fluids were 26 oz, which is less than (<) 30 oz, so the answer is no.

Cory is on an 1,800-calorie diet. He eats cereal with one-half cup of milk (150 calories) for breakfast and an apple (90 calories), a soft drink (170 calories), and a cupcake (250 calories) for lunch. How much has he consumed so far today?

$$
\begin{array}{r}
150 \\
90 \\
170 \\
+\ 250 \\
\end{array}
$$

The answer is 660 calories. Although Cory needs to evaluate the quality of his food, he has not exceeded his restriction of 1,800 calories (Check Up 6.1).

### Subtraction calculations

When solving math problems, work on any addition first and then move onto subtraction. In the earlier calorie example, Cory consumed 660 calories. If he has an 1,800-calorie restriction, how many calories can he consume for the rest of the day? To find out, subtract the 660 calories he has already consumed from the maximum of 1,800:

$$
\begin{array}{r}
1,800 \\
-\ 660 \\
\hline
1,140 \\
\end{array}
$$

The answer is that 1,140 calories remain before Cory hits his maximum of 1,800. This problem can be solved in two ways: one is to ask, "What number needs to be added to 660 to make 1,800?" and the other is simply to subtract 660 from 1,800 (Check Up 6.2).

$$660 + ? = 1,800$$
$$1,800 - 660 = 1,140$$

## CHECK UP 6.1: ADDITION PROBLEMS

Here are some addition problems for you to try.

| 250 | 3 | 1000 | 5 | 150 |
|---|---|---|---|---|
| + 150 | + 4 | + 480 | + 26 | + 26 |

## CHECK UP 6.2: SUBTRACTION PROBLEMS

Here are some subtraction problems for you to try.

| 250 | 500 | 21 | 35 | 90 |
|---|---|---|---|---|
| − 175 | − 300 | − 7 | − 8 | − 60 |

## Multiplication calculations

When you multiply numbers, you are adding them together a certain number of times.
   For example:

$$3 \times 4 \text{ is like saying } 4 + 4 + 4 \text{ (adding 4 three times)}$$
$$5 \times 6 \text{ is like saying } 6 + 6 + 6 + 6 + 6 = \text{ (adding 6 five times)}$$

If Sally takes three pills per day for 7 days, how many does she take in a week?

$$\text{Sunday Monday Tuesday Wednesday Thursday Friday Saturday}$$
$$3 + 3 + 3 + 3 + 3 + 3 + 3$$
$$\text{or } 7 \times 3 = 21$$

Multiplying $3 \times 7$ is usually easier than adding 3 seven times. Addition can be used to check multiplication: $3 + 3 + 3 + 3 + 3 + 3 + 3 = 21$ (Check Up 6.3). Table 6.1 provides more multiplication examples.

---

### CHECK UP 6.3: MULTIPLICATION PROBLEMS

Here are some multiplication problems for you to try.

| 4 | 2 | 3 | 30 | 100 |
|---|---|---|----|-----|
| × 10 | × 90 | × 7 | × 7 | × 3 |

---

**TABLE 6.1   Examples of the Practical Use of Multiplication**

If Alex Boles drinks six 12-oz sodas per day, how many sodas does he consume in 1 week?

$$6 \times 7 = ? \text{ sodas per week}$$
$$6 \times 7 = 42 \text{ sodas per week}$$

If each soda is 12 oz, how many ounces of soda does he consume in 1 week?

$$42 \text{ sodas} \times 12 \text{ oz each} = 504 \text{ oz}$$

If each soda has 150 calories, how many calories does he consume from soda in 1 week?

$$42 \text{ sodas} \times 150 \text{ calories} = 6{,}300 \text{ calories from soda per week}$$

---

## Division calculations

Division is the fourth of the basic math concepts (Check Up 6.4). In an earlier example, Corey was allowed 1,140 calories for the rest of the day. How can this amount be split evenly throughout the day? A possible solution is to divide the calories into two meals:

$$1{,}140 \div 2 = 570 \text{ calories during each of the two meals}$$

---

### CHECK UP 6.4: DIVISION PROBLEMS

Here are some division problems for you to try.

| 500 | 6 | 18 | 21 | 90 |
|-----|---|----|----|-----|
| ÷ 250 | ÷ 3 | ÷ 6 | ÷ 7 | ÷ 10 |

These examples of addition, subraction, multiplication, and division show that these functions are used daily in the health-care setting. The next section discusses fractions and how to add, subtract, multiply, and divide them.

# ■ WORKING WITH FRACTIONS

A **fraction** is simply a part of a whole. Understanding fractions is important because often a dose that must be administered is not a whole number. If we do not understand how fractions function, patients will be in danger of receiving the incorrect dosage.

Suppose you have a whole pizza and want to give some to your friends. You can divide the pizza in slices of varying sizes (Fig. 6-1). For example, you can divide the pizza into three pieces or four pieces; a slice of pizza from the three-piece division is larger than a slice of pizza from the four-piece division. In other words:

1/3 is greater than 1/4
1/4 is less than 1/3

The number on the top is called the **numerator.** It is part of the whole being divided. The **denominator** is the number on the bottom. It represents the total number of equal parts in the problem.

If the numerator is smaller than the denominator, the fraction is called a **proper fraction** (Fig. 6-2). In the pizza example, if you have three friends and divide the pizza into four pieces, each of your three friends will have a piece, and that leaves one piece (1/4) for you.

*CRITICAL THINKING*

What happens to the pizza slices when a numerator becomes larger? A denominator becomes larger? If you have trouble remembering this concept, ask yourself, what would happen if you and your siblings were inheriting money? The more brothers and sisters you have, the smaller your share would be.

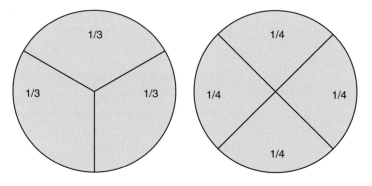

**FIGURE 6-1:** Fractions. Slices of a pie (represented as this circle) divided into three sections are larger than slices of a pie divided into four sections: 1/3 is larger than 1/4.

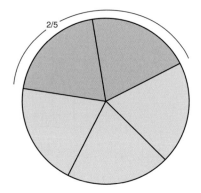

**FIGURE 6-2:** Proper fraction. This figure shows the proper fraction 2/5. It is a proper fraction because the numerator (top number) is smaller than the denominator (bottom number).

An **improper fraction** means that the numerator is larger than the denominator. It is top-heavy. For example, you divide a pizza into four pieces but have five friends (5/4). You will need to find another pizza or cut smaller pieces (Fig. 6-3 and Check Up 6.5 to 6.7).

## Least common denominators

A common denominator is a number that is a common multiple of two (or more) denominators. Finding the lowest number into which both denominators can be divided to keep the fraction small makes it easier to work with and is called the **least common denominator (LCD)**. To find the LCD of two or more fractions:

■ List the multiples of each denominator.

■ Compare the lists. Any numbers that appear on all lists are common denominators.

■ The lowest number that appears on all lists is the LCD.

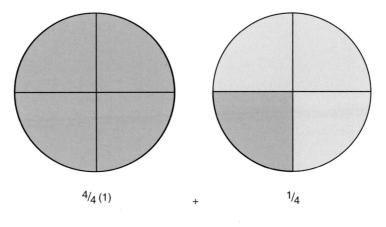

4/4 (1)  +  1/4

= 5/4 or 1 1/4

**FIGURE 6-3:** Improper fraction. If you divide a pie into four pieces but have five friends, you need to find another pie, be "improper," or cut smaller pieces. This illustration shows the improper fraction of 5/4. You can also write 1 1/4 because 5/4 = 4/4 (or 1) + 1/4.

---

### CHECK UP 6.5: FRACTION SIZES

Circle the fraction with the largest value in each listing. Then, using the same numbers, underline the lowest value in each listing.

4/25, 5/25, 10/25     1/75, 1/100, 1/125

1/300, 1/200, 1/100     4/8, 1/8, 2/8

5/3, 2/3, 4/3

Circle the fraction with the lowest value, and underline the highest.

1/10, 1/8, 1/6     2/16, 1/16, 4/16

3/6, 2/6, 5/6     2/12, 1/12, 6/12

1/25, 1/75, 1/50

## CHECK UP 6.6: SHADE THE PIZZAS

In each of the circles, divide the pizza into the denominator, and shade the numerator.

## CHECK UP 6.7: IMPROPER FRACTIONS

1.  Shade the circles to represent the improper fraction 16/5

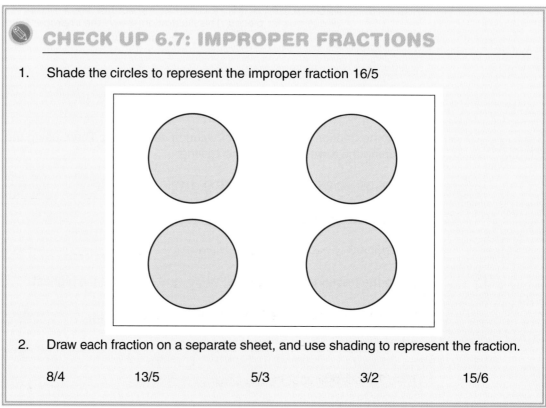

2.  Draw each fraction on a separate sheet, and use shading to represent the fraction.

   8/4        13/5          5/3          3/2          15/6

Example: 1/9 + 1/6

Write the multiples of each denominator:

9   »   9...**18**...27...36

6   »   6...12...**18**...24...36

As you can see, both 18 and 36 are common denominators of 9 and 6. However, 18 is the LCD. Once you have the LCD, it becomes the denominator of each fraction. Using this example, determine what number, when multiplied, would give you the LCD. In this case, if you multiplied 9 by 2, you would have 18, which would become the denominator.

$$9 \times 2 = 18$$

Next multiply 2 by the numerator, which is 1. Your fraction would then be 2/18. For the fraction of 1/6, the denominator is 6. You would multiply 6 by 3 to make 18, and then multiply the 1 by 3 and place it over 18. Thus:

$$1/9 + 1/6 = 2/18 + 3/18 = 5/18$$

In Check Up 6.8 and 6.9, test your knowledge of working with fractions.

## CHECK UP 6.8: LEAST COMMON DENOMINATORS

Find the least common denominator, and then work out the problem on a separate sheet.

1/15 + 1/45 = _____        4/5 + 5/12 = _____

1/3 + 3/8 = _____          5/6 + 3/5 = _____

5/12 + 1/10 = _____        1/2 + 1/19 = _____

1/4 + 1/5 = _____          3/25 + 4/75 = _____

3/8 + 1/6 = _____          1/4 + 3/16 = _____

## CHECK UP 6.9: TAKING FRACTIONS APART

Examine the fraction 3/4.

1.   What are the total equal parts in one whole? _____

2.   What is the size of each part? _____

3.   How many parts are being talked about? _____

4.   The numerator is _____.

5.   The denominator is _____.

## Mixed numbers and improper fractions

A **mixed number** is a whole number plus a fraction (for example: 5 1/2). You will need to know how to convert mixed numbers into improper fractions as you work with various medication orders and dosages. To do this:

■ Multiply the denominator by the whole number.

$$2 \text{ (denominator)} \times 5 \text{ (whole number)} = 10$$

■ Add the result from the first step to the numerator.

$$10 + 1 \text{ (numerator)} = 11$$

■ Keep the denominator.

$$11/2$$

The reverse is also necessary—learning how to convert improper fractions to mixed numbers. The process for this is as follows:

■ Divide the numerator by the denominator.

$$29 \text{ (numerator)} \div 5 = 5 \text{ (remainder of 4)}$$

■ The remainder becomes the numerator.

$$5 \ 4/5$$

■ The denominator stays the same.

$$29/5 = 5 \ 4/5$$

In Check Up 6.10 and 6.11, convert the mixed numbers to improper fractions and vice versa.

---

### CHECK UP 6.10: CONVERTING

Convert these mixed numbers to improper fractions.

3 1/3 = _____      10 2/5 = _____

9 1/2 = _____      1 1/6 = _____

6 1/4 = _____

---

### CHECK UP 6.11: CONVERTING

Convert these improper fractions to mixed numbers.

28/5 = _____      52/10 = _____

42/5 = _____      7/6 = _____

30/7 = _____

### Reducing to lowest terms

Because large numbers can be more difficult to work with, learning how to reduce a number to its lowest term is important. **Factors** (numbers multiplied together to make another number) are used to determine the largest common divisor (the biggest whole number that reduces multiple whole numbers) to divide the **dividend** (the number you want to reduce). In this case, both the numerator and denominator are divided.

To reduce a larger fraction such as 6/10 to its lowest term, follow these steps:

■ Determine the largest common divisor.

Determine the factors of each number:

$$6$$
$$1 \times 6 = 6$$
$$2 \times 3 = 6$$

Factors of 6 are therefore 1, **2**, 3, and 6.

$$10$$
$$1 \times 10 = 10$$
$$2 \times 5 = 10$$

Factors of 10 are therefore 1, **2**, 5, and 10.

Compare the two lists of factors, and determine the highest number common to both lists. In this instance, 2 is the highest number on both lists; thus, both 6 and 10 are divisible by 2.

■ Divide the numerator and denominator by this number to reduce it to its lowest terms (Check Up 6.12).

$$\frac{6 \div 2}{10 \div 2} = \frac{3}{5}$$

### Adding fractions

At times, a patient is required to take partial tablets. When computing a month's supply of medication, you must be able to calculate how many tablets the patient takes per day because pharmacies do not dispense partial tablets. Adding fractions is easy when they have the same denominator.

■ Add the numerators.

$$\text{Example: } 1/4 + 1/4$$
$$1 + 1 = 2$$

■ Place the sum (what you find when you add) over the denominator.

$$2/4$$

### CHECK UP 6.12: REDUCE THE FRACTIONS

Reduce these fractions to lowest terms.

2/6 = _____        15/50 = _____

8/10 = _____       36/12 = _____

3/9 = _____        21/27 = _____

5/10 = _____       6/10 = _____

2/8 = _____        100/300 = _____

■ Reduce to the lowest terms.

$$\frac{2 \div 2}{4 \div 2} = \frac{1}{2}$$

Adding fractions with different denominators:

■ Change fractions to an equal fraction with the LCD.

Example: 1/3 + 1/4 = LCD for both 3 and 4 is 12. Multiply this number by the numerator.

$$3 \times 4 = 12; \text{ so, } 4 \times 1 = 4/12$$
$$4 \times 3 = 12; \text{ so, } 3 \times 1 = 3/12$$

■ Add the numerators.

$$4 + 3 = 7$$

■ Place the sum over the denominator.

$$= 7/12$$

■ Reduce to the lowest terms.

The largest common divisor for 7 and 12 is 1; therefore, 7/12 constitutes the lowest terms (Check Up 6.13).

## Subtracting fractions

Subtracting fractions with the same denominator follows the same process as adding fractions.

■ Subtract the numerator.

■ Preserve the same denominator.

■ Reduce if necessary.

Example: 5/6 – 1/6 = 4/6 = 2/3

If the denominators are different, you must:

Example: 12/5 – 1/2

■ Find the LCD.

5 **10** 15 20 25 30
2 4 6 8 **10** 12 14 16

■ Change to equivalent fractions.

5 × 2 = 10; thus, multiply 12 × 2 = 24, which results in 24/10
2 × 5 = 10; thus, multiply 1 × 5 = 5, which results in 5/10

---

### ✐ CHECK UP 6.13: ADD THE FRACTIONS

Add the fractions with both a common denominator and a different denominator based on what you have reviewed.

1/2 + 1/3 = _____          1/4 + 1/6 = _____

1/10 + 2/5 = _____          1/9 + 2/3 = _____

5/8 + 3/7 = _____

■ Subtract the numerators.

$$24 - 5 = 19$$

■ Place the remainder over the common denominator.

$$19/10$$

■ Reduce if necessary (Check Up 6.14).

$$1\ 9/10$$

## Multiplying fractions

Multiplying fractions is also fairly straightforward. You do not have to worry about common denominators.

■ Multiply the numerators.
■ Multiply the denominators.
■ Reduce if necessary.

$$\text{Example: } \frac{2}{5} \times \frac{3}{4} = \frac{2 \times 3}{5 \times 4} = \frac{6}{20} = \frac{3}{10}$$

In Check Up 6.15, multiply the fractions.

---

### CHECK UP 6.14: SUBTRACT THE FRACTIONS

Subtract these fractions.

2/3 – 1/3 = _____          10/6 – 2/3 = _____

5/6 – 5/12 = _____          15 – 7 1/2 = _____

250/500 – 50/500 = _____

---

### CHECK UP 6.15: MULTIPLY THE FRACTIONS

Multiply these fractions.          Divide these fractions.

1/3 × 4/6 = _____          1/6 ÷ 1/2 = _____

1/8 × 5/10 = _____          15/30 ÷ 5 = _____

2/3 × 8/9 = _____          2/3 ÷ 3/2 = _____

5/6 × 1/6 = _____          6/2 ÷ 3/4 = _____

5/25 × 5/3 = _____          2/3 ÷ 6/8 = _____

*CRITICAL THINKING*

If you give 1/3 tablespoon of a medication four times daily, how much of the medication do you need per day?

### Dividing fractions

Division is multiplication in reverse. When you multiply 1/5 × 2/3, you have 2/15. Suppose you divide 2/15 by 1/3. You should have 2/3.

To reverse multiplication, **invert** the fraction you are dividing by (flip the numerator and denominator over), and change the process to multiplication instead of division.

$$\text{Example:} \quad \frac{2}{15} \div \frac{1}{5} \rightarrow \frac{2}{15} \times \frac{5}{1} = \frac{10}{15} = \frac{2}{3}$$

Therefore, the steps for dividing fractions are as follows:

■ Invert the second fraction.

■ Multiply the two fractions.

■ Reduce if needed.

In Check Up 6.15, try dividing the fractions.

*CRITICAL THINKING*

Sometimes we need to teach the patient how to break certain pills. For example, if Colleen Watkins takes 1 1/2 pills per dose, how long will 30 pills last?

## DECIMALS

A **decimal** is similar to a fraction, but with 10, 100, 1,000, and so on in the denominator. However, rather than writing it as a fraction, you can use a decimal point. Because drug doses often contain decimal points, it is important to understand decimals and how they work. Figure 6-4 illustrates how to identify units in numbers that have a decimal.

### Rounding decimals

Tablets are not usually dispensed in parts unless they are specifically **scored** (easily divisible into accurate doses) to do so. Capsules cannot be broken apart and separated evenly. Thus, you would usually round up or down if a dosage calculation does not produce a whole number. With fluids, you can give an

---

### CHECK UP 6.15: MULTIPLY AND DIVIDE

| Multiply these fractions. | Divide these fractions. |
|---|---|
| 1/3 × 4/6 = _____ | 1/6 ÷ 1/2 = _____ |
| 1/8 × 5/10 = _____ | 15/30 ÷ 5 = _____ |
| 2/3 × 8/9 = _____ | 2/3 ÷ 3/2 = _____ |
| 5/6 × 1/6 = _____ | 6/2 ÷ 3/4 = _____ |
| 5/25 × 5/3 = _____ | 2/3 ÷ 6/8 = _____ |

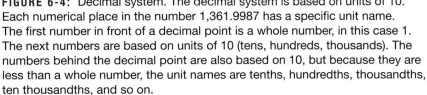

**FIGURE 6-4:** Decimal system. The decimal system is based on units of 10. Each numerical place in the number 1,361.9987 has a specific unit name. The first number in front of a decimal point is a whole number, in this case 1. The next numbers are based on units of 10 (tens, hundreds, thousands). The numbers behind the decimal point are also based on 10, but because they are less than a whole number, the unit names are tenths, hundredths, thousandths, ten thousandths, and so on.

exact decimal (e.g., 1.3 mL), but you may need to round up or down between 1.3 and 1.4 if the decimal is between those marks on the syringe or a measuring cup.

If a tablet is not scored, and you must round the amount:

For 0.04 to 1.49 → give one tablet
For 1.50 to 1.99 → give two tablets

For dosage calculations, it is rarely necessary to go past the hundredths place.

## Identifying decimal values

Determining whether you are giving a correct dosage requires a basic understanding of how decimals change the value of a number. Moving the decimal by one place increases or decreases the value of the number by 10; moving it two places changes the value by 100, and so forth. Those differences are significant in the amount of medication given to a patient. Thus, it is important to know how to compare numbers with decimals.

When decimal numbers contain whole numbers, the whole numbers must be compared to determine which is larger. For example, 5.8 is larger than 2.9, and 7.37 is larger than 6.39. When the whole numbers are the same or zero and the numbers in the tenths place are the same, the decimal with the higher number in the hundredths place is larger. For example, 0.66 is larger than 0.64, and 2.17 is larger than 2.15.

In Check Up 6.16, solve the problems regarding scored and unscored tablets.

The addition of zeros to the right of the end of a decimal does not alter its value, so these zeros are usually deleted. For example, if the number is 3.0, we would write 3 instead of 3.0. In addition, if the decimal is somehow missed (read as 30 instead of 3.0), an error would occur, resulting in a dosage 10 times too high. The zero to the left of the decimal point, however, is very important; it shows that the dosage is very small; 0.35 would be written instead of .35. Again, if the decimal point were missed (read as 35 instead of .35), this particular error would cause the patient to receive 100 times too much medication. Therefore, use of the decimal point in relation to zeros is a safety issue.

In Check Up 6.17, circle the larger number.

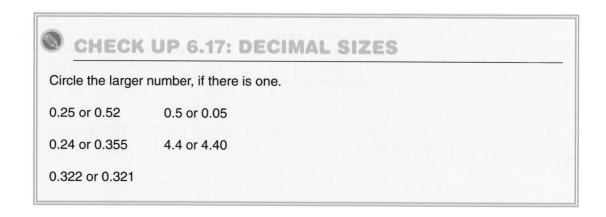

## CHECK UP 6.16: SCORE THE TABLETS

If you had a scored tablet, what would you give for each of the following doses?

1.1 = _____     2.1 = _____

1.5 = _____     2.49 = _____

1.0 = _____

If you had an unscored tablet, what would you give?

1.1 = _____     2.1 = _____

1.5 = _____     2.59 = _____

1.9 = _____

## CHECK UP 6.17: DECIMAL SIZES

Circle the larger number, if there is one.

0.25 or 0.52       0.5 or 0.05

0.24 or 0.355      4.4 or 4.40

0.322 or 0.321

*CRITICAL THINKING*

**Why is it important when writing a prescription to write the leading zero (e.g., 0.25 instead of .25)?**

### Adding decimals

To add decimals, line up the decimal points and add each column; carry over a number as necessary.

$$\begin{array}{r} \text{Example:} \quad 1.25 \\ +\ 2.56 \\ \hline 3.81 \end{array}$$

In Check Up 6.18, add the decimals.

### Subtracting decimals

To subtract decimals, line up the decimal points and subtract.

$$\begin{array}{r} \text{Example:} \quad 4.3000 \\ -\ 1.7942 \\ \hline 2.5058 \end{array}$$

In Check Up 6.19, subtract each of the decimal values.

CHECK UP 6.18: ADD THE DECIMALS

Add the following. You may want to rewrite them on top of each other.

0.3 + 0.07 = _____          5.44 + 60.66 = _____

219.8 + 14.02 = _____        8.774 + 0.26 = _____

9.07 + 19.1 = _____

CHECK UP 6.19: SUBTRACT THE DECIMALS

Subtract these decimals. You may want to rewrite them on the top of each other.

13.2 – 6.82 = _____          64.1 – 1.999 = _____

3.005 – 1.882 = _____        25.4 – 3.9 = _____

29 – 10.03 = _____

## Multiplying decimals

To multiply decimals, multiply as for whole numbers, and insert the decimal point into the product so that the number of places to the right is equal to the sum of the decimal places in the factors.

$$
\begin{array}{r}
\text{Example: } 21.4 \quad \rightarrow \text{ one place to the right of the decimal point} \\
\times\, 0.36 \rightarrow \text{ two places to the right of the decimal point} \\
\hline
1284 \\
642 \quad\; \\
\hline
7.704 \rightarrow \text{ three places to the right of the decimal point}
\end{array}
$$

To multiply a decimal by a power of 10 (10, 100, 1,000 ....), move the decimal point to the right the same number of places as there are zeros in the power of 10. This is important in case a prescriber orders a medication in a unit of measure different from what is on the label (Fast Tip 6.1). Chapter 8 discusses this issue in more detail.

In Check Up 6.20, multiply the decimal values.

## Dividing decimals

To divide decimals, follow these steps.

■ Move the decimal in the **divisor** (number doing the dividing) to the right of the decimal place to make the divisor a whole number. If you are dividing 100 by 0.5, 0.5 would become 5.0.

■ Move the decimal the same number of places in the dividend (number being divided). In this example, 100 would become 1,000.

■ Then do the long division. In this case, 1,000 ÷ 5 = 200.

In Check Up 6.21, divide the decimal values.

## Decimal and fractional forms

Have you noticed that decimals are really fractions? For example, 0.3 is simply 3/10, and 0.95 is 95/100.

# Activities

To make sure that you have learned the key points covered in this chapter, complete the following activities.

## Calculations

Find the answer to each of the following equations.

1. 90 ÷ 3 = _____

2. 3 × 7 = _____

3. 28 ÷ 4 = _____

4. 4 + 3 + 2 = _____

5. 50 – 28 = _____

Find the least common denominator.

1. 1/3 and 1/4 _____

2. 1/8 and 1/6 _____

3. 1/2 and 1/3 _____

4. 1/5 and 1/15 _____

5. 1/15 and 1/90 _____

6. 1/7 and 1/9 _____

7. 1/4 and 1/9 _____

8. 1/10 and 1/4 _____

9. 1/100 and 1/25 _____

10. 1/2 and 1/10 _____

Add the following.

1. 3/4 + 1/4 = _____

2. 1/5 + 2/5 = _____

3. 1/6 + 2/3 = _____

4. 1 1/3 + 1/3 = _____

5. 1 1/3 + 2/3 = _____

6. 8/17 + 6/17 + 2/17 = _____

7. 2/3 + 3/8 = _____

8. 2/5 + 1/3 = _____

9. 1/4 + 1/6 = _____

10. 1 1/3 + 1/2 = _____

Subtract the following.

1. 1 1/2 – 1/2 = _____

2. 15/7 – 8/7 = _____

3. 150/50 – 75/50 = _____

4. 21/1 – 3/1 = _____

5. 5/6 – 3/6 = _____

6. 3/4 – 2/4 = _____

7. 6/3 – 1 1/2 = _____

8. 3/4 – 1/4 = _____

9. 7/18 – 3/24 = _____

10. 4/6 – 1/6 = _____

Multiply the following.

1. 1/3 × 1/4 = _____

2. 250/1 × 1/500 = _____

3. 200/400 × 1/2 = _____

4. 5/1 × 1/4 = _____

5. 3/1 × 10/1 = _____

6. 1/2 × 90 = _____

7. 4/1 × 2 1/2 = _____

8. 3/7 × 3/9 = _____

9. 300/600 × 1 = _____

10. 150/450 × 2 = _____

Divide the following.

1. 4/4 ÷ 5/9 = _____

2. 5/10 ÷ 2/4 = _____

3. 1/6 ÷ 1/6 = _____

4. 9/10 ÷ 3/5 = _____

5. 6/9 ÷ 9/10 = _____

6. 6 ÷ 1/6 = _____

7. 1 2/3 ÷ 2/4 = _____

8. 3/5 ÷ 5/9 = _____

9. 100 ÷ 4 = _____

10. 6 ÷ 6/8 = _____

Reduce the following fractions.

1. 500/250 = _____

2. 600/3 = _____

3. 1,000/10 = _____

4. 100/4 = _____

5. 75/150 = _____

6. 240/3 = _____

7. 250/25 = _____

8. 50/500 = _____

9. 100/150 = _____

10. 15/150 = _____

Calculate these decimal problems.

1. 0.04 ÷ 0.2 = _____

2. 10.87 – 0.345 = _____

3. 100 × 9.8 = _____

4. Arrange from smallest to largest: 0.135, 0.13, 0.003 _____

5. Write 52 thousandths as a decimal. _____

6. Divide 17.25 by 0.85. Round to the nearest tenth. _____

7. Round to the nearest tenth: 18.75 _____

8. Convert to a decimal: 6 1/4 _____

9. Write as a decimal: 7 1/5 _____

10. 1.054 + 3.15 = _____

11. 0.05 + 0.005 = _____

12. 250.98 – 5.55 = _____

13. 250 × 0.2 = _____

14. 250 ÷ 500 = _____

15. 250 ÷ 0.5 = _____

Which is greater?

1. 0.12 or 0.012 _____

2. 4.4 or 0.44 _____

3. 0.15 or 0.16 _____

4. 1.6 or 0.16 _____

5. 0.05 or 0.50 _____

Answer the following questions.

1. What is 10% of a fraction? _____

2. What is 5/100 as a percentage? _____

3. What is 50% of 60? _____

4. What is 0.25 as a percentage? _____

5. What is 75 % as a decimal? _____

Convert these decimals to ratios.

1. 0.33 _____

2. 0.50 _____

3. 0.67 _____

4. 0.75 _____

5. 0.90 _____

Convert these ratios to percentages.

1. 1:2 _____

2. 2:3 _____

3. 1:4 _____

4. 2:5 _____

5. 4:6 _____

Convert these percentages to ratios.

1. 50% _____

2. 67% _____

3. 80% _____

4. 99% _____

5. 60% _____

Check whether the following ratios are correct. Write true or false.

1. 1:10::4:50 _____

2. 250:500::1:2 _____

3. 100:400::3:5 _____

4. 1:2::200:400 _____

5. 50:150::1:2 _____

Solve for the ? (unknown).

1. 1:10::3:? _____

2. 100:1::400:? _____

3. 200:400::2:? _____

4. 2:3::4:? _____

5. 1:2::?:8 _____

6. 100:300::?:3 _____

7. 100:300::?:6 _____

8. 100:200::?:4 _____

9. 200:1::400:? _____

10. 1:200::?:400 _____

11. 100:1::200:? _____

12. 1:3::2:? _____

13. 0.5:1::?:2 _____

14. 0.25 :1::25:? _____

15. 75:150::1:? _____

## Application Exercises

Respond to the following situations on a separate sheet.

1. One slice of bread contains 100 calories. How many calories do you reduce if you omit a slice of bread per day for 30 days?

2. One serving of crisp bread is 60 calories. If you ate three servings, how many calories did you eat?

3. A banana split has 550 calories. If you burn 350 calories, how many calories do you still have to burn to work off the banana split calories?

4. Jamie received 21 sample pills from her physician. If she has to take three per day, how many days will the pills last before she needs to fill the written prescription her physician gave her?

5. Jane weighed 102 lb at the end of January. He gained 4 lb in February and 2 lb in March. How much does he weigh at the end of March?

6. Joyce gives her daughter 1/2 T at each of three meals each day. How much does she give in 1 day?

7. Diana drank 2 1/2 cups of water, 1 1/4 cups of milk, and 1 cup of orange juice. How many cups did she drink?

8. At the beginning of the day, you have a 30-oz bottle of medication. If each dose is 1/2 oz, how many doses in total do you have?

9. Jasmine weighed 100 lb at the last visit. She has lost 4 1/2 lb this month. How much does she now weigh?

10. Annabelle is receiving 500 mL of fluid IV. A total of 250 mL has been used in 1 hour. How much is left?

11. Peter makes $12.00 per hour. If he works for 32 hours, how much does he make?

12. Colleen is feeling very drowsy on 50 mg of Zoloft. The nurse practitioner says to cut the prescription by 50%. How much should Colleen take?

13. Donnie made sales totaling the following this hour: $15.28, $77.42, $35.00, $10.00, $35.00, $98.99, and $17.44. How much in total did he make this hour?

14. Kelly owes a medical office $498.43 and pays $35.00. How much does she now owe?

15. Gary sees the physician four times this month. Each time he pays $35.50. How much does he pay in total?

16. Dr. Binderwald has allotted $240.60 in bonuses to be split equally among his six staff members. How much should each person receive?

17. In this medical office, the ratio of allied health professionals to patients is 1:3. If there are 60 patients, how many allied health professionals are needed at this time?

18. If there are 50 vials of flu vaccine in a box and you need 200 vials, how many boxes do you need?

19. If 3 grams of a drug are contained in 50 mL of solution, write the ratio.

20. Describe a 10% bleach solution as a ratio.

21. How much bleach is in the solution mentioned in question 20? How much water?

22. David weighs 50 lb. He is about one third of an adult's weight. How much of an adult dose should he receive?

23. Ian weighs 300 lb. If an adult dose is based on 150 lb and he is twice that size, how much of an adult dose should he receive of a medication with a dosage based on weight?

24. Judith is slicing a pie. She sliced six pieces for her three children. If the children are given equal shares, how many slices does each child receive?

25. Sheri Yamada is adding up her paychecks for this month. She received $355.60, $320.00, $440.00, and $350.40. How much did she make this month?

# Measurement Systems

*After reviewing the basic mathematics necessary to determine dosage calculations, the next steps are to examine and review the four systems of measurement used for drug dispensing: avoirdupois, apothecary, household, and metric.*

## LEARNING OUTCOMES

At the end of this chapter, the student will be able to:

7.1 Define all key terms.
7.2 Compare the four systems of measurement used for drug dispensing.
7.3 State the basic units of measurement in the metric system.
7.4 Use conversion methods for each system of measurement correctly and accurately.

### KEY TERMS

| Apothecary system | Avoirdupois system | Compound |
|---|---|---|

## MEASUREMENT SYSTEMS

Before the metric system was developed, pharmacists used to **compound,** or mix, and dispense drugs. Patients and their families often measured drugs with whatever utensils were handy, such as teaspoons, tablespoons, and cups of various sizes. Today, medications are ordered using the metric system. The four systems discussed here are the avoirdupois, apothecary, metric, and household systems.

### Avoirdupois system

The **avoirdupois system** is a measurement system in which all units are based on the pound. This system is used for measuring medications, as well as for general purposes. Most scales used to weigh patients measure weight in pounds and ounces. As a health-care professional, you need to learn how to convert pounds to kilograms to calculate drug dosages. Dosages of some medications are strictly based on a patient's weight, and others must be adjusted if the patient is either obese or very small. The two accepted conversion methods have results that differ slightly, as shown in the examples given here. The conversions for kilograms to pounds and for pounds to kilograms are as follows:

$$1 \text{ kg} = 2.2 \text{ lb}$$
$$1 \text{ lb} = 0.45 \text{ kg}$$

Therefore, if a patient weighed 95 lb and you needed to convert this weight to kilograms, you would multiply by 0.45:

$$95 \times 0.45 = 42.75 \text{ kg, rounded to } 43 \text{ kg}$$

An alternative would be to divide by 2.2:

$$95 \div 2.2 = 43.18 \text{ kg, rounded to } 43 \text{ kg}$$

### CRITICAL THINKING

> Harold French is seen in the office. He has a history of congestive heart failure and is concerned that he is gaining a lot of weight. You determine that he weighs 185 lb. When he asks you how much weight he has gained since his last check up the previous month, you check the chart and find that he weighed 79 kg. What will you tell him?

The foregoing conversions work well with whole numbers. However, suppose a pediatric patient weighs 9 lb 8 oz. In this case, to calculate accurately, you must know how many ounces are in 1 lb. Ounces are most commonly used when weighing infants and children, whose weight is typically much less than an adult's and in whom every ounce counts. In addition, as discussed in Chapter 8, because infants' body systems are not fully developed, infants are extremely susceptible to inappropriately high drug doses. The nervous system, kidneys, and liver of these small patients are not mature enough to process the medications as a healthy adult does. Therefore, we must be extremely precise when weighing infants and small children and again when converting their weights between systems, to ensure appropriate medication doses.

$$1 \text{ pound (lb)} = 16 \text{ ounces (oz)}$$

Example: The foregoing patient weighs 9 lb 8 oz; therefore:

$$\text{Divide } 8 \text{ by } 16 = 0.5$$
$$9.5 \text{ lb} \times 0.45 = 4.28 \text{ kg or } 4.3 \text{ kg rounded}$$

Or

$$9.5 \text{ lb} \div 2.2 = 4.31 \text{ kg or } 4.3 \text{ kg rounded}$$

### CRITICAL THINKING

> Sally Smitty brings her 3-month-old baby to the clinic because of a fever and possible ear infection. You find that the infant weighs 13 lb, 4 oz. The physician writes an order for you to give a dose of antibiotics based on the infant's weight in kilograms. Before you give the medication, you must convert the child's weight to kilograms. How will you do this, and what is her weight in kilograms?

Conversely, the scale used may be calibrated in the metric system, and you may need to convert kilograms to pounds and ounces for the patient or the patient's family. For example, if a patient is told that he lost 5 kg, this value may not mean as much to him as if you told him that he lost 11 lb. It is also more likely that a home scale will measure in pounds and not in kilograms. Parents of infants may also want to know their infant's weight in pounds rather than kilograms.

Example 1: The patient weighs 14 kg.

$$14 \times 2.2 = 30.8 \text{ or } 31 \text{ lb rounded}$$

Or

$$14 \div 0.45 = 31.1 \text{ or } 31 \text{ lb rounded}$$

Example 2: The patient weighs 4.3 kg.

$$4.3 \times 2.2 = 9.5 \text{ lb and}$$
$$9.5 \text{ lb} = 9 + (0.5 \times 16) = 9 \text{ lb } 8 \text{ oz}$$

Or

$$4.3 \div 0.45 = 9.5 \text{ lb and}$$
$$9.5 \text{ lb} = 9 + (0.5 \times 16) = 9 \text{ lb } 8 \text{ oz}$$

In Check Up 7.1, practice converting weights from pounds to kilograms

### CRITICAL THINKING

Would you rather be weighed in kilograms or pounds? Why?

## Apothecary system

The **apothecary system,** which uses fractions instead of decimals, is one of the oldest systems of measurement. In addition, Roman numerals are common in this system, as opposed to Arabic numerals used in all other systems. Pharmacists, or apothecaries as they were known, used this system for compounding drugs. The apothecary system is not used often because it is complicated and less accurate (rounding of numbers is necessary). However, some prescribers continue to use it, just as some patients continue to use nonmetric measuring utensils, so you must be familiar with it. Common drugs that follow the apothecary system of measurement are Tylenol (Tylenol gr V) and morphine (morphine gr 1/4), which may be ordered or available in grains. Chapter 8 discusses how to convert grains into metric measurements.

### Virtual Field Trip

Search Google (www.google.com) for "apothecary in Williamsburg." Print information about what it was like to work as an apothecary in Colonial Williamsburg.

## CHECK UP 7.1: POUNDS TO KILOGRAMS

Convert these weights from pounds (lb) to kilograms (kg).

195 lb = _____kg          300 lb = _____kg

55 lb = _____kg          125 lb = _____kg

40 lb = _____kg

Convert these weights from pounds (lb) to kilograms (kg).

2 lb 4 oz = _____kg          6 lb 12 oz= _____kg

7 lb 3 oz = _____kg          12 lb 6 oz= _____kg

4 lb 8 oz = _____kg

Convert these weights from kilograms (kg) to pounds (lb).

85 kg = _____lb          200 kg = _____lb

10 kg = _____lb          21 kg = _____lb

120 kg = _____lb

### Household system

At home, a patient may use available teaspoons, tablespoons, cups, glasses, teacups, or other utensils to measure medication. However, this practice is unsafe because household utensil sizes are not standardized. Encourage your patients to use the metric system or standardized measuring tools. Box 7.1 provides key equivalents of household measures.

---

#### A CLOSER LOOK: Apothecary Symbols and Abbreviations

Although symbols and abbreviations for some apothecary measurements are not recommended, some prescribers still use them, so you should be familiar with them.

| Unit | Abbreviation | Symbol |
|------|--------------|--------|
| Grain | gr | None used |
| Minim | — | ♍ |
| Dram | dr | ʒ |
| Ounce | oz | |

---

In Check Up 7.2, convert the measurements based on the content in Box 7.1.

### Equivalents between apothecary and household systems

Before discussing the metric system, it is important to understand the equivalents between the apothecary and household measuring systems. If a doctor writes an order in the apothecary system, you must convert it to the household system so that patients understand how much medication to

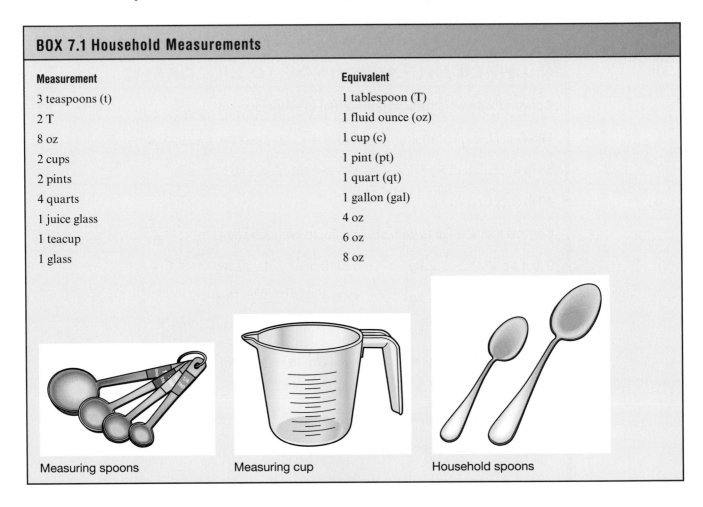

**BOX 7.1 Household Measurements**

| Measurement | Equivalent |
|-------------|------------|
| 3 teaspoons (t) | 1 tablespoon (T) |
| 2 T | 1 fluid ounce (oz) |
| 8 oz | 1 cup (c) |
| 2 cups | 1 pint (pt) |
| 2 pints | 1 quart (qt) |
| 4 quarts | 1 gallon (gal) |
| 1 juice glass | 4 oz |
| 1 teacup | 6 oz |
| 1 glass | 8 oz |

Measuring spoons          Measuring cup          Household spoons

## CHECK UP 7.2: HOUSEHOLD EQUIVALENTS

Write the equivalent household measurement.

1 juice glass = _____oz       1 cup = _____oz

1 teacup = _____oz            1 pint = _____cups

1 glass = _____oz             1 quart = _____pints

1 T = _____oz                 1 gallon = _____quarts

1 oz = _____t                 1 cup = _____pint

take. Think about the number of minutes your favorite television drama lasts. Most likely, it is 60 minutes. This association may help you remember that 1 dram (a measurement used for fluids) equals 60 minims.

Larger fluid measurements are pints, quarts, and gallons. Here are some equivalents that you may already know:

$$1 \text{ pint} = 16 \text{ fluid ounces}$$
$$2 \text{ pints} = 1 \text{ quart}$$
$$4 \text{ quarts} = 1 \text{ gallon}$$

Some equivalents are minute. In fact, these equivalents are so small that the number of tiny amounts in a larger amount can vary greatly, similar to grains of sand in a cup.

One drop (gt) is so small that 360 to 480 drops (gtt) = 1 oz.

There are 360 to 480 grains or minims in an ounce.

One drop (gt) = 1 grain = 1 minim because they are all about the same size.

In Check Up 7.3, write the equivalents based on the foregoing relationships.

## CHECK UP 7.3: MORE EQUIVALENTS

1 oz = _____dr                4 pints = _____quarts

16 dr = _____oz               8 fluid ounces = _____pint

1 dr = _____minims            1 gallon = _____quarts

120 minims = _____dr          360 gtt = _____oz

80 dr = _____oz               1 oz = _____grain

1 quart = _____gallon         1 gt = _____oz

1 pint = _____fluid ounces

How did you do? Be sure to familiarize yourself with these equivalents. Fast Tip 7.1 offers a quicker way to learn different measurements, with less to memorize.

---

### ✳ CRITICAL THINKING

Does it bother you that 1 oz is equivalent to something between 360 and 480 gtt, minims, or grains? What does this say about the accuracy of these systems?

---

Sometimes Roman numerals are used when ordering grains. The most common examples are Tylenol and morphine, as discussed earlier. For example, grains (gr) V = 5 grains. Table 7.1 provides a list of ways Roman numerals are used.

## The metric system

The metric system is based on the decimal system of places of 10 (10, 100, and 1,000). This system is used by many countries and most researchers, and it has become the standard for calculating drugs because it is the most accurate. The base units of measure are as follows:

Mass or weight = gram

Length = meter

Volume or fluids = liter

---

### ⬤ *Fast Tip 7.1* One-Ounce Conversions

The following may be an easier way to learn how different measurements relate to each other and how they relate to an ounce.

$$
\begin{aligned}
1\ oz &= 2\ T \\
&= 6\ t \\
&= 8\ dr \\
&= 360\ to\ 480\ gtt,\ grains,\ minims \\
&= 30\ mL
\end{aligned}
$$

If you memorize these relations, you can always move through the ounce for conversions.

---

### TABLE 7.1 Values of Roman Numerals

Roman numerals can be written one of three ways. The two most common ways are listed here. If you are unsure about the order written, always check with the prescriber.

| Value | Roman Numeral | Options |
|-------|---------------|---------|
| 1 | i | I |
| 2 | ii | II |
| 3 | iii | III |
| 4 | iv | IV |
| 5 | v | V |
| 6 | vi | VI |
| 7 | vii | VII |
| 8 | viii | VIII |
| 9 | ix | IX |
| 10 | x | X |

Dosage calculations do not usually involve very large or very small numbers. The most common metric units of measure are listed in Table 7.2. The prefixes in the table are added to the base unit to make the measurement. For example, the prefix "kilo-" means "thousands" of units; when it is added to "grams," the result is "kilograms" or 1,000 grams. When the prefix "deci-," which means 1/10 of a unit, is added to "liter," the result is "deciliter" or 1/10 of a liter. Each prefix provides a hint about the unit of measure.

In Check Up 7.4, determine how many units are in 1 gram. Use Table 7.2 for reference.

## Virtual Field Trip

Go to google.com, and search for the U.S. Metric Association. Write down one interesting fact about the metric system.

Dosage calculations predominantly use the base units of liters and grams because they are the units of weight and volume. Rarely is a unit of length needed when giving medication. For instance, a syringe is calibrated so 1 cubic centimeter (cc) of space holds 1 mL of fluid.

If a syringe is narrow, more length is needed to form 1 cc of length, depth, and width. If a syringe is wide, the plunger does not need to be pulled back as far to fill the syringe with 1 cc (Check Up 7.5).

Converting units within the metric system is a common task when administering medications. For instance, if a prescriber orders a medication and uses grams in the order, could you convert this order to milligrams, which is how the label usually states the drug amount? The following examples show what an order may contain and ways to convert the units to ascertain the correct dosage. Table 7.3 summarizes whether you need to multiply or divide when converting from one type of unit to another.

Example 1: A prescriber orders 0.2 grams; think of this as 0.200. Milligrams are 1/1,000 gram, so multiply 0.200 by 1,000.

$$0.200 \times 1,000 = 200 \text{ mg}$$

Example 2: Sometimes it is helpful to use fractions or ratios for the conversion.

$$\frac{0.500 \text{ gram}}{? \text{ mg}} = \frac{1 \text{ gram}}{1,000 \text{ mg}}$$

### TABLE 7.2  Common Metric Units of Measurement

| Prefix | Level of Measurement |
|--------|---------------------|
| Deci- | Tenths |
| Centi- | Hundredths |
| Milli- | Thousandths |
| Micro- | Millionths |
| Kilo- | Thousands |

## CHECK UP 7.4: GRAMS

Number the following measurements in order, from the smallest (1) to the largest (4).

Gram _____          Centimeter _____

Kilogram _____          Decimeter _____

Microgram _____          Meter _____

Milligram _____          Millimeter _____

CHECK UP 7.5: SHADE THE SYRINGES

Shade the syringes to show the amount of fluid indicated.

1.5 mL

3 mL

2.25 mL

You can cross-multiply to find the answer.

$$1 \times ? = 0.500 \times 1{,}000$$
$$? = 500 \text{ mg}$$

In Check Up 7.6, determine whether you need to multiply or divide to solve the problems. Use Table 7.3 for reference. How did you do? If you have trouble with this, it may help to create a chart, as shown in Box 7.2.

The prescriber may order a drug in grams or milligrams of weight, but this number must be converted into fluid, or milliliters, so the correct amount can be injected. In other words, a prescriber may order a dose of medication, but the medication comes in different sizes, strengths, and forms. It is up to you to find the correct medication and convert the order to the correct amount and form of the drug.

**TABLE 7.3   Simple Unit Conversions**

| | |
|---|---|
| Grams to kilograms | Divide by 1,000 |
| Grams to milligrams | Multiply by 1,000 |
| Kilograms to grams | Multiply by 1,000 |
| Milligrams to grams | Divide by 1,000 |
| Liters to milliliters | Multiply by 1,000 |
| Milliliters to liters | Divide by 1,000 |

### CHECK UP 7.6: CONVERSIONS

0.200 grams to milligrams _____         0.5 L to kilograms _____

200 mg to grams _____                   1 kg to grams _____

2 grams to kilograms _____

Convert the following orders into milligrams

0.35 grams _____         0.125 grams _____

0.5 grams _____

---

### BOX 7.2 Converting from One Unit to Another

Kilo- × 1,000 to get to unit → 1 km = 1,000 meters
Centi- ÷ 100 to get to unit → 100 cm = 1 meter
Milli- ÷ 1,000 to get to unit → 1,000 mm = 1 meter
Micro- ÷ 1,000,000 to get to unit → 1,000,000 mcm = 1 meter

---

For example, a physician may order 100 mg ampicillin to be given intramuscularly (IM). You go to the cupboard and find that you have a vial of ampicillin, but in powder form, which cannot be used "as is." Information on the label of the drug vial states exactly what and how much liquid to mix with the powder to transform the drug into an appropriate form. In addition, the label states the concentration of the resulting liquid if the directions are followed correctly. For the ampicillin example, the label on the vial states that 100 mg of drug is dispersed in 1 mL of fluid. To draw up 100 mg of the drug, you would need to fill the syringe with 1 mL of fluid, so you would pull back the syringe to 1 cc.

Once you have calculated the milliliters to administer, recall that 1 cc of space in the syringe is equal to 1 mL of fluid, so you do not need to convert to cubic centimeters.

#### CRITICAL THINKING

**Do you have trouble seeing the decimal point? Do you think pharmacists ever do? How can you be sure that a patient is given 0.5 gram instead of 5 grams?**

If you prefer to use words to visualize concepts, you may find this story helpful. There was once a king named Gram. He had 1,000 servants, called milligrams. He owned 15 grain fields (apothecary). In each grain field, 60 milligrams worked.

Repeat this story, and learn to draw the picture (conversion triangle) in Figure 7-1. The words in the story can help you understand whether to use 1/15 or 15 in the triangle.

You can also memorize these equivalents:

1 gram = 1,000 mg

1 gram = 15 grains

1 grain = 60 mg

Keeping in mind the story and triangle, consider the following more difficult example.

King Gram has 1,000 milligram servants. Each milligram is 1/1,000 of his workforce. If a milligram is sick one day, 1/60 of the workforce in the field is missing, because 60 milligrams work in each grain

**FIGURE 7-1:** King Gram's conversion triangle. Following the words of the story, there is one king (gram) who has 1,000 servants (milligram). The king owns 15 grain fields (grains). Each grain field (grain) has 60 servants (milligrams) working them. Thus, 1 gram = 1,000 mg, 1 gram = 15 grains, and 1 grain = 60 mg.

field. If King Gram gives away one grain field to his child as a wedding gift, he will give away 1/15 of his fields. Refer to Figure 7-2 as a guide.

As an alternate to relating conversions to the King Gram story, you can also memorize the conversions.

| | |
|---|---|
| 1 mg = 1/1,000 gram (g) | 1 g = 1,000 mg |
| 1 grain = 1/15 gram (g) | 1 g = 15 grains |
| 1 mg = 1/60 grain (gr) | 1 gr = 60 mg |

You must know these conversions to calculate drug dosages safely.

In Check Up 7.7, use the previous story and triangle or memorization tables to answer the questions.

**FIGURE 7-2:** King Gram's fractional conversion triangle. Following the words of the story, there is one king (gram) who has 1,000 servants (milligram). The king owns 15 grain fields (grains). Each grain field (grain) has 60 servants (milligrams) working them. If one servant (milligram is sick), the king is missing 1/1,000 of his work force, and the grain field (grain) is missing 1/60 of its workforce. If the king (gram) gives away one grain field (grain), he is giving away 1/15 of his fields. Thus, 1 mg = 1/1,000 gram, 1 mg = 1/60 of a grain, and 1 grain = 1/15 of a gram.

## CHECK UP 7.7: KING GRAM CONVERSIONS

1. How many servants did King Gram have? _____

2. How many milligrams are in a gram? _____

3. How many grain fields did King Gram have? _____

4. How many grains are in a gram? _____

5. How many milligrams worked in each field? _____

6. How many milligrams are in a grain? _____

### CHECK UP 7.7: KING GRAM CONVERSIONS—cont'd

7. If King Gram gives away 1 grain field, what fraction of his wealth has he given away? _____

8. A grain is _____ a gram.

9. Each milligram is what fraction of his workforce? _____

10. A milligram is _____ a gram.

11. A milligram is sick today. What fraction of the workers in the field is out sick?

   _____

12. A milligram is _____ of a grain.

## ●●● SUMMARY

Understanding units of measure and knowing how to convert them from one unit to another are critical when calculating dosages. This chapter describes the four measurement systems: avoirdupois, apothecary, household, and metric. The avoirdupois system is often used in weight measurements and is based on the pound. The apothecary system, which is the oldest, is seldom used today. The house-hold measurement system is based on the apothecary system and is the system with which patients are most comfortable and familiar. Because of inadequate standardization of measurements, however, it is not the safest method to use for medication. The most accepted measurement system is the metric system given that it is the most accurate and is based on units of 10.

The large amount of information presented in this chapter is critical to safe administration of med-ication to patients. Continue to work on learning this material; make flash cards, or use the CD that accompanies this textbook to practice further. As a future health professional, do not think you can learn this material, take a test, and then forget it. You will use most of this information on a daily basis and must become confident and competent in your practice.

## Activities

To make sure that you have learned the key points covered in this chapter, complete the following activities.

Fill in the blanks to show what you have learned.

1. 1 juice glass = _____oz

2. 1 teacup = _____oz

3. 1 cc = _____mL

4. 1 kg = _____lb

5. 1 oz = _____t

6. 1 lb = _____kg

7. 1 dr = _____minims

8. 1 oz = _____dr

9. 1 pint = _____oz

10. 1 oz = _____mL

11. 1 quart = _____pints

12. 1 oz = _____ gtt, minims, or grains

13. 1 gallon = _____quarts

14. 1 oz = _____gtt

15. 1 T = _____t

16. 1 cup = _____oz

17. 1 kg = _____gram

18. 1 gram = _____mg

19. 1 grain = _____mg

20. 1 gram = _____grain

21. 1 glass = _____oz

22. 1 oz = _____grain

23. 1 oz = _____T

24. 8 oz = _____mL

25. 2T = _____dr

26. 1,000 mL = _____oz

27. 12 oz = _____mL

Write Roman numerals two ways for the numbers 1 through 10.

1.

2.

3.

4.

5.

6.

7.

8.

9.

10.

Define the following on a separate sheet.

kilo-

micro-

deci-

milli-

centi-

## Application Exercises

Respond to the following scenarios on a separate sheet.

1. Faith calls the medical office. The label on over-the-counter cough syrup she is using lists the dose as 30 mL. She wants to know how many teaspoons to take. How would you respond?

2. Charlie weighs 110 lb. How many kilograms is this?

3. Doug has a fluid restriction of 1,000 mL/day. He has had 40 oz to drink today. Has he exceeded his restriction? Show your calculations.

4. Nancy is calculating a drug dose. The doctor ordered 0.500 gram. She calculates that as 500 mg. Is she correct?

5. Jaquan calls from the pharmacy. The physician ordered 1/15 gram, and he was given 2 grains. He wants to know whether he received the correct dose. Did he? Show your work.

# Dosage Calculations

*N*ow *that you have reviewed and learned the mathematical principles necessary to calculate dosages safely and the systems of measurement, this chapter identifies four methods by which to calculate dosages. Each method is independent of the others, so try them all, and select the one you prefer and perhaps another to check your work. In this chapter, you will learn dosage calculations for special circumstances, such as for the pediatric and geriatric patient, as well as calculations for parenteral medications and for dosages based on weight and body surface area. You will also learn how to reconstitute solutions and how to help patients calculate their intake and output.*

## LEARNING OUTCOMES

At the end of this chapter, the student will be able to:

8.1   Define key terms.

8.2   Learn and understand the four methods for calculating drug dosages.

8.3   Explain why certain calculations are considered special and which populations are affected.

8.4   Explain how to reconstitute powdered medication and calculate the desired dosage.

8.5   Discuss the factors to consider when calculating the dosages of parenteral medications and the two ways intravenous medications are administered.

8.6   Explain the calculation process for determining fluid intake.

---

### KEY TERMS

| | | |
|---|---|---|
| Available dose | Dimensional analysis | Infiltrate |
| Body surface area (BSA) | Diluent | Ordered dose |
| Conversion factor | Formula | Reconstitute |
| Desired dose | | |

---

# THE BASICS OF DRUG DOSE CALCULATION

Correctly calculating dosages is critical for safe administration of drugs. For instance, if you miscalculate a morphine dose, you could potentially cause a patient's death if you administer too much or fail to provide adequate pain relief if you administer too little.

The ratio and proportion method uses two ratios (comparisons between two things) and a proportion (statement saying those two ratios are equal). The formulation method involves inserting numerical values into a **formula** (rule prescribing how to calculate a dosage) to arrive at the correct dosage. Dimensional analysis is a method based on the premise that any number can be multiplied by one without changing its value. The fraction method uses two equivalent proportions to find the answer. The last method described is the word problem. All these methods are discussed in detail later in this chapter.

Regardless of the method chosen, you follow the same basic steps. The first step is conversion of numbers to the same unit of measurement. Second, using the preferred method, write the problem on paper. Finally, check and check again to confirm that your calculations are correct.

# METHODS FOR CALCULATING DRUG DOSAGES

When approaching mathematical problems, you may use multiple methods to find the correct answer. Some methods will be easier for you than others; decide which works best and stick with it. As mentioned earlier, there are four methods by which to calculate drug dosages for the nonparenteral (oral) route of administration:

**1.** Ratio and proportion method

**2.** Formulation method

**3.** Dimensional analysis

**4.** Fractions

You may choose one method of calculation and use another to check the accuracy of your results. Regardless of the method, you must first read the drug label accurately.

Figure 8-1 shows a sample drug label. The quantity is sometimes in tablets, capsules, milliliters, or another unit, and each label has its own equivalents. As discussed in Chapter 5, the manufacturer, lot number, and expiration dates are included on the label, as well as the name, dosage, form, and route of the drug. Most of this information is needed to calculate the dosage. The prescriber usually states the number of milligrams (or other unit of measurement) of a medication to administer, but unless you know what is in the container holding the ordered medication, you will not have the necessary numbers for the calculations. Now you are ready to learn how to calculate dosages.

**FIGURE 8-1:** Sample drug label. The drug label should include (A) the brand (trade) name, (B) generic name, (C, D) drug strength and drug form, route of administration if other than oral, total amount of medication in the container, directions for reconstitution if necessary, (E) manufacturer, (F) National Drug Code (NDC), (G) expiration date, and (H) lot number.

## Ratio and proportion method

The ratio and proportion method uses ratios, which are comparisons between two objects (numbers in this case). For example, if you have four pieces of pepperoni pizza and three pieces of cheese pizza, the ratio would be written as 4:3, or it may be written as 4/3. A proportion is a statement saying that two ratios are equal and, in this case, would be written as 4:3::8:6 or 4/3 = 8/6.

Example: The medication order is for 400 mg. The available medication is 300 mg in 1 mL.

■ Step 1: Write the ratio that you know (what is available).

$$\frac{300\ mg}{1\ mL}$$

■ Step 2: Write the ratio that you need to solve for.

$$\frac{400\ mg}{?\ mL}$$

■ Step 3: Write the proportion.

$$\frac{300\ mg}{1\ mL} = \frac{400\ mg}{?\ mL}$$

■ Step 4: Cross-multiply to discover what ? equals.

$$300\ ? = 400$$

■ Step 5: Divide both sides by 300 to isolate ?.

$$\frac{300?}{300} = \frac{400}{300}$$
$$? = 1.25\ mL$$

Use the means and extremes method discussed in Chapter 6 as a shortcut to solve problems if you prefer.
Example: The medication order is for 100 mg. The medication label reads "200 mg/mL."
Figure 8-2 illustrates the following calculation using the means and extremes method.

■ Step 1: Write what is on the label.

$$200\ mg: 1\ mL$$

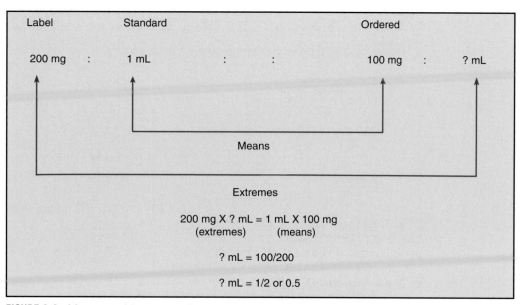

FIGURE 8-2: Means and extremes. To calculate, multiply the means (inner units) and relate them to the extremes (outer units).

■ Step 2: Write what you need to solve.

$$100 \text{ mg}: ? \text{ mL}$$

■ Step 3: Write the whole proportion statement. Both sides of the equation should have the same units (e.g., mg-mL or mg-tablets).

$$200 \text{ mg}:1 \text{ mL}::100 \text{ mg}:? \text{ mL}$$

■ Step 4: Using means and extremes, multiply the inner (means) numbers and outer (extremes) numbers.

$$1 \text{ mL} \times 100 = 200 \times ?$$
$$100 = 200 ?$$

■ Step 5: To isolate ? and discover the correct amount to administer, divide both sides of the equation by 200.

$$\frac{100}{200} = \frac{200?}{200}$$
$$0.5 \text{ mL} = ?$$
$$200 \text{ mg}:1 \text{ mL}::100 \text{ mg}:? \text{ mL}$$
$$\text{mL} \times \text{mg (means)}$$
$$\text{mg} \times \text{mL (extremes)}$$

Setting the calculation up in one of these two ways should help you determine ratios correctly (Check Up 8.1).

### The formulation method

The formulation method involves stacking units that are the same and multiplying by the unit requested. The **desired dose** equals the dosage that has been ordered or **ordered dose.** This dose must be the same units as the **available dose** (the dosage on hand). The following is an example of a calculation using the formulation method. If the physician orders 200 mg, and the label reads "200 mg = 1 tablet," you would give one tablet when following this formula, in which D is the

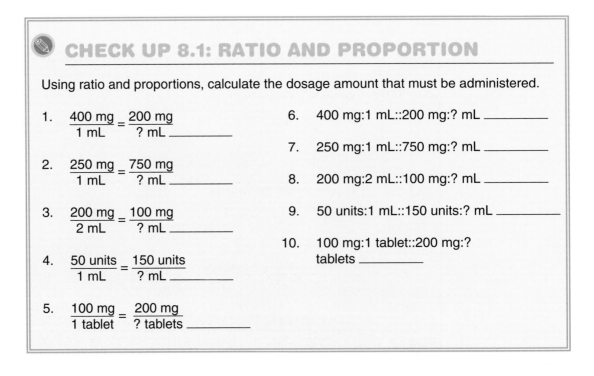

### CHECK UP 8.1: RATIO AND PROPORTION

Using ratio and proportions, calculate the dosage amount that must be administered.

1. $\dfrac{400 \text{ mg}}{1 \text{ mL}} = \dfrac{200 \text{ mg}}{? \text{ mL}}$ _____

2. $\dfrac{250 \text{ mg}}{1 \text{ mL}} = \dfrac{750 \text{ mg}}{? \text{ mL}}$ _____

3. $\dfrac{200 \text{ mg}}{2 \text{ mL}} = \dfrac{100 \text{ mg}}{? \text{ mL}}$ _____

4. $\dfrac{50 \text{ units}}{1 \text{ mL}} = \dfrac{150 \text{ units}}{? \text{ mL}}$ _____

5. $\dfrac{100 \text{ mg}}{1 \text{ tablet}} = \dfrac{200 \text{ mg}}{? \text{ tablets}}$ _____

6. 400 mg:1 mL::200 mg:? mL _____

7. 250 mg:1 mL::750 mg:? mL _____

8. 200 mg:2 mL::100 mg:? mL _____

9. 50 units:1 mL::150 units:? mL _____

10. 100 mg:1 tablet::200 mg:? tablets _____

desired dose, H is the on-hand or available amount in ordered units, and Q is the quantity in the units given (Fig. 8-3):

■ Step1: Set up the D/H $\times$ Q formula with known values.

$$\frac{D}{H} \times Q = \frac{200 \text{ mg (order)}}{200 \text{ mg (label)}} \times 1 \text{ tablet}$$

■ Step 2: Solve the formula.

$$\frac{200 \text{ mg}}{200 \text{ mg}} \times 1 \text{ tablet}$$
$$1 \times 1 \text{ tablet} = 1 \text{ tablet}$$

Example 2: The physician's order is for 400 mg. The label reads "200 mg/mL."

■ Step 1: Set up the D/H $\times$ Q formula with known values.

$$\frac{400 \text{ mg}}{200 \text{ mg}} \times 1 \text{ mL}$$

■ Step 2: Solve the formula.

$$\frac{400 \text{ mg}}{200 \text{ mg}} \times 1 \text{ mL}$$
$$2 \times 1 \text{ mL} = 2 \text{ mL}$$

Often, ordered units do not match the units on the drug's label. Here is how to proceed in such as case:
Example 1: The medication order is for 0.25 gram, but the label has "250 mg/mL."

■ Step 1: Convert grams to milligrams.

$$0.25 \text{ g} \times 1{,}000 \text{ mg (the number of milligrams in 1 g)} = 250 \text{ mg}$$

■ Step 2: Set up the D/H $\times$ Q formula.

$$\frac{250 \text{ mg (order)}}{250 \text{ mg (label)}} \times 1 \text{ mL}$$

■ Step 3: Solve the formula.

$$1 \times 1 \text{ mL} = 1 \text{ mL}$$

Example 2: The medication order is for gr X (10 grains), but the label states "300 mg per tablet" (Check Up 8.2).

■ Step 1: Convert grains to milligrams.

$$1 \text{ grain} = 60 \text{ mg; therefore, 10 grains would be } 10 \times 60 \text{ mg} = 600 \text{ mg}$$

**FIGURE 8-3:** Sliding formula method. Known values are plugged into this formula where D is the desired dose, H is the dose on hand, and Q is the quantity in which the dose is available.

---

### CHECK UP 8.2: FORMULATION METHOD

Calculate these dosages.

1. Physician's order: 500 mg
   Label: 250 mg/mL
   What would you give in milliliters? _____

2. Nurse practitioner's order: 100 mg
   Label: 200 mg/scored tablet
   How many tablets would you give? _____

3. Physician's order: 500 mg
   Label: 500 mg/capsule
   What would you give in capsules? _____

4. Physician assistant's order: 200 mg
   Label: 1 oz = 100 mg
   What would you give in ounces? _____

5. The patient weighs 100 lb. How many kilograms is this? _____

6. D = 1,000 units  H = 10,000 units  Q = 10 mL
   Milliliters to be given? _____

7. D = 200 mg  H = 400 mg  Q = 1 tablet
   Tablets to be given? _____

8. D = 250 mg  H = 500 mg  Q = 2 mL
   Milliliters to be given? _____

9. D = 700 mg  H = 0.35 gram  Q = 1 tablet
   Tablets to be given? _____

10. D = 1,000 mg  H = 1 gram  Q = 2 bottles
    Bottles to be given? _____

---

■ Step 2: Set up the D/H × Q formula.

$$\frac{600 \text{ mg}}{300 \text{ mg}} \times 1 \text{ tablet}$$

■ Step 3: Solve the formula.

$$2 \times 1 \text{ tablet} = 2 \text{ tablets}$$

### Dimensional analysis

**Dimensional analysis** uses the ordered amount of a drug to multiply with two equal quantities in different dimensions (units of measurement) to derive the answer. The physician or practitioner always includes both a quantity and a dimension in each medication order. If you focus on the dimension, rather than the numbers, you can create a template to use for every problem.

Dimensions (or units) vary depending on the circumstance. They may be tablets, capsules, bottles, milliliters (mL), ounces (oz), tablespoons (T), milligrams (mg), grams, grains, or something else. Calculating the dimension analysis can be done in four steps:

■ Step 1: Write the *units* of the dose ordered. For example, if the ordered dose is milligrams, write "mg" in the first position of the equation. If the order is in grams, write "grams." An order for 500 mg would be "mg."

■ Step 2: Write the *units* that are on the label and the *unit* that you plan to give to the patient. For instance, if a label shows that a drug is available in *milligrams*, and you want to give the drug in *milliliters*, you would place the unit of the ordered dose on the bottom of the **conversion factor** (formula to change from one unit of measurement to another). In this way, if you found that this unit of the ordered dose was mg, putting it on the bottom of this formula would cancel out the mg in the first position and leave you with the unit that is on the top. The desired unit is the unit that you want to give and is placed on the top of the conversion factor.

$$\text{Mg (ordered)} \times \frac{\text{mL}}{\text{Mg from label (ordered)}} = \text{mL (desired)}$$

The conversion factor effectively multiplies the other units by $1/1$ because the two values are equal but in different units. The answer to this equation is the desired dose.

Therefore, if 250 mg = 1 mL (from the label), then

$$\frac{250 \text{ mg}}{1 \text{ mL}} = \frac{1}{1}$$

Can you find equivalents?

$$\frac{1 \text{ oz}}{? \text{ mL}} = \frac{1}{1} \qquad \frac{1 \text{ gram}}{? \text{ mg}} = \frac{1}{1}$$

■ Step 3: Now fill in the numbers for each unit and cancel the ordered units.

$$500 \text{ mg} \times \frac{1 \text{ mL}}{250 \text{ mg (from label)}} = 2 \text{ mL}$$

Note: 1 mL = 250 mg (from label).

Check each label carefully; different vials may have different equivalents. Sometimes a label may not have a conversion of 1 mL; it may read "250 mg = 2 mL." You can reduce this fraction to be 125 mg = 1 mL or leave it as 250 mg = 2 mL for calculations. Both are equivalents.

■ Step 4: Check your work for accuracy sense.

Would you inject 2 mL? Yes, OK.

What if your calculations resulted in an answer of 20 mL? Would you inject that much fluid? No.

If no, then you would go back and check your calculations again. Are these values equivalents?

$$\frac{500 \text{ mg}}{2 \text{ mL}} = \frac{250 \text{ mg}}{1 \text{ mL}}$$

Yes.

In Check Up 8.3, try calculating drug amounts based on medication orders.

Dimensional analysis can be used to convert between measurement systems. For example, the nurse practitioner orders a 1,000-mL fluid restriction for Clark Castillo. Clark drank 50 oz of fluid today. Did he exceed the restriction?

■ Step 1: mL (units in which the fluid restriction is ordered)

■ Step 2:

$$\frac{\text{oz}}{\text{mL}}$$

$$\text{mL} \times = \text{oz (units for the fluid he drank)}$$

---

### CHECK UP 8.3: DIMENSIONAL ANALYSIS

Using the information in the box, calculate the amount in milliliters of drug you would give according to the following orders.

| Generic cough syrup |
| --- |
| 100 mg/1 mL |
| For oral use only |

1. 100 mg

2. 200 mg

3. 50 mg

4. 300 mg

5. 250 mg

---

■ Step 3:

$$1{,}000 \text{ mL} \times \frac{1 \text{ oz}}{30 \text{ mL}} = 33.3 \text{ oz}$$

Thus, 33.3 oz is less than 50 oz. If he drank 50 oz, he exceeded the 33.3-oz restriction.

■ Step 4: Check for common sense. Think of 1 liter (1,000 mL) as approximately a quart, which is 32 oz. Fifty ounces is larger than a quart. You may need to teach Clark not to drink more than a quart a day because he may not know what a liter looks like.

Dimensional analysis can also be used when dosages given are not in the unit on the label—if equivalent conversion units are used.

Example 1: The physician orders 1/2 gram of medication. The label says "250 mg = 1 capsule."

■ Step 1: Convert to the same unit of measure.

$$1/2 \text{ gram} = 0.5 \text{ gram}$$

■ Step 2: Use the dimensional analysis equation.

$$g \times \frac{mg}{grams} = capsule$$

■ Step 3: Plug in known values.

$$0.5 \text{ gram} \times \frac{1{,}000 \text{ mg}}{1 \text{ gram}} = 500 \text{ mg}$$

$$500 \text{ mg} \times \frac{1 \text{ capsule}}{250 \text{ mg}} = 2 \text{ capsules}$$

■ Step 4: Does a two-capsule dose make sense? Yes.

Example 2: Suppose you weighed a patient in pounds but needed to know the weight in kilograms to calculate a dosage. Could you use dimensional analysis? The patient weighs 70 lb. What is the equivalent in kilograms?

■ Step 1: Convert pounds to kilograms.

■ Step 2: Use the dimensional analysis equation.

$$lb \times \frac{kg}{lb} = kg$$

■ Step 3: Plug in known values.

$$70 \text{ lb} \times \frac{0.45 \text{ kg}}{1 \text{ lb}} = 31.5 \text{ kg}$$

■ Step 4: Does this answer make sense? If a pound is approximately 1/2 kg, the amount of kilograms should be approximately one half of the number of pounds.

70 lb × 1/2 = 35 kg
Is 31.5 approximately 35 kg? Yes (Check Up 8.4).

### Virtual Field Trip

Visit www.google.com, and find a tutorial on dimensional analysis. Print the information, and use it for practice.

## The fraction method

To use the fraction method for calculating dosages, the ordered dose and units given must be in the same proportion as the amount on the label. This method uses two equivalent proportions (the label and the desired dose) to find the missing number.

$$\frac{\text{Dosage on hand}}{\text{Dosage unit}} = \frac{\text{Desired dose}}{\text{Dose given}}$$

Example: If the label reads "200 mg of a drug is in 1 mL of fluid," the correct dosage must maintain that proportion.

$$\frac{100 \text{ mg}}{0.5 \text{ mL}} = \frac{200 \text{ mg}}{1 \text{ mL}} = \frac{300 \text{ mg}}{1.5 \text{ mL}} = \frac{400 \text{ mg}}{2 \text{ mL}} = \frac{500 \text{ mg}}{2.5 \text{ mL}} = \frac{600 \text{ mg}}{3 \text{ mL}} = \frac{700 \text{ mg}}{3.5 \text{ mL}}$$

### CHECK UP 8.4: DIMENSIONAL ANALYSIS

Using dimensional analysis, try solving the problem.
   A mother calls your office from home and says that she does not know how many teaspoons to give her child because the directions on the medication bottle read "Give 15 mL."

Step 1: Write the units ordered.

Step 2: Write the known equivalent (hint: teaspoons to milliliters).

Step 3: Calculate.

Step 4: Does the answer make sense?

If you worked out the answer like this, congratulations!

$$15 \text{ mL} \times \frac{1 \text{ teaspoon}}{5 \text{ mL}} = 3 \text{ teaspoons}$$

Suggestion: Make sure your patient uses a properly calibrated teaspoon because kitchen teaspoons can vary in size.

All these proportions are the same. Sometimes you may even be able to cancel to obtain a lower number. This is fine as long as you maintain the same proportion.

Example: If the label reads "100 mg/tablet," what dose would be given if 200 mg is ordered?

■ Step 1: To find the desired proportion, write the label ratio on one side, and the same units on the other.

$$\underset{\text{On hand}}{\frac{\text{mg}}{\text{tablets}}} = \frac{\text{mg}}{\text{tablets}} \quad or \quad \underset{\text{Desired}}{\frac{\text{mg desired}}{\text{mg on label}}} = \frac{\text{tablets desired}}{\text{tablets on label}}$$

■ Step 2: Write the same units on the other side of the equal sign.

$$\frac{\text{mg}}{\text{tablets}} = \frac{\text{mg}}{\text{tablets}}$$

■ Step 3: Insert the numbers.

$$\frac{100 \text{ mg}}{1 \text{ tablet}} = \frac{200 \text{ mg}}{? \text{ tablets}}$$

■ Step 4: Perform the calculation.

$$\frac{100 \text{ mg}}{1 \text{ tablet}} = \frac{200 \text{ mg}}{2 \text{ tablets}}$$

■ Step 5: Check for sense. Would it make sense to give two tablets? Yes (Check Up 8.5 and 8.6).

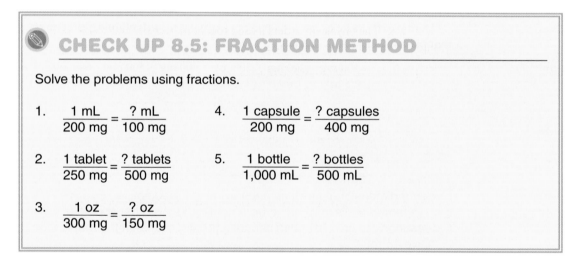

### CHECK UP 8.5: FRACTION METHOD

Solve the problems using fractions.

1.  $\dfrac{1 \text{ mL}}{200 \text{ mg}} = \dfrac{? \text{ mL}}{100 \text{ mg}}$

2.  $\dfrac{1 \text{ tablet}}{250 \text{ mg}} = \dfrac{? \text{ tablets}}{500 \text{ mg}}$

3.  $\dfrac{1 \text{ oz}}{300 \text{ mg}} = \dfrac{? \text{ oz}}{150 \text{ mg}}$

4.  $\dfrac{1 \text{ capsule}}{200 \text{ mg}} = \dfrac{? \text{ capsules}}{400 \text{ mg}}$

5.  $\dfrac{1 \text{ bottle}}{1,000 \text{ mL}} = \dfrac{? \text{ bottles}}{500 \text{ mL}}$

### CHECK UP 8.6: FRACTION METHOD TO VERIFY RESULTS

Using the fractions, check to see whether these dosage calculations are correct. You may reduce or cross-multiply. Write true or false next to each calculation

1.  $\dfrac{250 \text{ mg}}{1,000 \text{ mg}} = \dfrac{1 \text{ mL}}{3 \text{ mL}}$

2.  $\dfrac{100 \text{ mg}}{200 \text{ mg}} = \dfrac{1 \text{ mL}}{2 \text{ mL}}$

3.  $\dfrac{500 \text{ mg}}{250 \text{ mg}} = \dfrac{2 \text{ mL}}{1 \text{ mL}}$

4.  $\dfrac{700 \text{ mg}}{350 \text{ mg}} = \dfrac{1 \text{ mL}}{2 \text{ mL}}$

5.  $\dfrac{300 \text{ mg}}{100 \text{ mg}} = \dfrac{3 \text{ mL}}{1 \text{ mL}}$

*CRITICAL THINKING*

Does it make a difference if you align like units on one side and desired units on the other? Explain.

## SPECIAL CIRCUMSTANCES

Special calculations often include the special populations of pediatric and geriatric patients because their body systems are either immature (pediatric) or weakened by the aging process (geriatric). Other special calculations use the patient's weight or body surface area (BSA) to calculate for the correct dosage. For example, an order may be for a drug in milligrams per kilogram per day (mg/kg/day), which would require you to convert the patient's weight from pounds to kilograms and multiply that number by the number of milligrams to determine the daily dosage.

### Calculating pediatric dosages

In the **pediatric** (infants and children) population, weight is frequently used to calculate dosages because the body systems of a child have not matured. In addition, the total body water content is higher in a child than in an adult, and thus medication is absorbed differently and at a different rate. Children's bodies simply cannot tolerate an adult dose. Most drug references list a pediatric dosage for drugs approved for use in children. If a dose is not listed, the drug may not be indicated for children, and the reference will often state that the drug has not been approved for pediatric use. Consult with the physician who wrote the order or the pharmacist if you have any question regarding the safety of a prescribed medication for a child. A pediatric dosage can be calculated as follows.

Example: The physician orders a drug that has a recommended dosage of 30 mg/kg/*day*. How much would you give a 100-lb child each *day*?

■ Step 1: Convert 100 lb to kilograms.

$$100 \text{ lb} \times \frac{0.45 \text{ kg}}{1 \text{ lb}} = 45 \text{ kg}$$

■ Step 2: Multiply weight in kilograms by the order for 30 mg/*day*.

$$45 \text{ kg} \times \frac{30 \text{ mg/}day}{1 \text{ kg}} = 1{,}350 \text{ mg/}day$$

Note: If the drug is given bid (twice daily), divide the *daily* dose by 2.

$$\frac{1{,}350 \text{ mg}}{\text{day}} \div 2 = \frac{675 \text{ mg}}{\text{dose}}$$

If the dose is labeled qid (four times daily), divide the *daily* dose by 4. If the dose is labeled tid, which is three times daily, divide by 3.

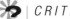 *CRITICAL THINKING*

Some dosages may be numbers that are difficult to decide how to administer. For example, when the dose is 337 mg/dose and the medication comes in 200-mg tablets, what would you do? How many tablets will you give? Who do you ask for advice?

Sometimes the ordered dose is given in milligrams per kilogram per *dose* (mg/kg/dose). To determine the total daily dose, multiply by the times per day the dosage is given.

Example: The patient weighs 100 lb. What is the total *daily dose* of a drug ordered as 20 mg/kg/*dose* to be given bid?

■ Step 1: Convert to kilograms.

$$100 \text{ lb} \times \frac{0.45 \text{ kg}}{1 \text{ lb}} = 45 \text{ kg}$$

■ Step 2: Plug in the known values. Solve.

$$45 \text{ kg} \times 20 \text{ mg}/dose = 900 \text{ mg}/dose$$

■ Step 3: To determine the total daily dosage and solve for bid, multiply by 2.

$$900 \text{ mg} \times 2 = 1,800 \text{ mg}/day$$

Other frequencies would change the total daily dose:

■ tid (three times daily): $900 \text{ mg} \times 3 = 2,700 \text{ mg}/day$
■ qid (four times daily): $900 \text{ mg} \times 4 = 3,600 \text{ mg}/day$

If the drug was available in 500-mg tablets, what would you give for each dose (Check Up 8.7)?

### Virtual Field Trip

Visit www.dogpile.com, and search for a site to instruct patients on pediatric dosages. Print a teaching tool, and bring it to class to share.

### Calculating geriatric dosages

**Geriatric** (aged) patients also need medications calculated very carefully because of the high risk for toxicity resulting from their aging body systems, particularly the renal (kidneys), hepatic (liver), and circulatory systems. The most common adjustments that must be made are to reduce the dosage.

---

## CHECK UP 8.7: PEDIATRIC DOSAGES

Answer these questions about pediatric dosages.

1. If a drug is ordered at 10 mg/kg/day, how much would a 20-lb patient need each day? _____mg/day

2. If the drug in question 1 is given tid, what would be the milligrams per dose? _____mg/dose

3. If a different drug is ordered at 20 mg/kg/day for the same patient, how much would he or she need each day? _____mg/day

4. If the 20 mg/kg/day drug is to be given qid, what would be the milligrams per dose? _____mg/dose

5. If a drug is ordered bid, how many doses do you give per day?

6. If the drug is ordered at 10 mg/kg/dose for a 50-lb patient, how much is given per dose? _____mg/dose

7. If the drug in question 6 is given tid, how much is given per day? _____mg/day

8. If the drug is ordered at 20 mg/kg/dose for a 50-lb patient, how much is given per dose? _____mg/dose

9. If the drug in question 8 is given qid, how much is given per day? _____mg/day

Unfortunately, no magic "formula" exists for safe administration of medications to geriatric patients. Thus, changes in adult dosage are made on an individual basis by the physician after evaluating the patient's organ function and body weight. In addition, each elderly individual reacts slightly differently (e.g., mental confusion, lack of appetite) to each medication and therefore must be assessed after each medication is begun or changes to doses implemented.

Another confounding factor is the complicated health of many elderly patients. These patients may be seeing a multitude of practitioners, each of whom treats a different health issue, as well as self-medicating with vitamins and herbal medications. Unless the primary care physician is keeping close watch on all drugs taken by the patient, the common problem of drug interactions, with unwanted and sometimes dangerous reactions in the patient, may occur. For example, a patient who is given two different medications that lower blood pressure may suffer a significant drop in blood pressure and risk falling.

### Calculation using body surface area

In some situations, knowing the exact size of a patient, both weight and height, is necessary. **Body surface area (BSA)** is a ratio of height to weight or the total surface area of the human body. This method is used most commonly in children, and it may also be used for administering chemotherapy to adults when dosage accuracy is critical. A patient's BSA is calculated by the prescriber and pharmacist to verify dosage. The allied health professional's role is primarily to obtain accurate measurements of the patient.

To find a patient's BSA, use the chart in Figure 8-4.

■ Find the patient's height on the left side of the chart, and put a ruler or piece of paper at that point.

■ Find the patient's weight on the right side (be sure to find it in kilograms or pounds, depending on how it was measured), and place the other side of the ruler or piece of paper at that point.

■ The ruler or paper cuts across the chart. The intersection point indicates the patient's BSA (Check Up 8.8).

## ■ RECONSTITUTING POWDERS

Powdered medications occasionally must be converted to liquid form to be administered. This process is called **reconstituting**. After adding a specified amount of sterile water or saline solution, use the conversion ratio on the drug label to calculate the dosage. You are looking for the concentration of the resulting solution (i.e., how much medication is contained in how much liquid). The amount of fluid, called the **diluent**, used to reconstitute the formula adds to the powder's volume, so the final solution (powder and fluid) may be greater than the volume of the diluent. Directions are on the label.

Example 1: A drug label indicates that you should mix 9 mL sterile water with 500 mg powder, which makes a total of 10 mL. To calculate the dosage after reconstituting, use the ratio 500 mg/10 mL.

If you had an ordered dose (D) of 300 mg, available dose (H) of 500 mg in quantity (Q) 10 mL:

$$\frac{300 \text{ mg}}{500 \text{ mg}} \times 10 \text{ mL} = 6 \text{ mL}$$

Example 2: A drug label indicates you should mix 74 mL of diluent to powder. After reconstitution, the resulting solution will provide 250 mg of medication in every teaspoon (5 mL). Therefore, the ratio for calculating the dosage is 250 mg/5 mL.

If you had an ordered dose of 200 mg:

$$\frac{200 \text{ mg}}{250 \text{ mg}} \times 5 \text{ mL} = 4 \text{ mL}$$

Example 3: A drug label indicates that you should add 3.4 mL diluent to powder containing 1 gram of antibiotic. The resulting solution will provide 250 mg medication per mL. Thus, the ratio for dosage calculations is 250 mg/1 mL (Check Up 8.9).

If you had an ordered dose of 300 mg:

$$\frac{300 \text{ mg}}{250 \text{ mg}} \times 1 \text{ mL} = 1.2 \text{ mL}$$

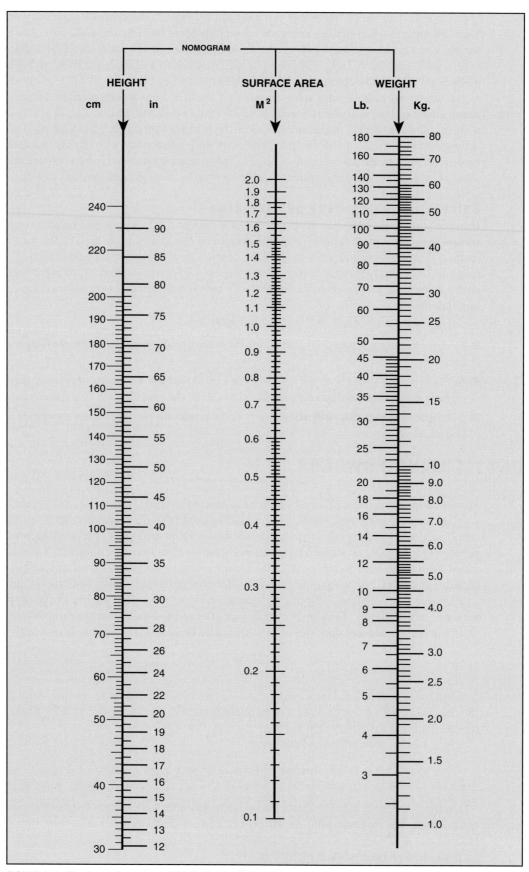

**FIGURE 8-4:** Body surface area (BSA) chart. This nomogram is used to determine the BSA of a patient. The chart is used primarily with medications that are particularly caustic, such as chemotherapy.

> ### CHECK UP 8.8: BODY SURFACE AREA (BSA)
>
> Using the BSA chart (see Fig. 8-4), determine the BSA of the patient. Be sure to note the dimensions (cm, kg, inches, lb).
>
> 1. 50 cm and 6 kg
>
> 2. 45 inches and 36 lb
>
> 3. 80 cm and 25 lb
>
> 4. 14 inches and 7.5 lb
>
> 5. 58 cm and 9 kg

> ### CHECK UP 8.9: RECONSTITUTION OF POWDERED MEDICATIONS
>
> Add 4 mL of sterile water. Resulting solution will contain 250 mg of medication/5 mL.
>
> 1. What amount of sterile water would you add to the vial?
>
> 2. What conversion factor would you use to calculate the dosage?
>
> Add 1.7 mL diluent. Resulting solution contains 250 mg medication/1 mL.
>
> 1. What amount of diluent will you add to the vial?
>
> 2. What conversion factor would you use to calculate the dosage?
>
> Add 33 mL diluent. Resulting solution will contain 500,000 units/mL.
>
> 1. How much diluent will you add to the vial?
>
> 2. What conversion factor would you use to calculate the dosage?
>
> Add 19 mL of sterile water for injection. Resulting solution contains 10 mg/mL of medication.
>
> 1. How much diluent will you add to the vial?
>
> 2. What conversion factor would you use to calculate the dosage?

## ■ PARENTERAL CALCULATIONS

Calculating dosages for parenteral (intravenous [IV]) administration is not as difficult as it would seem, but you must understand the equipment and the therapy, covered in Chapter 10. Dimensional analysis is the best way to calculate an IV drip rate because this method uses ratios as conversion factors and reduces the possibility of errors.

The laws related to IV therapy vary from state to state. Check with your state board of medicine to determine your legal responsibilities in terms of the scope of practice for your profession and what you are allowed to handle with parenteral therapy. Parenteral therapy policies also vary among organizations. Regardless of the scope of your responsibilities, you must know how IV dosages are calculated so you can double-check other health-care workers' calculations.

### Electronic regulator pumps

Electronic regulator pumps are machines that deliver and monitor IV fluids at a set rate. These pumps alert health-care professionals if a problem arises and allow them to perform other tasks. The physician or practitioner writes an order in milliliters to be infused over a certain period of time (e.g., 1,000 mL over

2 hours or 400 mL over 8 hours). The IV tubing, which is specific to the type of pump, is run through an electronic regulator; someone needs to program the rate for the regulator. The rate is expressed as follows:

$$\frac{\text{Total mL ordered}}{\text{Total time ordered in hours}} = \text{mL/hour (rounded to a whole number)}$$

Example: If the physician ordered 1,000 mL to be administered over 2 hours:

■ Step 1: Divide total fluid (mL) to be administered by time (hr)

$$\frac{1,000 \text{ mL}}{2 \text{ hours}} = \frac{500 \text{ mL}}{1 \text{ hour}}$$

■ Step 2: Does this seem reasonable? Cross-multiply to double-check (Check Up 8.10).

Sometimes a patient wants to know when the infusion will be finished. If the physician orders an amount over a certain number of hours, it is easy to calculate the completion time.

For example, a patient arrives at 10 a.m., and the physician orders 1,000 mL of IV fluid to be given over 3 hours:

$$10{:}00 + 3 \text{ hours} = 13{:}00, \text{ or } 1 \text{ p.m. } (13{:}00 - 12{:}00 = 1 \text{ p.m.})$$

At noon, the patient asks whether the infusion will be done on time. You see there are still 500 mL to be infused. The physician ordered 500 mL/hour.

$$\frac{500 \text{ mL}}{500 \text{ mL}} \times 1 \text{ hour} = 1 \text{ hour}$$

You can tell the patient that the infusion will be finished in 1 hour.

$$\text{Noon} + 1 \text{ hour} = 1 \text{ p.m.}$$

Suppose you looked up at noon and there were 750 mL left? When would the patient be finished?

$$\frac{750 \text{ mL}}{500 \text{ mL}} \times 1 \text{ hour} = 1.5 \text{ hours}$$
$$\text{Noon} + 1.5 \text{ hours} = 1{:}30$$

Not only will your patient be disappointed, but something may have malfunctioned. If the flow rate is not constant and correct, report it to your supervisor. Do not change the flow rate because the change may cause the fluid or medication to be infused too quickly, or the patient's IV may be **infiltrated**

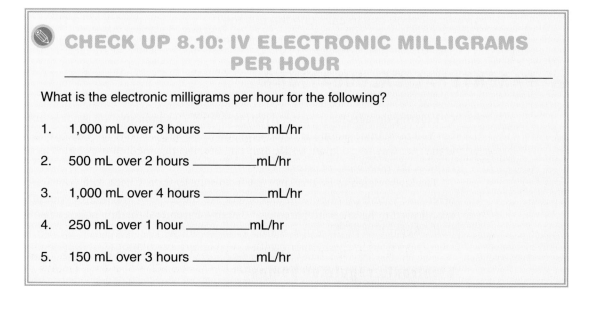

### CHECK UP 8.10: IV ELECTRONIC MILLIGRAMS PER HOUR

What is the electronic milligrams per hour for the following?

1. 1,000 mL over 3 hours _____mL/hr

2. 500 mL over 2 hours _____mL/hr

3. 1,000 mL over 4 hours _____mL/hr

4. 250 mL over 1 hour _____mL/hr

5. 150 mL over 3 hours _____mL/hr

(leakage of IV fluid or medication into the surrounding tissue). In either case, you could cause damage by increasing the flow rate.

---

### CRITICAL THINKING

In the foregoing case, in which the flow rate has not been consistent, you see that the IV insertion site is swollen. Would you increase the flow rate to make up the difference? What would you do?

## Manual IV sets

Manual IV sets use gravity to infuse a solution at a set rate. This means that you need to know the drop factor. The drop factor equals drops per milliliter (gtt/mL; how many drips are in 1 mL) and is stated on the package of the IV tubing. (The drop factor is built into electronic pumps because the tubing matches the pump). IV tubing has either a microdrip or a macrodrip chamber. The micro drip is 60 gtt/mL, and the macrodrip is either 10 or 15 gtt/mL, again as stated on the tubing packaging.

The health-care professional who starts the IV infusion establishes the rate by hanging the bag or bottle at a certain height and adjusting the number of drops per minute with the roller clamp. The IV set must not be moved (gravity changes how fast the drops fall) or adjusted; doing so could change the drip rate.

The formula for the IV flow rate is:

$$\frac{\text{Total volume (V) to be infused (mL)}}{\text{Total time in minutes}} \times \frac{\text{Drop factor (D) (gtt)}}{\text{mL}} = \frac{\text{Rate of flow (R) (gtt)}}{\text{min}}$$

or, more simply

$$\frac{V}{T} \times D = R$$

Example: The prescriber has ordered 500 mL to be infused over 4 hours. You have on hand 15 gtt/mL tubing. You need to determine the desired drip rate.

■ Step 1: Convert hours to minutes, and set up the equation.

$$60 \text{ minutes} \times 4 \text{ hours} = 240 \text{ minutes}$$

■ Step 2: Plug known values into the equation.

$$\frac{500 \text{ mL}}{240 \text{ minutes}} \times 15 \text{ gtt}$$

■ Step 3: Solve the equation.

$$\frac{32 \text{ gtt}}{\text{minute}}$$

If you were the health-care professional starting this infusion, you would count the drips in the drip chamber and adjust until you reached 32 gtt in 1 minute.

### Virtual Field Trip

Find three Web sites that manufacture IV tubing, and see what is used as gtt factor. Use each of these drip factors to solve the problems in Check Up 8.11 on manual IV rates.

**CHECK UP 8.11: MANUAL IV RATE CALCULATIONS**

For using a manual setup, calculate the following in drops per minute.

1. 1,000 mL NS over 24 hours. Tubing: 15 gtt/mL

2. 250 mL over 3 hours. Tubing: 10 gtt/mL

3. 50 mL penicillin IV over 1 hour. Tubing: 60 gtt/mL

4. 750 mL RL over 8 hours. Tubing: 15 gtt/mL

5. 40 mEq KCL in 100 mL NS over 1 hour. Tubing: 10 gtt/mL

*CRITICAL THINKING*

When you receive an order to infuse fluid and are using manual drip tubing, which would drip faster at the same hourly rate, macrodrip or microdrip tubing? Explain your answer (see Check Up 8.11).

**A CLOSER LOOK: Military Time**

Complete the following for 24-hour times.

Noon =
1 p.m. =
2 p.m. =
3 p.m. =
4 p.m. =
5 p.m. =
6 p.m. =
7 p.m. =
8 p.m. =
9 p.m. =
10 p.m. =
11 p.m. =
12 p.m. =

Some facilities use military time, which is based on a 24-hour clock. The hours pass from 0100 to 1200 and then continue the next sweep from 1300 (1 p.m.) to 2400 (12 midnight). To return to the 12-hour clock, simply subtract 1200 from the number: 1300-1200 = 1.

## CALCULATING FLUID BALANCE

Fluid balance is vital for life. Pediatric and geriatric (elderly) patients can easily suffer from dehydration, overhydration, or electrolyte imbalances because of the differences in their kidneys, as discussed earlier in this chapter. Calculating a patient's input and output of fluids can help you determine his or her fluid status and can guide treatment planning.

Fluid output is determined by measuring, in milliliters, either urine or emesis (vomit) caught in a special container that includes the unit of measure. Measuring or calculating fluid intake presents more of a challenge. Patients may comply easily with urinating into a plastic device placed on the toilet that allows correct calculation of output. However, because part of measuring input relies on a patient's remembering to complete a log of ingested fluids, it is more difficult to calculate, especially if a patient is cognitively impaired. Instruct patients on the importance of keeping an accurate log of both intake and output.

In addition, education of patients about fluid intake should clarify that coffee, caffeinated sodas, and beer have a diuretic effect on the kidneys, meaning that they increase urination. Although consumption of these fluids counts as hydration, these drinks are not the best choices when intake and output are important to the patient's health.

The physician's order will usually indicate fluid intake restrictions or goals in milliliters, so you may need to teach the patient how to convert household measurements into milliliters to measure input and output or to use metric tools. Because some patients forget how to do conversions, you must be able to convert household measurements to metric measurements. See Box 8.1 for a review of these common measurements and their conversions.

Example 1: Nita Page, who presents with dehydration, is required to drink 1,500 mL/day. Her fluid intake is as follows:

One 20-oz soda

One 8-oz glass of water

One 4-oz glass of orange juice

One 8-oz cup of milk

■ Step 1: Add all fluid in ounces: 40 oz.

■ Step 2: Set up the equation with known values.

$$40 \text{ oz} \times \frac{30 \text{ mL}}{1 \text{ oz}}$$

■ Step 3: Calculate the answer: 1,200 mL.

■ Step 4: Compare amounts to determine whether Nina met her requirement of 1,500 mL.

$$1{,}200 \text{ mL} < 1{,}500 \text{ mL}$$

No, she did not achieve 1,500 mL fluid intake.

### CRITICAL THINKING

**What instructions would you give to a child's parents about increasing the child's fluid intake to counteract dehydration?**

Example 2: Jeremy Jones is in heart failure and is restricted to a 1,000-mL fluid intake. Did he meet this requirement?

■ Step 1: Calculate total number of ounces of intake.

Two 6-oz cups of herbal tea: $2 \times 6 = 12$

One 8-oz bowl of milk in cereal: $1 \times 8 = 8$

One 4-oz glass of prune juice: $1 \times 4 = \dfrac{4}{32 \text{ oz}}$

■ Step 2: Set up the equation with known values. Remember 30 mL = 1 oz.

$$32 \text{ oz} \times \frac{30 \text{ mL}}{1 \text{ oz}}$$

■ Step 3: Multiply and solve the equation.

$$32 \text{ oz} \times \frac{30 \text{ mL}}{1 \text{ oz}} = 960 \text{ mL}$$

■ Step 4: Compare amounts to determine whether Jeremy met his restriction of 1,000 mL.

$$960 \text{ mL} < 1,000 \text{ mL}$$

Yes, Jeremy should be praised (Check Up 8.12).

---

### CHECK UP 8.12: INTAKE CALCULATIONS

Solve these problems.

1.  John Elliott has a 1,000-mL fluid restriction. He drank two 10-oz lemon-lime sodas, one 8-oz glass of milk, and one 8-oz cup of decaffeinated coffee. Did he exceed his restriction? Show your work.

2.  Kathy Thomas is dehydrated. Her physician ordered her to drink at least 1,200 mL/day. Did she achieve this goal if she drank two 12-oz decaffeinated sodas, one 8-oz cup of decaffeinated coffee, and one 8-oz glass of water? Show your work.

---

### SUMMARY

Calculating dosages is instrumental in providing quality care to your patients. You have learned how to use the medication label to determine the conversion factor of the available medication needed to calculate dosages. You have learned four methods for calculating dosages: ratio and proportion method, the formulation method, dimensional analysis, and the fraction method. Any method will work; use the one you prefer. Always check your answer to be sure it is accurate and reasonable. Pediatric and geriatric medication dosages are calculated differently from the average adult dose. Infants and children are given medications based on their body weight, whereas older adults are given medication after evaluation by their physician on an individualized basis depending on numerous factors (e.g., organ function, individual reactions to medications, body size). In addition, you have learned about reconstitution of powdered medications and calculation of IV drip rates. Finally, you have learned about special situations in which medication dosages are calculated using BSA, as well as calculation of fluid intake and output.

# Activities

To make sure that you have learned the key points covered in this chapter, complete the following activities.

Using ratio and proportion, calculate the following.

1. 100 mg:1 tablet::200 mg:? tablets

2. 1,000 units:1 mL::10,000 units:? mL

3. 1 gram:1,000 mL::500 mg:? mL

4. 1 oz:30 mL::? oz:90 mL

5. 2 T:1 oz::? oz:90 mL

6. 1 oz:8 drams::3 oz:? drams

7. 4 oz:1 oz::? mL:30 mL

8. 250 mg:500 mg::? mL:1 mL

9. 1,000 units:10,000 units::? mL:1 mL

10. 500 mg:250 mg::? mL:1 mL

Use the formulation method to calculate the following.

| D | H/Q |
|---|---|
| 1. 1.5 g | 500 mg/capsule |
| 2. 90 mL | 30 mL/oz |
| 3. 200 mg | 100 mg/tablet |
| 4. 0.5 g | 1,000 mg/bottle |
| 5. 160 mg | 80 mg/tablet |
| 6. 600 mg | 100 mg/capsule |
| 7. 200 mg | 100 mg/tablet |
| 8. 750 mg | 250 mg/tablet |
| 9. 125 mg | 250 mg/mL |
| 10. 25 mg | 100 mg/mL |

Calculate the following using dimensional analysis.

1. Order: 100 mg        Label: 50 mg/mL

2. Order: 2 oz        Label: 1 oz/30 mL

3. Order: 10,000 units        Label: 1,000 units/mL

4. Order: 500 mg        Label: 250 mg/tablet

5. Order: 300 mg                 Label: 100 mg/capsule

6. Order: 125 mg                 Label: 250 mg/mL

7. Order: 125 mg                 Label: 75 mg/mL

8. Order: 250 mg                 Label: 1,000 mg/bottle

9. Order: 250 mg                 Label: 125 mg/mL

10. Order: 1 g                   Label: 500 mg/capsule

Calculate the following using fractions.

| Order | Label |
| --- | --- |
| 1. 200 mg | 100 mg/2 mL |
| 2. 250 mg | 500 mg/tablet |
| 3. 160 mg | 80 mg/capsule |
| 4. 350 mg | 70 mg/mL |
| 5. 75 mg | 150 mg/mL |
| 6. 1,000 units | 500 units/mL |
| 7. 250 mg | 125 mg/mL |
| 8. 25 mg | 50 mg/tablet |
| 9. 0.5 g | 500 mg/mL |
| 10. 1 gram | 500 mg/tablet |

Give the flow rate for an IV solution that is being infused through an electronic pump.

1. 50 mL over 2 hours

2. 2,500 mL over 4 hours

3. 1,000 mL over 8 hours

4. 500 mL over 3 hours

5. 1,000 mL over 2 hours

Give flow rates in gtt/minutes for a solution that is being infused through a manual IV setup.

1. 100 mL D5RL over 8 hours                 set: 15 gtt/mL

2. 500 mL NS over 4 hours                   set: 10 gtt/mL

3. 1,500 mL RL over 6 hours                 set: 60 gtt/mL

4. 2,500 mL NS over 10 hours                set: 15 gtt/mL

5. 1,000 mL D5 and 1/2 NS over 6 hours set: 60 gtt/mL

6. 90 mL NS over 1 hour set: 15 gtt/mL

7. 50 mL over 40 minutes set: 10 gtt/mL

8. 200 mL NS over 2 hours set: 10 gtt/mL

9. Kefzol 0.5 gram in 50 mL D5W over 30 minutes set: 60 gtt/mL

10. 250 mL 1/2 NS over 5 hours set: 60 gtt/mL

## Application Exercises

Respond to the following situations on a separate sheet.

1. Dr. McCauley orders 400 mg. The label reads "100 mg is found in 1 mL." How many cubic centimeters (cc) do you inject?

2. Dr. Palmer orders 10,000 units of a drug. On hand you have 1,000 units. The quantity is 1 mL. How many milliliters do you give?

3. Dr. Seiler orders 500 mg. The label says "250 mg/mL." What do you give?

4. The examination question says:

   100 mg:1 mL::250 mg:? mL

   What is your answer?

5. You are asked to make a large quantity of 10% bleach solution. If you need 20 mL of total solution, how much bleach do you need?

6. Emily weighs 44 lb. If the doctor orders a medication for 10 mg/kg/day, how much should she receive per day?

7. If the patient in question 6 was ordered a drug for 20 mg/kg/dose with two doses per day, how much would she receive per day?

8. When Maria goes to the drug cabinet, she notes that there is 1 gram of medication in a bottle. She adds 4 mL of sterile water. This yields 250 mg/mL. If the ordered dose is 500 mg, what should she give?

9. Mr. Belcher calls to try to understand how to compute his child's fluid intake. All he has at home are regular cups, glasses, and mugs. What would you suggest?

10. Matthew has a 1,000-mL fluid restriction. Does he exceed it if he drinks two 20-oz sodas, one 8-oz glass of milk, and one 4-oz glass of orange juice? Show your work.

11. You notice that a nurse has not set the correct IV drip dose for an electronic pump. What would you do or say?

12. Kathy is having an infusion. She needs to pick up her children by 4:30 p.m. at the day-care center. If the infusion begins at 10 a.m. at 125 mL/hour and she needs 750 mL, will she be able to pick up her children on time? Show your work.

13. Gloria is having an IV infusion. She is supposed to be finished in 2 hours at 150 mL/hour, and the infusion bag has 450 mL left. Is it infusing correctly? Show your work.

# Administration of Medications

# 9

# Enteral Medications and Administration

*B*uilding on the review of basic calculations and an understanding of the methods for correct dosage calculation, you are ready to learn the different routes of administration and the medications associated with them. This chapter discusses those medications forms associated with the enteral route and covers oral, buccal, sublingual, and rectal medications, their uses, and procedures for administering them to patients. Each of these routes and forms of medication has specific considerations related to administration.

## LEARNING OUTCOMES

At the end of this chapter, the student will be able to:

9.1 Define all key terms.

9.2 List the forms in which medications are manufactured for the enteral route.

9.3 Differentiate how the different forms of drugs affect the body.

9.4 Describe the possible enteral routes for administering medications.

9.5 Describe how to administer oral medications safely.

9.6 Discuss the methods for administering medications through nasogastric or gastric tubes.

9.7 Explain why prescribers choose certain forms and routes over others.

---

### KEY TERMS

| | | |
|---|---|---|
| Buccal | Enema | Sublingual |
| Buffered | Enteric-coated | Timed-release |
| Delayed action | Mortar and pestle | |

---

# ■ ENTERAL MEDICATIONS

Enteral medications include any medications that involve the gastrointestinal tract such as capsules, tablets, enemas, suppositories, and many others. The most common enteral route of administration is the oral route. Most common medications are given orally and include antibiotics, antacids, and antihypertensives to treat infections, heartburn, and hypertension, respectively, as well as vitamins to supplement the diet. Although absorption is slower compared with the parenteral route, oral administration is less invasive and is well tolerated by patients. In addition, because it requires little to no equipment, it is one of the least expensive routes of medication administration. For these reasons, the oral route is preferred. These are some of the advantages. Disadvantages include the risks of choking and possible aspiration of the medication into the lungs, thus leading to infections or even death. Another disadvantage is that stomach acid destroys or inactivates many medications. The most common medication that cannot be given by mouth is insulin. The stomach acid destroys insulin and renders it useless to the body. In addition, the patient's cooperation is necessary for this route to work.

Medications given via the oral route are absorbed at different points in the digestive tract. Some medications are absorbed directly from the mucosa of the stomach. Others are coated to protect them from stomach acid or to allow timed released and thereby eliminate the need for frequent doses. Many medication-related considerations arise with regard to food. Sometimes, it is important to take a medication on an empty stomach to ensure the most rapid action. Certain other medications are very irritating to the gastric mucosa and lead to nausea and vomiting, so patients are advised to take these medications with a glass of milk or food. Sometimes, patients are advised to take medications with a full glass of water, which will also prevent stomach irritation. In other instances, plenty of water is indicated to prevent dehydration. The guiding principles are familiarity with the medication and an awareness of dietary guidelines to teach the patient.

Contraindications to the oral route include nausea, vomiting, and difficulty swallowing. In addition, the oral route should not be used for medications that become inactivated by stomach acids or in patients who are not conscious and alert. Precautions include close monitoring of any patient with difficulty swallowing or a questionable level of consciousness. In addition, care must be taken to make sure that patients actually swallow the medication and do not hide it or throw it away.

### Oral solid medications and administration

Oral medications can be either solid or liquid. Solid forms include tablets and capsules. Tablets are disks of compressed medication in distinctive shapes and colors (Fig. 9-1). Oral drugs are frequently poured out of a bulk (multiple-dose) bottle first into the cap of the bottle and then into a medicine cup (Fig. 9-2). Frequently, pills come prepackaged in individual doses, referred to as unit-dose. A group of unit-doses may be contained in a blister pack, which must be opened gently by pressing on the tablet so that the pill falls into the medicine cup. Always wash your hands before administering medications, and avoid touching the pill to prevent transfer of microbes to the patient.

**FIGURE 9-1:** Tablets. Tablets come in a variety of sizes, colors, and shapes. Oblong tablets are known as caplets.

**FIGURE 9-2:** Medication cup. Both liquid and solid medications are placed in a cup for the patient.

Sometimes, a tablet must be crushed before it is administered; these tablets can be mixed with food or a liquid to make it easier for patients to swallow. A pair of devices called **mortar and pestle** is used to crush pills and tablets (Fast Tip 9.1). However, not all pills can be crushed. For example, pills coated to slow the release of the drug (enteric-coated tablets) and timed-release capsules should not be crushed. If in doubt, contact a pharmacist, or check drug resources to see whether a tablet can be crushed.

Because tablets can be difficult to swallow, given their chalk-like consistency, some medications are also available as gelatin-coated capsules (Fig. 9-3). These capsules can be easily pulled apart to mix the drug into food for patients with difficulty swallowing pills. This should be done only if approved by the pharmacy, and the contents of a capsule should be mixed only with small amounts of food to ensure that the entire dose is consumed. Tablets can be coated to improve swallowing or prevent release in the stomach. **Enteric-coated** drugs are released not in the stomach but in the intestines; they are especially useful for patients with stomach ulcers or sensitivity. **Buffered** tablets have added antacids to prevent stomach irritation. Tablets can be scored (marked in half) for easy separation if half of a tablet is needed (Fig. 9-4). Caplets (see Fig. 9-1) are similar to tablets but may be easier for some patients to swallow because of the oblong shape.

A capsule can be in a **timed-release** or **delayed action** form that prevents it from being broken down in the acidic environment of the stomach. Instead, the capsule breaks down in the more alkalotic environment of the small intestine. Adderall XR is an extended-release capsule used to treat attention deficit

---

● *Fast Tip 9.1* Special Forms of Tablets

Tablets can be coated to improve swallowing or prevent release in the stomach (enteric-coated tablets), or they can be in a timed-release form. Enteric-coated drugs are released not in the stomach but in the intestines, so they are especially useful for patients with stomach ulcers or sensitivity. Buffered tablets have antacids added to them to prevent stomach irritation. Caplets are similar to tablets but may be easier for some patients to swallow because of the shape.

---

**FIGURE 9-3:** Capsules. Capsules are available in variety of sizes and colors.

**FIGURE 9-4:** Scored tablets. Tablets are marked to allow for easy splitting.

hyperactivity disorder. This medication is given only one time, in the morning, and the timed-release action allows the patient to take it less often. Timed-released capsules cannot be opened or crushed because doing so releases the drug all at once or causes an overdose. Steps for administering solid oral medications are outlined in Procedure Box 9.1.

### Oral liquid medications and administration

At times, solid medication is not the best option for oral medication administration. Patients may have difficulty swallowing solid medication, or the medication needs to start working sooner than the solid form allows. Liquid medications are easier to swallow and are more quickly absorbed than are solid forms, and they are available in a variety of compositions (Fig. 9-5). For instance, effervescent salts are granules or coarse powders containing one or more medicinal agents, as well as tartaric acid or sodium bicarbonate. When dissolved in water or other liquids, effervescent salts produce carbonation. An example is Alka-Seltzer, which is a medication used for heartburn. The advantage of taking it in effervescent salt form is that the medication is already dissolved and does not have to wait for the stomach to dissolve it before the medication begins to work. Disadvantages of this form are the same as those of most other medications. Because of possible allergy to inactive ingredients, patients must read the ingredient list carefully before using this form of liquid medication.

---

**Procedure Box 9.1** *Administration of Solid Medications*

- Observe the seven "rights" of medication administration.
- Read the medication order, and compare it with the medication container.
- Wash hands.
- Compare the medication order with the container a second time. Check the expiration date.
- Assemble equipment needed: medication, medication cup, order, and cup of water to help swallow medication.
- Identify the patient, and explain what you will be doing.
- Compare the order and container a third time.
- Without touching the medication, gently tap the correct amount into the cap of the container.
- If the medication is scored and must be cut, place it (without touching it) into a scoring device, and cut correctly.
- Place solid medication in a medicine cup.
- Give the medication to the patient with a glass of water.
- Instruct the patient to swallow the medication completely. (Never leave until you witness patient taking medication.)
- Assess the patient for any negative response (e.g., choking).
- Wash hands.
- Document medication administration and the patient's response.

*Example:*
*11/15/2012 8:15 a.m.: 500 mg ampicillin given PO. No problems noted. CJ Watkins RN, MSN*

**FIGURE 9-5:** Liquid medication. Liquid medications are easiest for most patients to swallow and are more rapidly absorbed than are solid medications.

Another form of liquid medication is an elixir, named because it contains alcohol (ETOH) in the preparation. The alcohol helps to dissolve the medication and makes it more palatable. Dimetapp Elixir used for cold symptoms is an example. Elixirs must be kept tightly capped to prevent evaporation of the alcohol because this would change the concentration of the medication in the elixir, and dosing errors could occur. Elixirs are used less often because of the detrimental effects of alcohol, the potential for interaction with many other medications, and the development of new medication delivery systems. Elixirs should not be given to children or to anyone suffering from alcoholism or diabetes (the liver converts alcohol to sugar). Other liquid forms include the following: emulsions, which are liquid drug preparations that contain oils and fats in water; magmas, which are liquid and fine particles in water, such as Milk of Magnesia; and powders, which are finely ground forms of an active drug, sometimes given for pain relief. Goody's powder, for example, is placed on the tongue and absorbed into the bloodstream for pain relief. Other powders, such as bulk laxatives, are added to large amounts of liquid and are taken orally.

Occasionally, oral liquid medications are given as a solution. This means that the medication is evenly distributed throughout a liquid and will not separate. For this reason, solutions do not need to be shaken. The first milliliter in the bottle should contain the identical amount of medication as the last milliliter. An example is normal saline solution (NSS) used to irrigate eyes. Conversely, suspensions are medications dispersed in a liquid, but because the medication may not have been evenly distributed, it must be shaken before it is administered. Read the directions to help you tell the difference. Additionally, a suspension separates into different layers of liquid, thus indicating the misdistribution of medication. An example of a suspension that must be shaken before administration is Pepto-Bismol, which is used for stomach discomfort.

Syrups are medications added to highly sweeten liquids, and they are popular with children. Robitussin cough syrup is an example. Medications that are made more appealing to children can encourage these young patients to consume more than the recommended dose and can lead to an overdose; therefore, all medications must be removed from a child's reach.

To administer a liquid medication, a calibrated medicine cup is used. It is important to place the medicine cup on a flat surface and pour the liquid into the cup to ensure accurate dosing. The cup must be at eye level for reading the measurement. The patient may need some water after swallowing a thick or bad-tasting medication; however, if the medication is used to coat the throat, do not offer water.

Procedure Box 9.2 outlines the necessary equipment and steps to take to administer liquid oral medications safely.

## Procedure Box 9.2 *Administration of Liquid Medications*

- Observe the seven "rights" of medication administration.
- Read the medication order, and compare it with the medication container.
- Wash hands.
- Compare the medication order with the container a second time. Check the expiration date.
- Assemble equipment needed: medication, order, calibrated medication cup.
- Identify the patient, and explain what you will be doing.
- Shake the bottle if needed.
- Compare the order and the container a third time.
- With the container on a flat surface, pour the correct amount of medication. The top of the fluid (**meniscus**) should be at the calibration line ordered. If you pour too much, you must dispose of the excess. Do not return the excess to the stock bottle.
- Give the patient the liquid medication.
- Instruct the patient to swallow the medication completely. (Never leave until you witness the patient taking medication.) If medicine is thick or tastes bad, offer patient water afterward.
- Assess the patient for any negative response (e.g., choking).
- Wash hands.
- Document medication administration and the patient's response.

*Example:*
*03/02/2013 3:45 p.m.: 125 mg Tylenol drops given PO. Patient tolerated well. CJ Watkins RN, MSN*

## Nasogastric tube medications and administration

Most liquid oral forms of medications can be administered through a nasogastric (NG) tube, which leads from the nose to the stomach, or a gastric tube, which a surgeon places directly into the patient's stomach under sterile conditions (Procedure Box 9.3). These tubes are used for patients who, for various reasons, have trouble swallowing or ingesting an adequate diet for optimal health.

## Procedure Box 9.3 *Administration of Medications by Nasogastric or Gastric Tube*

- Observe the seven "rights" of medication administration.
- Read the medication order, and compare it with the medication container.
- Wash hands.
- Compare the medication order with the container a second time. Check the expiration date.
- Assemble equipment needed: syringe, medication, flushing fluid, order.
- Compare the order and the container a third time.
- Identify the patient, and explain what you will be doing.
- Elevate the patient's head,
- Hold end of tube up, and remove the clamp, plug, or adapter.
- Attach an empty syringe (without a needle) to the port.
- Verify the tube is in the stomach (see Fast Tip 9.2).
- Use the syringe to flush the tube with NSS.
- Use the syringe to administer medications.
- Place more critical medications into the tubing first, so it is less likely that a crucial medication will be vomited out of the tube.
- After medication has been administered, flush the tubing with NSS.
- Clamp the tube with your fingers by pinching it.
- While the tube is closed, remove the syringe, and reattach the securing device.
- Assess the patient.
- Wash hands.
- Document medication administration and the patient's response.

*Example:*
*12/01/2012 12:25 p.m.: 15 mg Reglan liquid administered via NG. Tube placement checked X2. Patient tolerated well. CJ Watkins RN, MSN*

---

● *Fast Tip 9.2*  Checking Tube Placement

You can check that the nasogastric (NG) tube is in the stomach either by injecting air into the tube while listening with a stethoscope for the sound of air in the stomach or by drawing back on a syringe attached to the tube and checking whether stomach contents flow backward into the syringe.

---

Only liquids or tablets that have been crushed and mixed in water can be delivered through the tube. Before the drug is given, the NG tube must be checked to ensure proper placement. NG tubes may become displaced, with the tip in the respiratory system, and this can lead to aspiration pneumonia or death if fluid is administered by this route. Be sure to flush the tube with NSS before and after medications are administered to keep the tube patent (Fast Tip 9.2).

---

### A CLOSER LOOK: Special Situations for Administering Medications by Mouth

Liquid medications: If the patient is a small child or has trouble swallowing a liquid medication, the medication can be drawn up into a syringe (without a needle) and injected slowly and gently into the buccal pouch (cheek). This helps to prevent aspiration if the medication were injected directly toward the back of the throat. The infant should also be in a semireclined position, not flat on the back, for this reason.

Crushing medications: In some instances, the tablets must be crushed (or capsules opened), so that the medication may be mixed in liquid or small amounts of food for ease of swallowing or to insert into a tube (liquid only) in the stomach. Be sure that the medication is not a timed-release or delayed-release drug. If it is a tablet, you need a mortar and pestle to crush the medication. Then add it to a spoonful of soft, thick food, such as ice cream or applesauce, and give it to the patient. The patient must swallow all the food and medication on the spoon. If administering via a gastric tube, mix the medication with a sufficient amount of water, and administer it according to agency protocol.

---

### The buccal route of medication administration

The **buccal** pouch, or cheek, is a good route for applying medication in the mouth or throat to ease local inflammation. Troches (a lozenge) can be held in the cheek. They are usually pleasant tasting and melt slowly over time, to coat the throat and mouth. For patients with a sore throat, this route is ideal. It is important to tell the patient not to swallow or bite the buccal medication because it will not work as planned. In addition, liquid medication may be used to coat the interior of the mouth and cheeks. The patient is instructed to swish the medication around and then spit it out. One example is nystatin, used for fungal infections. Another example is a lidocaine solution, which is used in patients who are receiving chemotherapy and have resulting lesions in the mouth. The patient may need to refrain from drinking for 15 to 20 minutes after taking the buccal medication, to maximize the effect and prevent the medication from being washed away.

### The sublingual route of medication administration

**Sublingual** means under the tongue. The many capillaries under the tongue provide a rich blood supply for quick absorption of a medication. For that reason, nitroglycerin, which improves heart function, is placed sublingually for immediate relief of chest pain or during a heart attack. Although slower than an injection into a vein, the sublingual route delivers medication quickly without having to pass completely through the digestive system.

### Rectal medications and administration

Some medications, such as suppositories, enemas, suspensions, or ointments, must be administered rectally. This route is sometimes necessary because the patient has severe nausea or vomiting or is not alert enough to swallow. Some may ask why the medication cannot be given by the intravenous (IV) route. The reason is that some medications do not come in parenteral forms (e.g., Tylenol), or the patient may not have IV access. Many medications, such as Tylenol (fever, pain) and Phenergan (nausea and vomiting), are available as suppositories. They have a glycerin or cocoa butter base containing the medication. Because suppositories soften when warm to release the medication, they must be kept cool before administration. Be sure to insert a rectal suppository immediately after opening it or it will melt in your hand. **Enemas** are liquids administered through the rectum to soften stool, cleanse bowels, or deliver medication. Enemas are rarely given in the ambulatory setting, but many patients must administer them at home as a preparation for bowel procedures or surgery or as treatment for constipation. For these reasons, patients must be taught how to use them. To administer a rectal suppository or enema, follow the instructions in Procedure Box 9.4.

Other medications that may be given rectally include rectal suspensions (e.g., mesalamine, used as a gastrointestinal anti-inflammatory medication) and ointments (e.g., Preparation H, used to treat hemorrhoids). Both these types of medications are usually administered through an applicator tip placed into the rectum.

 *CRITICAL THINKING*

Why is the gastrointestinal a popular route for taking medication?

---

#### Procedure Box 9.4 *Rectal Administration*

- This procedure can be used for a rectal suppository or an enema.
- Observe the seven "rights" of medication administration.
- Read the medication order, and compare it with the medication container.
- Wash hands.
- Compare the medication order with the container a second time. Check the expiration date.
- Identify the patient, and explain what you will be doing.
- Compare the order and the container a third time.
- Have the patient remove his or her underwear.
- Assist the patient to lie on the left side.
- Place waterproof sheeting under the patient.
- Drape the patient for privacy.
- Put on gloves.
- Open the suppository wrapping, or remove the cover from the enema bottle.
- Gently separate the patient's buttocks.
- Apply a water-based lubricant to the tip of the enema bottle or suppository.
- Insert the suppository with one finger into the patient's rectum, or insert the tip of the enema bottle past the anal sphincter, and squeeze contents slowly into the rectum.
- Remove your finger or the tip of bottle from the patient's rectum.
- Assess the patient.
- Ask the patient to lie still for approximately 30 minutes.
- Clean the patient and the patient's area.
- Remove gloves.
- Wash hands.
- Document medication dosage and the patient's response.

*Example:*

*04/5/2013 3:30 p.m.: temperature 103.2 rectal. grV Tylenol PR. Patient tolerated procedure well. CJ Watkins RN, MSN*

*04/5/2013 4:00 p.m.: temperature now 100.2 rectal. CJ Watkins RN, MSN*

## S U M M A R Y

This chapter describes many different ways to give medications through the gastrointestinal tract and the different forms of these enteral medications. The most common and acceptable (to patients) method is the oral route; other routes include the buccal, sublingual, and rectal. The medication and its form, as well as the patient's condition, help to determine the route of medication administration. Knowing which medication forms can be used by which route is an important aspect of pharmacology.

# Activities

To make sure that you have learned the key points covered in this chapter, complete the following.

## True or False

Write true if the statement is true. Beside the false statements, write false, and correct the statement to make it true.

Sublingual is the most common enteral route used by patients. _____

A troche is a lozenge that is placed in the cheek (buccal pouch) and allowed to dissolve. _____

Patients should be instructed to rinse the mouth after being given a buccal medication. _____

Patients should be encouraged to lie quietly for 30 minutes after being given a suppository. _____

Insulin is a common medication given by mouth (oral). _____

A suspension never needs to be shaken. _____

Elixirs contain alcohol and therefore should not be given to children. _____

Effervescent salts must be mixed with carbonated water to create bubbles. _____

Solution never needs to be shaken. _____

A troche should be chewed completely within 5 minutes for maximum effect. _____

## Multiple Choice

Choose the best answer for each question.

**1. Which of the following is an example of a GI route?**

A. IV

B. Nasal

C. Oral

D. ID

**2. Suppositories are administered through which of the following routes?**

A. IV

B. Inhalation

C. ID

D. Rectal

**3. Which of the following contains alcohol?**

A. Capsule

B. Magma

C. Emulsion

D. Elixir

**4. Which must be added to a liquid before administering?**
   A. Effervescent salts
   B. Magmas
   C. Foams
   D. Troches

**5. Which of the following is given orally?**
   A. Syrups
   B. Emulsions
   C. Suspensions
   D. All of the above

**6. Which of the following is a term that means a tablet can be easily divided into two parts?**
   A. Scored
   B. Divided
   C. Marked
   D. None of the above

**7. A blister pack is _____.**
   A. Bubble wrap to ship medication
   B. The way that effervescent salts are packaged
   C. A common way that individual medication doses are packaged together
   D. None of the above

**8. The reason NG tube placement must be checked before the administration of medication is to verify that the tip is correctly placed in the _____.**
   A. Lung
   B. Esophagus
   C. Bowel
   D. Stomach

**9. Medications that may be administered via an NG tube include _____.**
   A. Liquid medication
   B. Tablets that are crushed and mixed with water
   C. Both of the above
   D. None of the above

**10. What type of oral medication consists of a gelatin coating containing a powdered form of medication?**
   A. Capsule
   B. Tablet
   C. Caplet
   D. None of the above

## Application Exercises

Respond to the following situations on a separate sheet.

1. To aid your memory, you decide to make a chart to help you remember the content of this chapter. Use books and resources as needed to complete the chart.

**Reference Guide for Routes**
Complete the following table.

| Route | When Used | Example |
|-------|-----------|---------|
| Buccal | | |
| Oral | | |
| Rectal | | |
| Sublingual | | |

2. Your patient does not understand why his medication cannot be given orally. Discuss the advantages and disadvantages of the gastrointestinal route.

3. Your physician has asked you to assemble the following drugs in case of an emergency and store them in the crash cart. By what route is each drug given, and for what is it used?

   A. acetaminophen

   B. aspirin

   C. diphenhydramine

   D. Compazine

   E. digoxin

   F. furosemide

   G. nitroglycerin

4. You notice that your colleagues at work do not wear gloves when handling medications. For what routes must gloves be worn? Defend your answer.

5. You need to give a dose of liquid Tylenol to a 3-month-old baby. Explain how you would accomplish this and what equipment you would need.

# Parenteral Medications and Administration

*T*his chapter describes the routes known as parenteral, the forms of medication used, the supplies needed, and the proper procedures for administering medication. The parenteral routes include transdermal or topical, nasal, inhaled, ophthalmic, otic, and vaginal, and the types of injectable medications are intramuscular (IM), subcutaneous (SC), intradermal (ID), and intravenous (IV). In this chapter, you will also learn the multiple factors that determine the route of administration, including chemicals used, necessary response time, and desired effect (whether local or systemic).

## LEARNING OUTCOMES

At the end of this chapter, the student will be able to:

10.1 Define all key terms.

10.2 Describe how to apply transdermal patches and other topical medications correctly.

10.3 Indicate how to administer ophthalmic, otic, and nasal medications correctly.

10.4 Describe how to insert vaginal medications safely.

10.5 List precautions for the safe administration of inhalation therapy.

10.6 Choose the correct needle and syringe for parenteral injections.

10.7 Indicate how to inject IM, SC, and ID medications safely.

10.8 Indicate how to prepare the patient for IV therapy.

10.9 Distinguish among the solutions used in IV therapy.

---

### KEY TERMS

| | | |
|---|---|---|
| Ampule | Infiltration | Phlebitis |
| Calibrated | Intradermal (ID) | Subcutaneous (SC) |
| Emboli | Intramuscular (IM) | Thrombus |
| Gauge | Lumen | Vial |

# PARENTERAL MEDICATIONS

Parenteral medications include all medications that are not ingested or introduced into the gastrointestinal system. They include topical, ophthalmic, otic, vaginal, nasal, inhaled, and injectable (intradermal [ID], intramuscular [IM], subcutaneous [SC], and intravenous [IV]) medications. The reasons for choosing a particular route, the forms of medication that can be administered parenterally, and the correct procedure for each parenteral route are discussed. When giving any medication, you must wash your hands, observe the seven "rights" of medication administration (right patient, right drug, right dose, right time, right route, right documentation, and right technique), compare the order with the container three times, and document the administration of the drug. The patient needs to know what the procedure entails before you administer the medication. Safely administering medications requires strict adherence to the protocols listed in this chapter or in your facility's procedure manual.

# TOPICAL MEDICATIONS AND ADMINISTRATION

Topical medications are applied directly to the skin as a patch, ointment, cream, lotion, or gel and are absorbed transdermally (through the skin). Topical medications are sometimes used if patients have difficulty swallowing or cannot take oral medications because of severe nausea. In addition, many conditions of the skin are treated by directly applying medication to the affected areas. Some medications are applied topically to achieve a systemic effect by maintaining continuous release of therapeutic doses of the drug.

### Semisolid preparations

Topical drugs come in several types of preparations. Semisolid preparations include creams, ointments, gels, and plasters and are applied to the surface of the skin. Ointments are petroleum based and work to keep the medication in contact with the skin. For this reason, before additional doses are applied, the remaining ointment should be wiped away to avoid cumulative effects of medication (overdose). Common ointments include antibiotic ointments such as Bactroban ointment placed on a wound and hydrocortisone cream used for itchy skin patches.

Creams are medications in a water base that absorb into the skin and disappear. Kwell (lindane) is a prescription cream used for the treatment of lice and scabies. Another cream is Oxy 10 Balance medicated cream, used on existing blemishes.

Gels are semisolid suspensions. This means that particles of drug are suspended in a thickened water base. An example is MetroGel for acne.

Plasters are medicated preparations that adhere to the skin with materials such as paper, linen, moleskin, or plastic. Examples include salicylic acid plaster, which is used for warts, and bandages that are saturated with antibiotics. These plasters are used to hold the medication directly against the lesion or wound to be treated. Other plasters are used to administer pain medication for arthritis or diabetic neuropathy and must be placed on healthy, intact skin only. Examples of these types of plasters are capsaicin plaster and 5% lidocaine medicated plaster.

Most of the previously mentioned medicated preparations contain significant doses of medication, and care must be taken when they are combined with oral medications so that overdosage does not occur. In addition, ingredients must be checked carefully to avoid exposing patients to allergens.

Liniments (or salves) and lotions are also semisolid preparations. Liniments are rubbed on the skin. They have an ingredient (usually camphor, wintergreen, or alcohol) that irritates the skin. This irritation (patients feel burning or pain) causes blood flow to increase to the affected area and decreases pain. Examples are Bengay and Icy Hot, used for sore muscles.

Lotions are used externally for skin disorders, such as the itchy skin associated with chickenpox or poison ivy. Lotions are similar to creams in that they are water based. Creams are basically 50% water and 50% oil, whereas lotions contain more water than oil, thus making them lighter and less greasy. They are patted on, not rubbed into, the skin, to allow the medication to stay on the target area and not absorb into the skin. An example is calamine lotion, which must be shaken and applied with a cotton ball or other applicator because of its thin consistency.

### Solid preparations

Topical medications are also available in solid form, such as a powder or patch. Powders are often applied to the skin to treat fungal disease or reduce moisture. One example is Desenex (miconazole nitrate), a powder to put on toes to prevent or treat athlete's foot. Gold Bond Extra Strength Medicated Powder is used to reduce moisture anywhere on the body, but most commonly the feet and toes.

A transdermal patch holds a specific amount of medication over a specific area and delivers medication over time (Fig. 10-1). Patches are often used to relieve nausea, provide pain relief, alleviate nicotine addiction, and control angina, as well as provide hormonal treatment such as birth control and hormone replacement therapy.

Advantages of using the transdermal patch include ease of application and removal, effectiveness over time, and reliable results based on even drug distribution in the body. Disadvantages include difficulty keeping the patch in place. Some patients' skin is not ideal because of excessive dryness or oiliness, which can cause the patch to fall off. Failure to wipe away leftover medication at the site when changing patches can lead to medication overdose. If patches are not disposed of properly, pets finding the patches in the garbage may be exposed to the medication and become very sick.

An example of a transdermal patch is NicoDerm, which delivers very small amounts of nicotine through the skin to help curb nicotine cravings when a person is trying to quit smoking. Another example is nitroglycerin, which is used to treat and prevent angina (chest pain caused by decreased blood flow to the heart). Nitroglycerin is a vasodilator that helps the coronary blood vessels open up and allows more efficient blood flow to the heart.

Most patches come from the manufacturer ready for administration. Wear gloves so medication from the patch does not enter your body. Remove the sticky backing on the patch, and apply the patch to an appropriate location on the body (Fig. 10-2). Be sure the area is free of tattoos, scarring, and redness because these features may alter absorption of the medication. Teach the patient to rotate sites to prevent skin irritation.

To remove the patch, apply gloves to avoid contact of the remaining medication with your own skin. Then fold the patch inward, and dispose of it carefully so that children or pets are not inadvertently exposed to the medication. See Procedure Box 10.1 for administration of a transdermal patch.

Clear backing   Drug reservoir

Drug-release membrane

Contact adhesive

Patch

Skin

**FIGURE 10-1:** Transdermal administration. In a transdermal delivery system, the medication is contained in a drug reservoir, which is released through a membrane when the patch is applied to the skin by an adhesive backing.

**FIGURE 10-2:** Removing a transdermal patch. Remove the sticky backing on the transdermal patch, and apply it to an appropriate location on the body.

---

### Procedure Box 10.1 *Transdermal Patch Administration*

Safety Precautions: Avoid touching medication to bare skin. Care should be taken when disposing of an old patch or wrapping of a current patch to avoid exposure of housekeepers, children, or animals to medication.

Supplies: Order, patch, gloves, teaching materials

Steps:

1. Observe the seven "rights" of medication administration.
2. Read the order, and compare it with the label on the medication container.
3. Wash hands.
4. Compare the medication order with the container a second time. Check the expiration date.
5. Identify the patient, and explain what you will be doing.
6. Compare the order and the container a third time.
7. Put on gloves.
8. Inspect the application site, and make sure that it is clean, dry, and free of lesions.
9. Carefully remove the adhesive backing from the patch.
10. Place the patch on the selected site, and make sure that all edges of the adhesive adhere securely to skin.
11. Remove gloves and wash hands.
12. Document medication dosage, location, and the patient's response.

*Example:*

*02/20/2013 6:45 p.m.: fentanyl 25 mcg/hr patch placed to left upper quadrant of abdomen. Patient advised to be cautious with change of positions to avoid falls. Pt. states understanding of side effects to report and activities to avoid. CJ Watkins RN, MSN*

---

There are still a few patches that you may have to prepare on your own. The most common patch you will need to make is nitroglycerin, although the use of these patches has declined in favor of commercially prepared patches. To make a transdermal patch, take an empty patch that marks the area of measurements on the application area. The medication order will be for centimeters or inches. Squeeze the tube of medication to place a specified measure on the ruled area. The more slowly you squeeze and move the tube, the thicker the line of medication will be. Therefore, the amount given is variable.

**CRITICAL THINKING**

What would be the effect of cutting a transdermal patch? Is it advisable?

## OPHTHALMIC MEDICATIONS AND ADMINISTRATION

Ophthalmic medications are placed directly in the eye for infections, for glaucoma treatment and prevention, and to facilitate examination and treatment. These medications can be given as drops or ointments. Eye drops may be used to lubricate the eye or treat other conditions through absorption in the inner canthus of the eye. Ophthalmic ointments are thickened drug solutions that are applied to the inside lower eyelids. Ocular inserts are small transparent membranes that contain medication. These inserts have the advantage of prolonging contact of the medication with the surface of the eye. One reason for using this method would be to treat chronic dry eye with an insert such as Lacrisert® (hydroxypropyl cellulose). Inserts are also in different stages of development for the treatment of infections and glaucoma. They are placed between the eye and lower conjunctiva and release medications over a period of time. Always keep ophthalmic preparations sterile, to avoid infection (Procedure Box 10.2).

Many patients are anxious about having medicine dropped into their eyes, so be sure to keep the patient informed at all times. When placing medication in a patient's eye, wear gloves and be careful not to touch the dropper to the eye itself, to avoid the spread of infection or contamination. Have the patient look upward as you drop in the exact number of drops ordered (Fig. 10-3). After the drops are

## Procedure Box 10.2 *Administration of Ophthalmic Medication*

Safety Precautions: Maintain sterility of applicator tips to avoid infection. Be sure to have assistance for uncooperative children, to avoid injury to the eye.

Supplies: Medication, order, gauze, gloves, teaching materials

Steps:

1. Observe the seven "rights" of medication administration.
2. Read the medication order, and compare it with the medication container.
3. Wash hands.
4. Make sure that the medication is at room temperature, not cold.
5. Compare the medication order with the container a second time. Check the expiration date.
6. Put on gloves.
7. Identify the patient, and explain what you will be doing.
8. Compare the order and the container a third time.
9. Ask the patient to look upward.
10. Drop the medication by dropper into the affected eye, or apply ointment by placing a line of ointment on the inner aspect of the lower eyelid, as ordered. REMEMBER: Drops BEFORE ointment if both are ordered.
11. Assess the patient.
12. Remove gloves and wash hands.
13. Document dosage, site of placement, and the patient's response.

*Example:*

*03/21/2013 09:30 a.m.: 2 drops gentamicin ophthalmic solution administered to left eye. Patient tolerated procedure well. CJ Watkins RN, MSN*

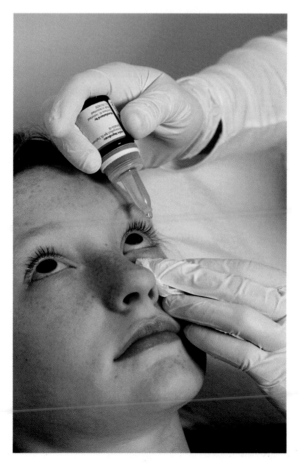

**FIGURE 10-3:** Ophthalmic administration.

instilled, have the patient close his or her eyes. This helps prevent the medication from entering a tiny tube called the nasolacrimal duct, which runs from the inside corner of the eye to the nose. Applying light pressure with a finger on the inner part of the closed eyelid after administration of the medication also helps to keep the drug from leaking into the nasolacrimal duct.

Some eye medications come in the form of an ointment, which is applied to the inside of the bottom eyelid. Be sure not to touch the tube to the eye or eyelid. If you have orders to administer both eye-drops and ointment, always administer the drops first because ointment forms a barrier that will not allow drops to penetrate.

## OTIC MEDICATIONS AND ADMINISTRATION

Otic medications are placed directly into the ear canal to treat infections of both the inner and outer ear, as well as impaction of cerumen (ear wax). To decrease discomfort, ear medications should be maintained at room temperature before they are given. Instill the exact number of drops ordered. Although ear medications do not leak as easily as ophthalmic medicines, the patient must keep the affected ear upright for a few minutes to allow maximum absorption of the medication.

Pull on the outer ear (pinna) to adjust the ear canal for best access. Adults should pull the pinna up and back; the outer ear should be pulled down and back in children, to straighten the ear canal for best absorption. See Procedure Box 10.3 for administration of otic medications.

## VAGINAL MEDICATIONS AND ADMINISTRATION

Vaginal medications are usually used for a local effect and are available in several forms: foams, gels, jellies, and lotions. Foams deliver medications via aerosolized foam. An example is VCF (vaginal contraceptive foam), which is sold over the counter. Gels and jellies are solid particles of medication in viscous (thick) suspensions. The thickness of the suspension keeps the medication from leaking. An example is metronidazole vaginal gel, used to treat bacterial infections of the vagina. Creams (lotions),

---

### Procedure Box 10.3 *Administration of Otic Medication*

Safety Precautions: Have patient remain lying down after administration, to avoid balance issues.

Supplies: Medication, order, cotton ball, gloves, teaching materials

Steps:
1. Observe the seven "rights" of medication administration.
2. Read the medication order, and compare it with the medication container.
3. Wash hands.
4. Make sure that the medication is at room temperature, not cold.
5. Compare the medication order with the container a second time. Check the expiration date.
6. Assess the patency of the ear dropper.
7. Identify the patient, and explain what you will be doing.
8. Compare the order and the container a third time.
9. Put on gloves.
10. Ask the patient to place his or her head on a counter or to lie down on the examination table with the affected ear upward.
11. Pull the pinna in the proper direction (up and back for adults, down and back for children).
12. Drop the medication by dropper into the affected ear.
13. Ask the patient to remain still for a few minutes.
14. Assess the patient.
15. Remove gloves and wash hands.
16. Document dosage, site of placement, and the patient's response.

*Example:*
*8/10/2012 3:10 p.m.: 3 drops of Ciprodex otic drops to right ear as ordered. Patient tolerated with complaints of minimal pain. CJ Watkins RN, MSN*

## Procedure Box 10.3 *Administration of Otic Medication—Cont'd*

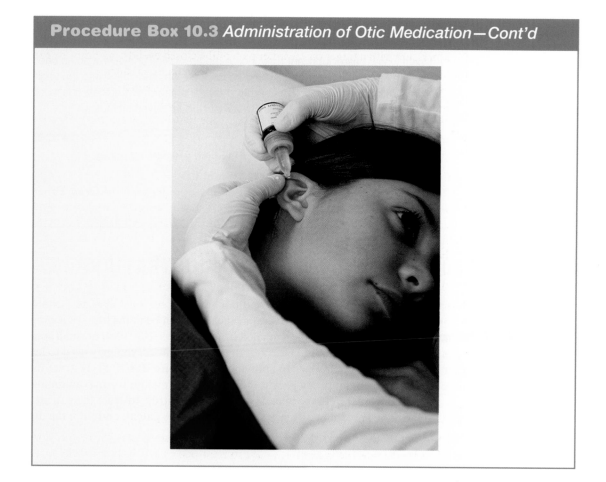

jellies, and gels are all products that can release hormones for contraceptive purposes. Antifungal creams are often used to treat yeast infections and are delivered via an applicator inserted high up into the vagina. An intrauterine device (IUD) is a contraceptive device implanted into the uterus by an advanced practitioner; some devices are coated with and release the hormone progesterone.

Vaginal medications such as suppositories and foams are often self-administered and do not require an allied health-care workers' assistance unless the patient is young or impaired. The patient should wash her hands and lie on her left side to make it easier to insert the foam or suppository. See Procedure Box 10.4 for administration of a vaginal medication.

## Procedure Box 10.4 *Vaginal Administration*

Safety Precautions: Assist patient on and off the examination table, to avoid falls.

Supplies: Medication, order, gloves, teaching materials

Steps:

1. Observe the seven "rights" of medication administration.
2. Read the medication order, and compare it with the medication container.
3. Wash hands.
4. Compare the medication order with the container a second time. Check the expiration date.
5. Identify the patient, and explain what you will be doing.
6. Compare the order and the container a third time.
7. Put on gloves.
8. Ask the patient to assume a relaxed, supine position with legs spread apart.
9. Drape the patient for privacy.
10. Remove the medications from the container.

*(continued)*

> ### Procedure Box 10.4 *Vaginal Administration—Cont'd*
>
> 11. Use a water-based lubricant to lubricate the applicator or medication as needed.
> 12. Use the applicator (if needed) or fingers to insert the medication into the vagina.
> 13. Remove the applicator or fingers from the vagina after the medication is inserted.
> 14. Ask the patient to close her legs and remain still for several minutes.
> 15. Assess the patient.
> 16. Remove gloves and wash hands.
> 17. Document dosage, site of placement, and the patient's response.
>
> *Example:*
> *04/06/2013 7:15 p.m.: miconazole 200 mg vaginal suppository administered. Patient tolerated procedure well. CJ Watkins RN, MSN*

## NASAL ROUTE OF MEDICATION ADMINISTRATION

Nasal medications are used to treat conditions such as seasonal allergies, asthma, congestion due to colds, and other sinus conditions. Nasal medications can be in the form of a spray, inhaler, or instillation. Nasal sprays are fine droplets inhaled from droppers (Fig. 10-4) or small spray bottles. If a patient requires nasal drops, perhaps to clear out the nose or sinuses, you may need to help the patient administer these drops with a dropper or spray mist (Procedure Box 10.5). Instruct the patient to blow the nose before giving nasal drops because this clears the mucosa for maximum absorption. Administer according to the order in the correct nostril or both nostrils. Instruct the patient to tilt the head backward to facilitate absorption. Be sure that the dropper is patent, and rinse the dropper afterward.

**FIGURE 10-4:** Medication dropper.

> ### Procedure Box 10.5 *Nasal Administration*
>
> Safety Precautions: Assist patient on and off the examination table, to avoid falls.
>
> Supplies: Medication, order, gloves, teaching materials
>
> Steps:
> 1. Observe the seven "rights" of medication administration.
> 2. Read the medication order, and compare it with the medication container.
> 3. Wash hands.
> 4. Compare the medication order with the container a second time. Check the expiration date.
> 5. Assess the patency of the nose dropper.
> 6. Identify the patient, and explain what you will be doing.
> 7. Compare the order with the container a third time.
> 8. Put on gloves.

**Procedure Box 10.5** *Nasal Administration—Cont'd*

9. Ask the patient to tilt his or her head backward.
10. Draw up medication into the dropper, as ordered.
11. Insert the dropper with medication into the nostril, as ordered.
12. Squeeze the dropper.
13. Ask the patient to maintain head tilt while you squeeze the nostril for a few moments, to prevent medication from leaking.
14. Assess the patient.
15. Remove gloves and wash hands.
16. Document dosage, site of placement, and the patient's response.

*Example:*

*07/14/2012 2:20 p.m.: Nasonex 50 mcg nasal spray 1 spray administered to each nostril as ordered. Patient tolerated procedure well and verbalizes understanding of procedure. CJ Watkins RN, MSN*

The same technique is used with a spray inhaler, except instead of drops, mist is sprayed into the nose via a pump. You do not rinse spray bottles, and you never use them for more than one patient.

## ■ INHALED MEDICATIONS AND ADMINISTRATION

Administering medications through inhalation into the respiratory system is a quick and effective way to access blood vessels. Techniques for administration include cannulas, masks, and a continuous positive airway pressure (CPAP) machine, as well as inhalers and nebulizers.

Sometimes a medication must be applied directly to the lungs or absorbed directly into the body through the lungs. Patients who have asthma especially benefit from inhaled medications because parts of their lungs are inflamed, and inhaling a medication directly into their lungs relieves this inflammation. Special devices, such as metered-dose inhalers (MDIs), are used to ensure that as the patient inhales, the medicine enters the lungs. This rapid method of administration is ideal for delivering certain kinds of drugs that break up congestion in the lungs, such as Mucomyst (acetylcysteine), and other medications, such as albuterol, that dilate the airways to assist a patient in breathing. Powders are more easily inhaled if sterile water or sodium chloride is added to be aerosolized with the medication.

### Metered-dose inhalers

MDIs are used to deliver specific doses of medication through a hand-held inhalation device. Some medications are prescribed for respiratory system conditions because these drugs are easily inhaled and begin working almost immediately at the site of distress. Hand-held inhalers fit into a patient's pocket or purse (Fig. 10-5). Spacers are used to allow the patient some control over when the medication is inhaled. A spacer is an extension tunnel that attaches to an inhaler and allows the medication to be held and administered whenever the patient can inhale, rather than escaping into the air if the patient exhales instead of inhaling. Spacers are especially useful for children and for adults who are cognitively impaired or disabled.

Patients should have their own inhalers for administering a specific dose of medication. Be sure to instruct the patient to take the medication exactly as ordered. The prescribed medication should be inserted into the plastic inhaler, so the opening on the prescription is inserted into the hole in the bottom of the chamber. Instruct the patient to put his or her mouth around the plastic inhalation device opening and depress the medication vial as he or she inhales for the number of puffs prescribed (see Fig. 10-5). Patients should not use another person's inhaler. Besides being unsanitary, the prescription dosages may be different. The plastic inhaler mouthpiece (not the prescription bottle) can be cleaned with soap and water after each use, to prevent infection (Procedure Box 10.6).

**FIGURE 10-5:** Metered-dose inhaler. **A,** Inhaler only. **B,** Inhaler with a spacer/chamber.

## Procedure Box 10.6 *Administration of Medication by Metered-Dose Inhaler*

Safety Precautions: Monitor the patient for elevation in heart rate, and report significant elevations to the physician.

Supplies: Medication, order, teaching materials

Steps:

1. Observe the seven "rights" of medication administration.
2. Read the medication order, and compare it with the medication container.
3. Wash hands.
4. Compare the medication order with the container a second time. Check the expiration date.
5. Identify the patient, and explain what you will be doing.
6. Compare the order and the container a third time.
7. Insert medication in the inhaler.
8. Gently shake the inhaler to ensure that the medication is aerosolized.
9. Ask the patient to exhale.
10. Instruct the patient to inhale slowly and deeply through mouth.
11. Insert the inhaler into the patient's mouth; depress the container when the patient inhales, and instruct the patient to hold his or her breath for approximately 10 seconds, to allow medication to reach the airway.
12. If more than one puff of medication is ordered, wait 1 to 5 minutes between puffs to allow for full distribution of medication.
13. Assess the patient.
14. Wash hands.
15. Document dosage, site of placement, and the patient's response.

*Example:*

*06/14/2013 11:15 a.m.: Atrovent MDI 2 puffs administered. Patient instructed on proper use and care of inhaler. Patient states understanding of instructions. Patient states relief of symptoms 5 minutes after administration. CJ Watkins RN, MSN*

## Nebulizers

Sometimes powders or drugs in solution are added to special equipment called a nebulizer. This equipment introduces the medication by using compressed air or oxygen to aerosolize or suspend medication into small particles in a fine mist for inhalation into the lungs through a face mask or mouthpiece. This form of treatment is common among asthmatic patients to help ease their breathing by administering medicine that, when inhaled, opens and relaxes the air passages to the lungs. Patients with cystic fibrosis also use this treatment method to deliver medication to break up the abnormally thick secretions in their lungs and allow them to be exhaled. Nebulizers are fairly portable (Fig. 10-6). Place the liquid medication in the chamber attached to the nebulizer tubing and pump. Once the pump is turned on, the mist will start to form, and the patient can begin to inhale the aerosol as prescribed through a special mouthpiece or mask. Procedure Box 10.7 explains the proper way to administer a medication via nebulizer.

**FIGURE 10-6:** Nebulizer. This machine is used to administer aerosolized medication to patients.

### Procedure Box 10.7 *Nebulizer Administration*

Safety Precautions: Observe the patient for elevation in heart rate, and report significant elevations to the physician.

Supplies: Medication, nebulizer machine, order, teaching materials

Steps:

1. Observe the seven "rights" of medication administration.
2. Read the medication order, and compare it with the medication container.
3. Wash hands.
4. Compare the medication order with the container a second time. Check the expiration date.
5. Identify the patient, and explain what you will be doing.
6. Compare the order and the container a third time.
7. Place the liquid medication in the chamber of the nebulizer tubing.

*(continued)*

## Procedure Box 10.7 *Nebulizer Administration—Cont'd*

8. Turn on the nebulizer machine, and wait for mist to begin forming.
9. Place a mouthpiece in the patient's mouth (or put on a facemask), and instruct the patient to breathe slowly and deeply through the mouth.
10. Wait 1 to 5 minutes between puffs to allow for full distribution of medication.
11. Assess the patient during treatment.
12. Wash hands.
13. Document dosage, site of placement, and the patient's response.

*Example:*
*04/28/2013 07:45 a.m.: 10 mg albuterol via nebulizer treatment. Patient tolerated procedure well. Pulse ox reading 99% 15 minutes after completion of treatment. Patient resting comfortably. CJ Watkins RN, MSN*

Not as portable as a nebulizer or MDI is a CPAP machine, which forces room air or oxygen into the lungs, even when the patient forgets to breathe. A CPAP machine is ideal for patients with sleep apnea, in which the patient stops breathing for short periods of time while asleep. Oxygen from a tank or out of a special wall port is considered a medication and requires an order from a doctor or other licensed health-care professional for the number of liters to be delivered each minute. This order is usually written as "L/minute."

Oxygen can be given to the patient through a nasal cannula or a mask (see Fig. 10-7). The prongs of the nasal cannula fit into a patient's nose. Although a nasal cannula is more comfortable for a patient than a mask, only lower concentrations (levels) of oxygen can be delivered. A mask is used to deliver high concentrations of oxygen, but it can be frightening to small children and patients who are disoriented and do not know where or who they are. These patients may feel like they are being suffocated. Teaching the patient what to expect or placing the mask near, but not on, the face may help ease the fear.

The use of CPAP, a nasal cannula, and a mask used over periods of time requires the air to be moisturized to avoid drying out the skin and mucosa. Patients should add distilled water to special chambers in the CPAP machine to humidify the air. Unlike tap water, distilled water does not add chemicals to the machine.

### CRITICAL THINKING

What would happen if a patient used a CPAP machine with a mask for 30 minutes without having added water to the inhaled air?

**FIGURE 10-7:** Oxygen administration. Oxygen is most commonly administered through a nasal cannula or a face mask.

# INJECTABLE MEDICATIONS

Injectable medications are available from the manufacturer in liquid or powder form. Powders must be mixed with sterile water or bacteriostatic sodium chloride solution. Liquids, however, may be diluted in this way or given as is. The medication is administered via needle and syringe and is drawn up from ampules or vials.

## Types of injectable medications

Four different routes of administration can be used with injectable medications.

- Intradermal
- Intramuscular
- Subcutaneous
- Intravenous

The **intradermal (ID)** site is just below the epidermis, in the dermis itself. ID injections are used for tuberculosis (TB) and allergy testing, so they need to be given immediately under the epidermis for easy evaluation.

The health-care worker selects the proper needle length and gauge and adjusts the angle of injection to reach the appropriate tissue level (Fig. 10-8). The usual sites for ID injections are the inner aspect of the forearm and the upper back. After preparing the site with an alcohol swab, the health-care professional holds the skin taut and inserts the needle just under the epidermis at a 10° to 15° angle. Usually, a short, small- gauge (diameter) needle is used. If the injection is administered properly, a wheal will form (Fig. 10-9).

Procedure Box 10.8 outlines ID injection protocol. At a 10° to 15° entry angle, be sure you gently push the needle just under the skin. Do not aspirate for blood return. Instead, slowly inject the medication, thus forming a **wheal** (slight elevation of the skin). Gently remove the needle, and do not massage the site. If some of the medication leaks or a wheal does not form, you will have to repeat the procedure.

### ? CRITICAL THINKING

Can you think of a way to make it more pleasant for a child to receive an ID injection?

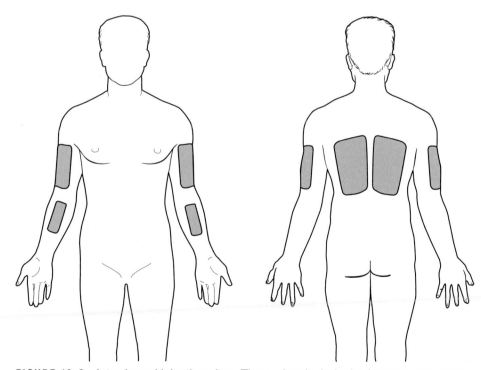

**FIGURE 10-8:**  Intradermal injection sites. These sites include the forearm and upper back.

**FIGURE 10-9:** Wheal. If the medication is administered properly, a wheal will form on the skin.

## Procedure Box 10.8 *Administration of Intradermal Injections*

Safety Precautions: Immediately dispose of sharps after administration.

Supplies: Medication in appropriate syringe with appropriate needle, alcohol wipe, cotton ball, gloves, order, teaching materials, sharps container

Steps:
1. Observe the seven "rights" of medication administration.
2. Read the medication order, and compare it with the medication container.
3. Wash hands.
4. Compare the medication order with the container a second time. Check the expiration date.
5. Identify the patient, and explain what you will be doing.
6. Compare the order and the container a third time.
7. Put on gloves.
8. Position the patient comfortably.
9. Locate the site.
10. Clean the selected site with a disinfectant wipe in a circular motion.
11. Allow disinfectant to dry.
12. Pull the skin taut.
13. Insert a needle at a 10° to 15° angle, bevel up, for about 1/4 inch.
    **Note:** Do not aspirate for blood because it would traumatize tissue.
14. Slowly inject all medication to produce a wheal (slight elevation under the skin).
15. Remove the needle and syringe quickly at the same angle of insertion, and place a cotton ball at the insertion site.
16. Do not massage the site.
17. Dispose of the needle and syringe immediately in a sharps container. **Do not recap**.
18. Remove gloves and wash hands.
19. Observe the patient for reaction for 15 minutes, because allergic reactions are more likely with ID wheals than with other types of drug administration.
20. Document dosage, site of placement, and the patient's response.

*Example:*
*03/01/2013 9:50 a.m.: Tuberculin ppd (mantoux) 0.1 mL to left inner forearm with wheal formation. Patient tolerated procedure well. CJ Watkins RN, MSN*

**Intramuscular (IM)** injections allow medications to be absorbed quickly into the bloodstream because of the plentiful blood supply to muscles. For example, if a patient presents with a serious streptococcal throat infection, the physician may order a dose of Rocephin (antibiotic) to be administered as an injection to start the healing process rapidly. The patient may then continue on an oral antibiotic regimen at home. This type of injection is also preferred for vaccinations and pain medications. The onset of drug action usually occurs within 10 to 15 minutes. IM injections are inserted at a 90° angle into a muscle. Although the injection may hurt when the needle is inserted, the patient does not usually experience great pain at the injection site if care is taken to select the correct site and the solution is injected slowly. Sites for IM injections must be identified accurately. Damage to major blood vessels, bones, and nerves can occur if an inappropriate site or improper technique is used. In addition, sites should be rotated to avoid damaging the muscle.

Sites for IM injections depend on the viscosity of the liquid, the size and development of the muscle, and, to a certain extent, the patient's preference. Be sure not to inject into a scar or tattoo because the tissue under these areas may have an inadequate blood supply. In addition, any injection site should be healthy (free of rashes, lesions, or other injuries). The following is a list of possible IM injections sites.

- Deltoid: The deltoid is a triangular muscle in the upper arm that is usually well developed and easily accessible (Fig. 10-10A). Because the deltoid tends to be small, the general rule of thumb is that 1 mL is the maximum amount of fluid to inject, and the length of the needle should not exceed 1 inch.

- Dorsogluteal: The dorsogluteal muscle is located in the buttocks. If a larger amount of medication (more than 1 mL) is needed or the patient has a very small deltoid muscle, the buttock is an alternative site. This site is safe for all patients older than 2 years. The danger in using this site is hitting the sciatic nerve, which runs medially (in the middle of) in the buttock, with possible nerve damage leading to pain and/or weakness in the affected hip and leg. To avoid this nerve, the safest area of injection is the upper, outer quadrant (Fig. 10.10B). To locate this site, a line is drawn between the greater trochanter of the hip and the posterior superior iliac spine. The injection is then given slightly above this line.

- Ventrogluteal: The ventrogluteal site is used when the patient cannot stand and, instead, lies on his or her side. This site is not as commonly used, but it is considered safe for all patients older than 2 years. To locate this site, place the heel of the hand over the greater trochanter of the patient's hip with your thumb pointing toward the patient's umbilicus. Your index finger should be on the patient's anterior iliac spine. Spread your middle finger back as far as possible. The injection is then given in the center of the triangle formed by your index and middle fingers (Fig. 10-10C).

- Vastus lateralis: The deltoid muscle is not well developed in infants and small children, so a better site is the vastus lateralis thigh muscle. As the name suggests, it is a large muscle on the side of the thigh. This site can be used in all age groups and is the site of choice in infants and small children. To locate this site properly, place one hand on the patient's upper thigh (just below the greater trochanter) and the other hand on the patient's lower thigh (just above the knee). The injection is given between your hands and the slightly lateral (toward the outer edge) aspect of the muscle (Fig. 10.10D). The procedure for IM injections is described in Procedure Box 10.9.

A different method is used when a medication is very irritating to the skin or may cause skin discoloration. This is called the **Z-track** method (Fig. 10-11). If a health-care professional does not use the Z-track method with a medication such as Imferon, the patient may have permanent discoloration of the skin at the site. It is important to follow the directions for Z-tracking closely, or the needle may break in the skin (Procedure Box 10.10).

A **subcutaneous (SC)** injection may be prescribed if the medication must be absorbed more slowly than it does with an IM injection. The SC route places the medication into the fat under the skin. SC injection enters the fatty layer of the skin (Fig. 10-12), where medications are absorbed more slowly than when administered by the IM route. Insulin is one example of a medication that is administered by the SC route. Because fat does not have as generous a blood supply as muscle and also has fewer nerve endings, patients rarely complain of pain at the site, which rarely bleeds after injection. The most common medications given by this route are insulin and heparin.

*(Text continues on page 180)*

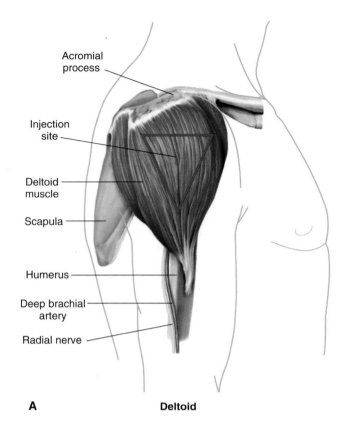

Acromial
process

Injection
site

Deltoid
muscle

Scapula

Humerus

Deep brachial
artery

Radial nerve

**A** **Deltoid**

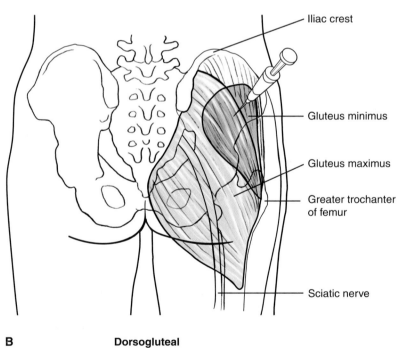

Iliac crest

Gluteus minimus

Gluteus maximus

Greater trochanter
of femur

Sciatic nerve

**B** **Dorsogluteal**

**FIGURE 10-10:** Intramuscular injection sites: (A) deltoid, (B) dorsogluteal,

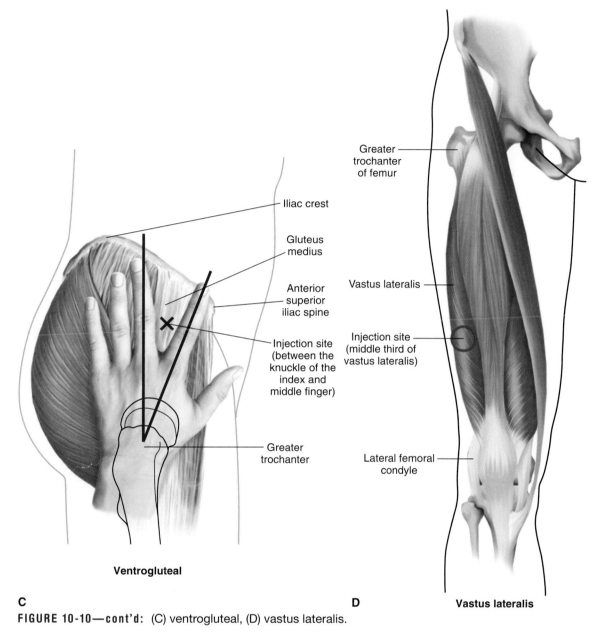

Ventrogluteal

**C**

**D**                                                  **Vastus lateralis**

**FIGURE 10-10—cont'd:** (C) ventrogluteal, (D) vastus lateralis.

## Procedure Box 10.9 *Administration of Intramuscular Injections*

Safety Precautions: Immediately dispose of sharps after administration. Use extreme care in locating landmarks for injection sites to avoid injury to muscles, nerves, and bones.

Supplies: Medication in appropriate syringe with appropriate needle, alcohol wipe, cotton ball, adhesive bandage, gloves, order, teaching materials, sharps container

Steps:

1. Observe the seven "rights" of medication administration.
2. Read the medication order, and compare it with the medication container.
3. Wash hands.
4. Compare the medication order with the container a second time. Check the expiration date.

*(continued)*

## Procedure Box 10.9 *Administration of Intramuscular Injections—Cont'd*

5. Identify the patient, and explain what you will be doing.
6. Compare the order and the container a third time.
7. Put on gloves.
8. Position the patient comfortably.
9. Locate the site using appropriate landmarks.
10. Clean the selected site with disinfectant wipe with circular motion.
11. Allow disinfectant to dry.
12. Remove the needle cover by pulling straight up.
13. Hold the skin taut at the selected, cleansed site.
14. Use a dart-like motion to insert the needle at a 90° angle completely to the hub.
15. Release the skin.
16. Aspirate for blood return (accidental placement in a blood vessel) by pulling backward on the plunger.
17. If no blood is noted, gently and slowly inject all medication. (If blood is noted, withdraw the needle, discard the syringe and needle, and start the procedure over with clean needle/syringe.)
18. Remove the needle and syringe quickly at the same angle of insertion, and place a cotton ball at the insertion site.
19. Massage the site if the organization's policy suggests massage, or ask the patient to move a muscle.
20. Dispose of the needle and syringe immediately in a sharps container. **Do not recap**.
21. Assess the patient and injection site.
22. Cover the wound with an adhesive bandage.
23. Remove gloves and wash hands.
24. Document dosage, site of placement, and the patient's response.

*Example:*

*07/10/2012 3:15 p.m.: 200 mg Rocephin IM to left vastus lateralis. Patient tolerated procedure well. CJ Watkins RN, MSN*

FIGURE 10-11: Z-track method. This method is used to administer medications that are caustic or will stain the skin.

## Procedure Box 10.10 Z-Track Administration

Safety Precautions: Immediately dispose of sharps after administration. Use extreme care in locating landmarks for injection sites, to avoid injury to muscles, nerves, and bones.

Supplies: Medication in appropriate syringe with appropriate needle, alcohol wipe, cotton ball, adhesive bandage, gloves, order, teaching materials, sharps container

Steps:

1. Follow all steps from Procedure Box 10-9 up until actually inserting the needle.
2. Before inserting the needle, pull the skin laterally 1 ½ inches away from the injection site (see Fig. 10-15).
3. Insert the needle at 90°, as for all IM injections.
4. Aspirate for blood return (accidental placement in a blood vessel) by pulling backward on the plunger.
5. If no blood is noted, gently and slowly inject all medication. (If blood is noted, withdraw the needle, discard the syringe and needle, and start the procedure over with a clean needle and syringe.)
6. Wait 10 seconds before removing the needle, to allow medication to be absorbed deeply.
7. Remove the needle and syringe quickly at the same angle of insertion, and place a cotton ball at insertion site.
8. Quickly release traction on the Z-track position (see Fig. 10-15). This prevents medication from leaking back into more superficial tissues.

*(continued)*

---

**●** *Fast Tip 10.1*   Rotating Sites for Regular SC Injections

Be specific when you instruct the patient to rotate sites. For example, you could draw a chart: Sunday, above the naval; Monday, right thigh; Tuesday, below the navel; Wednesday, left thigh; Thursday, right side of the navel; Friday, left side of the navel; Saturday, back of the left arm. There are more than enough injection sites to provide variety.

---

## Intravenous medications and administration

Finally, the IV route, which involves injecting the drug directly into a vein, is the most rapid method for administering medication into the bloodstream. IV medications are immediately absorbed and available for the body to use. The advantages of the IV route are not only rapid absorption, but also quick relief of symptoms. This route is the fastest method in an emergency. IV fluids and medications are administered directly into a vein to treat illness, to prevent illness, as part of a diagnostic procedure, or to provide nutrition and hydration. State and organizational policies differ on which allied health professionals can start IV infusions, so you may not be asked to perform this procedure. It is likely, however, that because so many patients are discharged from the hospital with IV lines in place, and because so many patients are receiving long-term infusion therapy, you may be asked to assess these patients and be familiar with IV supplies in case you are asked to help prepare them. These supplies include special bags filled with solutions that may or may not contain additives (medications, electrolytes, and vitamins), tubing, and IV catheters.

---

### A CLOSER LOOK 10.1: **Advantages and Disadvantages of IV Therapy**

Advantages

- It provides several options for medication and fluid delivery: direct injection or continuous or intermittent infusion.
- Patients can avoid multiple injections.
- An indwelling (in the vein) catheter with tubing or a port can be used. Ports are more comfortable for patients.

Disadvantages

- Medications may be incompatible. The health-care provider should check compatibility before combining any drugs in an IV line.
- A risk of complications exists, such as infiltrations, embolus, and infection.
- It costs more than other types of parenteral administration.
- Clots can form in an IV catheter or port, thus making it useless.

---

Sometimes a patient just needs fluids, and at other times the patient may need additives, total parenteral nutrition (TPN), or blood. The three main types of fluids or solutions are as follows:

1. Dextrose: A dextrose solution is a sugar and water solution. Dextrose 2.5% in water (D2.5W), 5% in water (D5W), and 10% in water (D10W) are the most popular. Dextrose can also come in combinations of 20% to 70%, but these are for patients with extremely low blood glucose levels, such as diabetic patients, infants, and severely malnourished patients, and are given only under very controlled circumstances, usually in an emergency room or intensive care unit.

2. Saline: If sugar is not needed, a saline, or sodium chloride (salt), solution may be prescribed. Sodium is a vital electrolyte for the body because it helps cells function normally along with other electrolytes such as potassium and magnesium. The usual solution, 0.9% sodium chloride (NaCl), is called normal saline solution (NSS). Also available is 1/2 NSS, which is 0.45% NaCl. NSSs can be added to dextrose solutions, such as D5NS, or D10/0.45 NaCl.

**3.** Lactated Ringer's: Lactated Ringer's solution was created by Sidney Ringer, an English physiologist who mixed dextrose, potassium chloride, sodium, lactate, and calcium to form an especially healthful mixture for patients. Other names for these mixtures include Ringer's lactate (RL) and dextrose 5% in lactated Ringer's (D5LR).

These three solutions are examples of crystalloids, which are simple solutions used to increase fluid volume when a patient is dehydrated or possibly in shock from bleeding. All these solutions are usually stored in dark cabinets because they can deteriorate if exposed to light for long periods of time. IV solutions look similar, so it is important to check the label against the order three times, as for any other medication.

Drugs administered by the IV route are given in one of three ways: infusion, piggyback line, or IV push. Infusion is slow IV administration of a large volume of fluid. The solution can contain additives such as medications, electrolytes, or minerals. IV fluid is usually packaged in a 250- to 1,000-mL bag or bottle. The allied health professional hangs the bag on a pole that is raised higher than the patient's heart. The fluid then flows into the vein by gravity or via an infusion pump. Some pumps strictly monitor the infusion rate, whereas others push the fluid into the patient's vein while regulating the infusion rate and the pressure it takes to infuse the fluid. Patient-controlled analgesia (PCA) pumps allow patients to push a button and receive medication, usually pain medication (such as morphine or Demerol), on demand within parameters ordered by the physician. Typically, licensed health professionals program these pumps and then lock them.

The possible complications of IV therapy are many, and as an allied health professional, you should be comfortable recognizing a problem, even if you are not responsible for implementing and administering the IV therapy. In some states and some facilities, allied health professionals can insert IV lines, hang IV fluids, disconnect IV lines, or flush indwelling ports. In other facilities and localities, these tasks are considered solely nursing functions. Become familiar with your state and facility parameters for your role so that you do not practice out of your permitted area. However, it is helpful to understand IV therapy, and you should be prepared to assess patients for signs and symptoms of infection and other problems associated with their IV lines.

---

### A CLOSER LOOK 10.2: Dialysis: Not for Veins

An IV treatment solution option for patients who have kidney problems is dialysis. If you work at a dialysis clinic, you need to understand the process. Dialysis refers to the passage of small particles through membranes. Electrolytes and drugs move from areas of high concentration to areas of lower concentration (osmosis). During this process, waste products are removed from the blood and then from the body. Normally, the kidneys perform this function, but when they are not working correctly, a machine must be used.

Dialysis solutions are never put directly into patients' veins, but they can be placed in a dialysis machine or across a membrane such as the peritoneum. If the patient lacks the electrolyte needed, it crosses from the solution into the blood. If the patient has too much of an electrolyte, it crosses from the blood into the dialysis solution.

---

Sometimes a patient needs medications or electrolytes several times per day over short periods of time. In such cases, a piggyback solution is used. A piggyback solution consists of a separate IV bag and tubing connected to the primary IV tubing. The piggyback may contain, for example, an antibiotic or potassium that is given every 4 hours in 100 mL of fluid. Vitamins can be added to IV solutions, especially when patients are unable to process vitamins in their gastrointestinal system.

An IV push refers to quick delivery of a small amount of medication in a syringe. An IV push cannot be used for drugs that can potentially irritate the vein, for drugs that may be fatal if given too quickly, or for a large amount of medication. Only a licensed health-care professional can administer IV push medication.

TPN is given when the patient's digestive system needs a complete rest. This treatment is also known as hyperalimentation. TPN is a nutritional solution infused (flowed) directly into the veins to give the patient complete nutrition. The solution is placed directly into a large vein because of the risk of damage to the vein or tissues surrounding a peripheral vein. TPN provides the patient with a well-rounded supply of fluid and electrolytes, in addition to calories from fats, protein, and vitamins. TPN fluids require the use of special long-term IV catheters placed by a physician, usually in the subclavian vein. The end of the catheter lies in the superior vena cava.

---

### A CLOSER LOOK 10.3: Types of IV Lines

Peripheral lines are IV lines placed in veins in the arms, hands, or sometimes the feet or scalp of a small child. Central lines are IV lines inserted in large veins such as the subclavian vein or internal jugular vein. These catheters terminate in the superior vena cava; that is, the tip of the catheter lies in the superior vena cava, just above the heart, to allow the medication and fluids to mix with a larger amount of blood. Central lines are used to give additives that irritate small veins, such as total parenteral nutrition. Peripherally inserted central catheter (PICC) lines are similar to central lines in that they terminate in a large vein close to the heart, but they are inserted from a peripheral site such as the lower arm.

---

Lipids, or fats, may also be added to IV solutions. Commercial lipid solutions contain substances such as soybean or safflower oil, which is added to water, glycerin, and egg yolks. These lipids increase the caloric source for patients who need it. Lipids, like TPN, usually require a special line.

Blood and blood products can be administered through an IV line. A licensed health-care professional administers blood, but everyone on the team must understand the types of blood products. Whole blood provides complete correction of blood loss in that it restores not only the fluid volume lost, but also the components, such as platelets and white blood cells, that were depleted. One unit of whole blood is 500 mL. Blood products provide various portions of whole blood based on a patient's needs. Patients with hemophilia, for example, require only clotting factors and platelets, not whole blood.

Before blood or a blood product is given, the patient's blood type must be checked against what is to be administered. This process, called "type and cross," ensures that patients do not have a transfusion reaction to blood that does not match their own.

A transfusion reaction is a serious negative response to the administration of blood or blood products. Signs and symptoms of a reaction include a rapid change in vital signs, dyspnea, restlessness, fever, chills, blood in the urine (hematuria), and pain in the chest, back, or flank. To discontinue a blood transfusion, the health-care worker first clamps the line infusing the blood and opens the line infusing NSS that is hung like a "Y" with the blood (Fig. 10-14). You should closely watch the patient's vital signs, including pulse, temperature, respiratory rate, and blood pressure, when transfusing blood products.

### Injectable medication supplies

Ampules, vials, needles, and syringes, as well as IV-related items, including bags or bottles of solutions, tubing, needles, and catheters, comprise some of the equipment you will need to know how to use if you are preparing an injection for administration or will be administering one.

An **ampule** is a small glass container that holds only one dose of a medication in solution for injections (Fig. 10-15). The ampule is broken by placing gauze around the neck of the container, to protect the hand and to keep glass from falling into the medicine. It is best to draw the solution from the ampule into a syringe with a filtered needle (needle with a filter built into it) and then change to a different needle to inject the solution into the patient; this reduces the chance that broken glass will enter the patient.

Most injectable solutions are supplied in vials instead of ampules. **Vials** are glass or plastic containers sealed on top with rubber stoppers. This makes the inside of the container sterile because it does not have to be opened or broken. Occasionally, the vial contains powder, and fluid (e.g., bacteriostatic sodium chloride or water) is added to reconstitute (mix) the solution. Once the solution is reconstituted, the vial should be used fairly quickly, according to the drug manufacturer's instructions, because the powder is more durable when it is stored without the fluid. Vials are either multiple-dose or unit-dose.

NSS

Blood

Line to be clamped

Clamp to be released

**FIGURE 10-14:** Blood administration setup. To discontinue a blood transfusion, the health-care professional first clamps the line infusing blood and opens the line infusing normal saline solution, which is hung like a "Y" with the blood.

**FIGURE 10-15:** Ampule. This small glass container holds only one dose of medication.

Multiple-dose vials contain several doses. After the first dose, the top of the stopper should be cleaned with an alcohol swab or other disinfecting swab before a needle is inserted into the vial for another dose. Multiple-dose vials should also be discarded within a specified time period after use, according to the manufacturer's recommendation, and labeled with the time and date of first use. Unit-dose vials contain just one dose of medicine and are discarded after use.

### CRITICAL THINKING

Why do you think vials are used more than ampules?

### Needles and syringes

When an injection is given, needles are used to puncture the skin and underlying layers, to deliver medication to the desired location. When an IV infusion is started, a needle is used to puncture the skin and place a plastic catheter. The needle is then removed, and the plastic catheter is left in place to deliver the IV fluid or medication. Choosing a needle is based on two measurements: length and circumference. Needle length ranges from 3/8 inch to 2 inches (Fig. 10-16). A shorter needle is used for ID injections, and a longer one is used for IM injections. Typically, a small needle is used in children or in adults with small muscles. Longer needles are used in large adults or in patients with large muscles.

The needle's **gauge** is determined by the width or circumference of the **lumen,** the inside of the needle (Fig. 10-17). Gauges vary from 14 (largest) to 27 (smallest): the higher the number, the smaller the lumen. The viscosity (thickness) of the fluid given determines the gauge. Drug resources or the instructions that come with the medications help determine the proper gauge of needle for viscous fluid. Thin fluid can pass through a 27-gauge needle, whereas a 20-gauge needle may be needed for thick fluid (e.g., blood).

Safety devices are frequently attached to needles because the Occupational Safety and Health Administration (OSHA) of the Department of Labor requires that employers protect employees from accidental needle sticks. These devices make needles more costly, but safer. Accidental needle sticks can result in the transfer of blood-borne pathogens (bacteria and viruses) from the patient to the person administering the medication.

Needle protectors either retract the needle before it is pulled out of the patient or cover the needle after use (Fig. 10-18). The easiest way to become familiar with the various types of needle protectors is to practice with them on a mannequin. Ideally, a needle is never recapped by hand. After the injection, the needle and syringe should be thrown away immediately in a biohazard sharps container (Fig. 10-19). However, after medication has been prepared, the needle may be recapped so it can be taken to the patient for administration of the medicine. The safest procedure is called the "scoop" method, in which you lay the cap on a flat surface and scoop it onto the needle.

A — 3/8"
B — 1/2"
C — 1"
D — 1 1/2"

**FIGURE 10-16:** Various needle lengths: (A) 3/8 inch, (B) 1/2 inch, (C) 1 inch, (D) 1 1/2 inch.

A — 27 gauge
B — 21 gauge
C — 18 gauge

**FIGURE 10-17:** Various gauges of needles: (A) 27 gauge, (B) 21 gauge, (C) 18 gauge.

**FIGURE 10-18:** Needle protector. The syringe has a needle protector covering the needle after use.

The last item to prepare for injection is the syringe, which holds the fluid to be administered. A syringe has the following parts: barrel, tip, and plunger (Fig. 10-20). The barrel is the hollow part of the syringe that holds the liquid medication and through which the plunger passes. The needle is attached to the tip of the syringe. Finally, the plunger is the part that pushes the medication through the barrel and the needle to deliver the medication to its intended site.

The three basic types of syringe are tuberculin (TB), insulin, and standard (Fig. 10-21). For TB testing or other ID injections, little fluid is injected, and therefore a narrow, finely **calibrated** (divided into accurate measurements) syringe known as a **tuberculin** syringe is used. Tuberculin syringes are calibrated to a hundredth of a milliliter (0.01 mL). These syringes are frequently used for newborns and children because doses of medicine for these patients are small.

An insulin syringe is calibrated in units instead of milliliters (Fig. 10-22). It can hold no more than 1 mL. The standard U-100 insulin syringe has 100 units calibrated on the barrel, and each line usually equals 2 units. Insulin syringes are also available with 30- and 50-unit capacity, used primarily for small children or when small amounts of insulin are needed. Because this insulin syringe has less capacity, each mark equals 1 unit, not 2. All insulin syringes are used solely for insulin because an error in measurement can be fatal. In addition, for this reason, no other syringe should ever be used to administer insulin. Regardless of manufacturer, these syringes generally have orange in the coloring (usually the needle cap) to identify them as insulin syringes. Facilities may have a policy that all insulin doses must be checked by two people before the injection is administered.

Standard, or **hypodermic,** syringes are available in sizes ranging from 3 to 60 mL. Even if the needle is attached or packaged together with the syringe, a different gauge or length needle may be necessary, especially if the patient is small or is a child. Prepackaged needles can be replaced with smaller needles in most cases. The calibration of these syringes depends on the size. Syringes holding 3 mL are calibrated in 0.1-mL increments, whereas larger syringes are calibrated in 0.2-mL increments.

Syringes are available without needles to deliver medication into the mouth. They can be purchased without needles, so separate needles can be attached according to the length and gauge desired for the specific task. The various types of syringes are summarized in Table 10.1. Table 10.2 summarizes the different types of injections and the needles and syringes used for them. Procedure Box 10.12 explains how to draw up medication by using the information you have learned regarding ampules, vials, needles, and syringes.

During an emergency, there is little time to prepare medication for injection. To expedite receipt of necessary medication and to ensure accuracy in a critical situation, some drugs are available in a prefilled cartridge that can quickly be attached to a special cartridge holder (Fig. 10-23). After the cartridge is used, do not throw the holder away. Simply dispose of the glass or plastic cartridge, and retain the holder for future use.

## Virtual Field Trip

1. Go to www.osha.gov, and research the Occupational Safety and Health Administration regulation for needle safety. Be prepared to discuss the consequences to the employer of not following these regulations.
2. Google a minimum of two medical suppliers, and investigate the various safety devices offered for needles. Decide which two you think would be most effective in the workplace, and defend your answers.

*CRITICAL THINKING*

Why is it dangerous to recap a needle? With so many safety devices available, why may there continue to be problems with needle sticks?

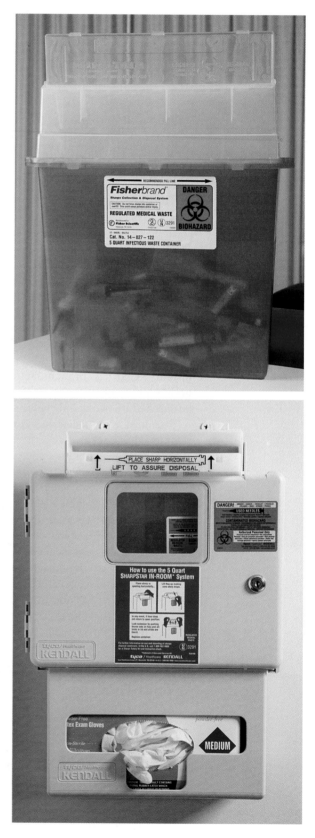

**FIGURE 10-19:** Biohazard sharps container. Dispose of used needles, syringes, or any other sharp object such as a broken medication vial in a biohazard sharps container.

**FIGURE 10-20:** Parts of a syringe: (A) needle, (B) hub, (C) tip, (D) barrel, (E) plunger.

**FIGURE 10-21:** Three types of syringes: (A) tuberculin (TB), (B) insulin, (C) hypodermic.

One side of U-100 insulin syringe

Other side of U-100 insulin syringe

U-50 insulin syringe

U-30 insulin syringe

**FIGURE 10-22:** Insulin syringe. These syringes are available in the following sizes: U-100, U-50, and U-30.

## TABLE 10.1   Syringes and Uses

| Syringe Type | Calibration and Capacity | Sample Use |
|---|---|---|
| Tuberculin | One line = 0.01 mL<br>Capacity = 1 mL | Tuberculin testing or other ID injections<br>Newborn and pediatric dosages |
| Insulin | One line = 2 mL<br>Capacity = 100 units | Insulin administration |
| Standard | Varies with size | IM injections |

## TABLE 10.2   Parenteral Injections

| Type | Depth | Injection Volume | Usual Needle Size | Angle |
|---|---|---|---|---|
| IM (Deltoid) | Muscle | 0.5–1 mL | 23–25 gauge<br>5/8 inch | 90° |
| IM (Ventrogluteal) | Muscle | 1–2 mL | 18–23 gauge<br>1 1/4-3 inch | 90° |
| IM (Vastus lateralis in adult) | Muscle | 1–2 mL | 20–23 gauge<br>1 1/4 - 1 1/2 inch | 90° |
| IM (Vastus lateralis in child) | Muscle | 0.5–1 mL<br>(Maximum 1 mL in infants and 2 mL in child) | 23-25 gauge<br>5/8 inch–1 inch | 90° |
| IM (Dorsogluteal) | Muscle | 1–2 mL | 18–23 gauge<br>1 1/4 - 3 inch | 90° |
| SC (Various sites) | Subcutaneous tissue | Up to 1 mL | 25–29 gauge<br>5/8 inch | 45° |
| ID (Various sites) | Under the epidermis | 0.1–0.2 mL | 25–27 gauge<br>5/8 inch | 10°–15° |

Note: this information addresses the typical patient. Make adjustments based on individual patient assessment.

### Procedure Box 10.12 Drawing Up Medication

Safety Precautions: Maintain sterility of the equipment. Work in a quiet, well-lit area free of distractions.

Supplies: Medication, alcohol wipe, appropriate syringe, appropriate needle, order

Steps:

1. Observe the seven "rights" of medication administration.
2. Read the medication order, and compare it with the medication container.
3. Wash hands.
4. Calculate the dosage correctly.
5. Compare the order and the container a second time. Check the expiration date.
6. Compare the order and the container a third time.
7. Remove the cap from the vial. If the vial has been used before, check for a discard date, and wipe with a disinfectant wipe. If using an ampule, break it carefully by using a piece of gauze.
8. Remove the cover from the needle by pulling it straight off.
9. If the drug is in an ampule, insert the needle into the ampule, and draw up the fluid into the syringe. Make sure to use a filtered needle (see Fig. 10-19). Change the needle after drawing up the medication.
10. If a vial is used, draw up an amount of air equal to the amount of fluid to be withdrawn. The air you inject will help to prevent a negative vacuum from occurring when you withdraw medication. Insert the needle into the vial, and inject the air (see the figure).

**Procedure Box 10.12** *Drawing Up Medication—Cont'd*

11. Turn the vial upside down, and withdraw the ordered amount of medication into the syringe. If bubbles appear, tap the syringe with your fingernail, or pull the plunger down farther and then push it back to the ordered calibration to push air above the medication and back into the vial.

12. Remove the needle and syringe from the vial, and carefully recap the needle using the scoop method.

13. You are now ready to inject the medication into the patient. Immediately proceed to administer the medication. Do not leave the medication sitting unattended.

Inject air

Withdraw medication

**FIGURE 10-23:** Prefilled medication cartridge. Many commonly used medications are available in prefilled cartridges and are placed into a cartridge holder such as this.

## Intravenous setup

Most IV lines and setups have the basic components illustrated in Figure 10-24. The health-care worker *spikes* the IV bag or bottle and attaches it to the IV tubing. He or she does this by inserting the end of the tubing into the outlet port of the bag or bottle. The cap on the spike section of the IV tubing is removed just before it is inserted into the IV container, to keep the spike sterile. An IV bottle may have an air vent located below the spike. The health-care worker must remove a diaphragm to let air in and release the vacuum. The vent allows air to enter the bottle as fluid flows out of it.

Bags collapse as the solution flows out, and therefore venting is not an issue. Bottles maintain their shape as they empty. Calibration marks on the bag or bottle show how much IV solution has been administered and how much is left (see Fig. 10-24).

B IV solution bag

A Poie

C Spike

D Injection port

E Drip chamber

F Flow regulator clamp

G Tubing

H Filter

I Needle adapter with protective cap

**FIGURE 10-24:** IV lines and setup: (A) pole, (B) IV solution, (C) spike, (D) injection port, (E) drip chamber, (F) flow regulator clamp, (G) tubing, (H) filter, (I) needle adapter with protective cap.

Below the spike (see Fig. 10-24C) (allows tubing to puncture the IV fluid container) is a drip chamber (see Fig. 10-24E). The drip chamber allows the flow of fluid from the bag after it has been primed (emptied of air) by squeezing it. The purpose of the drip chamber is to encourage any air in the line to remain in the chamber while only the solution flows down to the patient. The flow rate is set by counting the drops entering the drip chamber.

On the IV tubing (see Fig. 10-24G), the flow regulator adjusts the flow through the line (see Fig. 10-24F). The ports in various places along the line allow IV medications to be infused through them. The IV needle enters the patient's vein but is usually removed, thus leaving a flexible catheter in the vein. A protective cap covers the needle until it is ready for use (see Fig. 10-24I).

The length of the IV tubing varies from 6 to 120 inches, depending on need. The amount of fluid needed for priming (filling the tubing with fluid and removing air) the tubing varies, depending on the length of the tubing. A filter (see Fig. 10-24H) may be present to capture any air bubbles or particles or dirt or debris present in the IV fluid.

IV sets are individually wrapped and sterilized, to ensure a sterile pathway for the fluids. Damaged packages are not used because sterility may be compromised. Rigid parts of the IV set are made from plastic or polymerized chloride. Only plastic sets may be used for nitroglycerin, which interacts with polymerized chloride.

The most common needle sizes for IV infusions are 14 (largest) to 24 (smallest) gauges. The needle can be the winged "butterfly" type (Fig. 10-25) or a straight needle within a catheter, called an Angiocath (Fig. 10-26). Table 10.3 compares the two types of needles.

To begin IV therapy, the health-care worker assembles the necessary equipment, including a bag or bottle of the IV solution ordered, IV tubing, and a needle and cannula set to insert into the vein. Placing

**FIGURE 10-25:** Butterfly needle. These IV needles are used for small and fragile veins. The metal needle remains in place.

**FIGURE 10-26:** Angiocath. The IV needle is removed, leaving a flexible plastic catheter in place.

## TABLE 10.3   Comparison of Winged and Straight IV Needles

| Winged | Straight |
| --- | --- |
| Short-term use | Long-term use |
| Easy to insert | More difficult to insert |
| More likely to lead to infiltration (leakage of fluid from the vein into the tissue) | Inadvertent vein puncture less likely |
| Uncomfortable | More comfortable once placed |

the IV needle and cannula into the patient is similar to drawing blood, and only an indwelling cannula is left in the patient when the needle is removed. Procedure Box 10.13 shows how to insert an IV line. Never insert an IV line unless you are legally authorized to do so. See Fast Tip 10.2 for more information on the use of a tourniquet. After inserting the IV line, the following information must be documented:

■ Size and type of device

■ Date and time inserted

### Procedure Box 10.13 *Insertion of an IV Line*

Safety Precautions: Maintain sterility of the equipment. Dispose of the needle as soon as possible after an attempt is made.

Supplies: Tourniquet, needle and catheter, IV bag and tubing, disinfectant swab, adhesive tape

Steps:

1. Observe the seven "rights" of medication administration.
2. Read the medication order, and compare it with the medication bag.
3. Wash hands.
4. Compare the order and the bag a second time. Check the expiration date.
5. Identify the patient, and explain what you will do.
6. Compare the order and medication bag a third time.
7. Assess the appropriate site.
8. Apply gloves.

*(continued)*

## Procedure Box 10.13 *Insertion of an IV Line—Cont'd*

9. Place a tourniquet 6 to 8 inches proximal to the site to be used (top left).
10. Ask the patient to close his or her fist four to six times; if necessary, gently tap the vein.
11. Cleanse the site with circular motion, and use a disinfecting swab, either povidone-iodine or alcohol (top right).
12. Stabilize the vein by stretching skin 1 inch from the insertion site.
13. Insert the IV needle and catheter with the bevel upward at a 30° to 45° angle directly into the selected vein; then advance the catheter, and remove the needle (middle left).

    **Note:** Advance the catheter (without a needle) into a vein at a 10° to 15° angle.
14. Connect the IV tubing that has been primed (fluid runs out of the end to flush air out) (middle right).
15. Turn on the IV infusion using the flow regulator or slide clamp (bottom left).
16. Secure the site with an occlusive, waterproof dressing and tape (bottom right).
17. Some organizations require certain information be written on the dressing, such as your initials and the date and time.
18. Assess the patient.
19. Remove gloves and wash hands.
20. Document medication administration and the patient's response.

*Example:*

*06/21/2012 10:00 a.m.: #22 Angiocath placed to left hand after 1 unsuccessful attempt. D5LR started at 75 mL/hr as ordered. Patient tolerated procedure well. Patient advised of signs and symptoms to report to staff and states understanding. CJ Watkins RN, MSN*

---

**Fast Tip 10.2   Tourniquets**

Wrapping a constricting band (tourniquet) around the arm helps the vein become more visible. The tourniquet should never be placed on the patient for more than 2 minutes. If it takes longer to find a suitable site, release the tourniquet and begin elsewhere. Check your organization's policy, and call for assistance if you cannot insert the IV line after two attempts.

---

- Site location
- Type of solution
- Name of health-care provider who inserted the IV catheter or hung an IV bag
- Any additives added to the IV solution
- Flow rate
- Number of attempts at insertion (successful and unsuccessful)
- Complications, if any, and your interventions
- Patient teaching

Allied health professionals are sometimes allowed to stop IV therapy. To do so, put on gloves and then loosen the securing tape. Gently pull out the needle or catheter, and properly dispose of it. Apply pressure to the site with a sterile 2 × 2 gauze pad until the bleeding stops. Be sure to assess the patient and document the removal, including the time and date. Follow your organization's policy for assessing the site, changing sites, flushing, and changing tubing.

Health-care professionals may be asked to flush an indwelling IV device that is not attached to a running IV line. Follow the organization's policy by flushing with heparin or NSS as ordered and at the frequency specified. Also make sure that your agency's policy allows you to do this procedure. Clean the port with an antiseptic wipe, and enter the port with the needleless adapter and syringe drawn up with the ordered flush solution following your agency's procedure manual. Even if you are not allowed to flush a line, you should assess the patient who has an indwelling port for signs and symptoms of infiltration, infection, and other problems.

As an allied health professional, you must observe the IV site on a regular basis. If you see redness and swelling, feel unusual warmth at the site, hear the patient complain of tenderness or pain, or note that the site feels like a firm rope or that the cannula is no longer in a vein, notify your supervisor immediately. The supervisor may ask you to stop the IV infusion quickly, although do not remove the IV line without permission.

Complications of IV therapy include bleeding, infection, phlebitis, infiltration, catheter dislodgment, occlusion, vein irritation, severed catheter, hematoma, venous spasm, thrombosis, thrombophlebitis, circulatory overload, nerve, tendon, or ligament damage, systemic infection, air embolism, allergic reaction, incompatibility of medications, and irreversible medication error. The most common complications include the following.

- **Infiltration** occurs when the IV catheter becomes displaced and allows IV fluids and medications to leak into the tissue surrounding the vein. This complication can cause a varying degree of injury from discomfort to permanent damage to the tissue, depending on how quickly the problem is discovered and how caustic the medication is to the tissue.

- **Thrombus** (blood clot) or **phlebitis** (vein inflammation) can result from extremes in solution pH, needle or catheter trauma, particulate material, irritating drugs, or selection of a vein too small for the volume of solution infused. Check the vein for signs of inflammation (e.g., redness, swelling, and warmth to the touch) or pain.

- Air **emboli** (bubbles released into the bloodstream) can occur if air enters the vein. Small amounts of air in veins are not usually harmful, but rapidly injecting air into the vein can be fatal. Be careful to purge all air from the IV tubing before securing the line in the patient. Assess the patient's respiratory status, and report and document any changes.

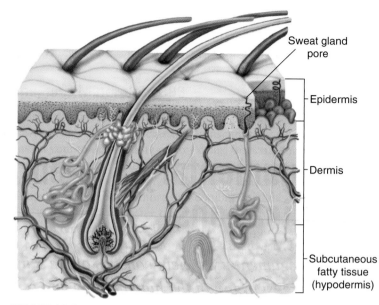

FIGURE 11-1: Layers and structures of the skin.

## INTEGUMENTARY SYSTEM: VULNERABLE BARRIER

The skin is the largest organ of the body. Skin has only a few openings, such as the eyes, ears, and nose. The skin is the only barrier our bodies have to the outside world, and it is particularly vulnerable to external injury. Injuries such as abrasions, blisters, calluses, cracks, cuts, irritated areas, inflamed areas, lesions, scrapes, sores, rashes, and sunburn can damage the skin and provide an opening for infection for bacteria, fungi, parasites, or viruses.

Some patients are more susceptible to skin irritations and/or tumors because of a genetic predisposition: their skin may be more delicate. People who have fair skin that has repeated exposure to the sun are more vulnerable to skin damage. Other environmental hazards may be responsible for causing the following skin conditions:

- Skin discoloration
- Alopecia (hair loss)
- Seborrhea (oily skin lesions)
- Psoriasis (scaly patches)
- Verrucae (warts caused by viruses)
- Nevi (moles)
- Tumors

Skin disorders are classified as infectious, inflammatory, or cancerous. The medications used are based on the diagnosis in that classification. These medications are given either topically or systemically, depending on the severity of the skin disorder (see the Master the Essentials table for descriptions of the most common integumentary system drugs).

### Skin infections and medications

As mentioned earlier, bacteria, parasites, viruses, and fungi can invade the body through a skin injury. Different types of medications treat skin infections either topically or systemically, depending on the ailment. Generally, antibiotics fight bacteria, whereas antifungal medications treat fungi, antiviral medications fight viruses, and pediculicides and scabicides fight parasites.

## Master the Essentials: Dermatologic Medications

This table shows the various dermatologic medications and key side effects, contraindications and precautions, interactions, and examples of each classification.

| Class | Side Effects | Contraindications and Precautions | Interactions | Examples |
|---|---|---|---|---|
| Benzoyl peroxide | Peeling, erythema, edema | Hypersensitivity | Tretinoin | Benzoyl peroxide (Benzagel, Benzox, PanOxyl) |
| Retinoids | Photosensitivity, local reactions (topical); depression, suicidal ideation, pseudotumor cerebri, pancreatitis, visual changes, hepatotoxicity, hyper-triglyceridemia (oral) | Hypersensitivity, pregnancy | Other topical products, photosensitizers | Tretinoin (Retin-A, Renova, Avita), tazarotene (Tazorac) |
| Scabicides and pediculicides | Eczema, rash, redness, itching, burning, headache | Hypersensitivity | Oils, pentobarbital, diazepam | Lindane (Kwell, Nix, Rid-X) |
| Keratolytics | Burning, irritation, tinnitus, dizziness, ototoxicity, headaches (oral) | Hypersensitivity, prolonged use, irritated skin, moles, birthmarks, or warts with hair growth, mucous membranes | Usually none with topical use | Salicylic acid (Compound W, Clearasil, Stri-Dex), ammonium lactate (Lac-Hydrin lotion) |
| Topical antifungals | Burning, stinging, pruritus, erythema | Hypersensitivity | None reported | Clotrimazole (Mycelex, Lotrimin, Gyne-Lotrimin), ketoconazole (Nizoral), nystatin (Mycostatin) |
| Topical corticosteroids | Burning, itching, irritation | Hypersensitivity (use on the face, groin, or axillae), pregnancy | None reported | Hydrocortisone (Westcort, Cortaid), dexamethasone (Decadron) |
| Topical Immunomodulators | Burning, pruritus | Hypersensitivity, pregnancy, breastfeeding | Formal studies not performed | Pimecrolimus (Elidel), tacrolimus (Protopic) |
| Antipsoriatic agents | Irritation to surrounding skin; discoloration of skin, hair, or fabrics | Hypersensitivity, use on the face, renal disease, pregnancy, breastfeeding, hypercalcemia (calcipotriene) | Topical corticosteroids | Coal tar (T/Gel, Neutrogena), anthralin (Dritho-Scalp, Psoriatec), cyclosporine (Gengraf, Neoral), etanercept (Enbrel), methotrexate (Trexall) |
| Topical fluorouracil | Erythema, burning, vesicle formation, insomnia, photosensitivity, malaise | Hypersensitivity, pregnancy | None reported | Fluorouracil (Efudex, Fluoro-plex, Carac) |

## Bacteria

Several bacterial infections can wreak havoc on the skin, the most common example being acne. **Acne** is an inflammatory disorder that affects the sebaceous glands. Acne occurs most commonly in adolescents due to an increase in androgens (male hormones present in both men and women). Bacteria can also cause acne, which affects adolescents and adults. Hormonal changes that occur during puberty cause **seborrhea,** a condition caused by an overproduction of skin oils. Abnormal **keratinization,** or hardening of the epithelial tissue, also occurs. A bacterium, *Propionibacterium acnes,* grows inside the sebaceous glands and makes an irritating, acidic substance. The skin produces inflamed bumps, called pustules, in response to this irritation.

Open **comedos,** or blackheads, are oil glands plugged with melanin granules. Closed comedos, or whiteheads, are white rather than black because they are produced just below the skin and lack melanin. Deeper lumps called **nodules** involve inflammation deep below the skin. Severe inflammation and pus can cause pain, deformity, and eventual scarring.

**Rosacea** is a type of skin irritation without pus. Small bumps, or papules, redden the skin. Even though these papules do not contain pus, they may produce pain because of the thickening and swelling. The patient with rosacea appears flushed, especially on the nose and cheek. Sunlight, stress, and hot temperatures can aggravate rosacea, as can alcohol, spicy foods, and hot beverages.

Medications used to treat acne and rosacea can be applied topically to the irritated areas, frequently the face, back, and neck. The active ingredient in these medications may be vitamin A, an acid, or an antibiotic. Over-the-counter (OTC) medications, such as a cream, gel, or lotion, usually contain benzoyl peroxide. Benzoyl peroxide is bacteriostatic (inhibits bacterial growth).

Retinoids contain vitamin A, which increases the body's resistance to infection by reducing the oil production that clogs the pores. Retinoids reduce both the function of the sebaceous glands and keratinization. Because of serious associated side effects (birth defects, emotional problems), oral retinoids are reserved for patients with severe acne who do not respond to other topical agents. For severe acne, salicylic acid, sulfur, or resorcinol may be used topically to remove the infected skin through shedding. Systemic antibiotics such as tetracyclines are sometimes necessary in extreme cases.

Oral contraceptives have also been effective in decreasing the symptoms of acne and are sometimes prescribed for this purpose. The hormones in some oral contraceptives can help stop acne from forming by reducing androgen production.

Another bacterial infection is **impetigo.** This most commonly occurs in children. A common example is a child with an upper respiratory infection who is constantly wiping his or her nose until the skin breaks down and allows entry of bacteria. This condition is treated with topical antibiotics, topical corticosteroids, and, if the infection is severe, systemic antibiotics.

## Parasites

Scabies is a parasitic infection caused by human itch mites that burrow into the skin and lay their eggs. This condition usually occurs in the webbing of the fingers and toes as well as the neck, axillae, and groin. Lice, which cause pediculosis (infestation of head, body, or pubic lice), live in hair and feed on blood. Scabicides and pediculicides are used to treat itch mite and lice infestations, respectively. These drugs are applied directly to the area of infestation.

Lice lay eggs called **nits.** After applying a pediculicide, the hair where the nits live should be combed with a special fine-toothed comb and the site inspected for at least 1 week to be sure all the nits are dead. Because bedding and clothing may hold eggs, they must be thoroughly cleaned daily for 1 week. Pediculicides are neurotoxins and may cause neurological side effects; therefore, they should be used only as prescribed.

### Virtual Field Trip

Using your favorite search engine, go to your local health department or similar Web site. Use the information there to create a patient teaching aid on lice infestation removal, and bring it to class to share.

### Viruses

Viruses are the smallest of microorganisms, and because they depend on a host cell for survival, eradicating them can be difficult without killing the host cell. Some examples of viruses that affect the skin are the human papillomavirus (HPV), herpes simplex virus type 1 (HSV-1), and herpes simplex virus type 2 (HSV-2). HPV causes venereal warts and most of the cervical cancer in women, and it can become problematic and difficult to eliminate. Warts on the genitals are called condylomas; otherwise, warts are called verrucae. HPV can lie dormant in the system and flare up if it is not completely treated. The goal of wart treatment is to destroy affected skin superficially at the site of growth. Cryosurgery with liquid nitrogen or topical products containing salicylic acid may be necessary to remove persistent or prolific warts.

HSV-1 typically causes cold sores, or fever blisters, on the mouth and lips. HSV-2 is a sexually transmitted virus and usually affects the genital mucosa. Both HSV-1 and HSV-2 are treated with oral antivirals. Herpes zoster, or shingles, is a reactivation of the varicella-zoster virus that causes chickenpox. This is also treated with oral antiviral medications, which are covered in Chapter 17, Immunologic System Medications.

### Fungi

Fungal infections that affect the integumentary system include tinea and candidiasis. In tinea infections, dermatophytes invade keratin and can infect the hair, nails, and skin. Topical antifungals, such as clotrimazole (Lotrimin) or terbinafine (Lamisil), may be used when the infection is present on the trunk, extremities, groin, or feet. If the infection is on the scalp, oral agents may be needed.

Candidal infections, also known as yeast infections, are caused by *Candida albicans.* This infection is associated with a pruritic red rash that may be painful. When it occurs in the mouth, this infection is commonly known as **thrush;** white plaques are usually present on the oral mucosa. Topical antifungals such as nystatin may be ordered.

## Inflammatory conditions and medications

Inflammatory conditions of the skin include burns, atopic dermatitis, and psoriasis. The most common treatments for burns are anesthetics and antibiotics. Atopic dermatitis is treated with corticosteroids, immunomodulators, and antihistamines. Antipsoriatic agents and ultraviolet (UV) therapy are used to treat psoriasis.

### Burns

Burns damage the skin by removing water from it, by causing it to blister, or by removing it entirely. Burns are classified as first-, second-, or third-degree (Fig. 11-2).

The most common first-degree burn is sunburn. The skin becomes red and painful to touch. People with few melanocytes (darkening cells), and thus fair skin, are especially vulnerable to sunburn.

Nonpharmacological treatment for sunburn includes application of cool water for 20 minutes and of an herb called aloe vera. A former practice by the layperson of applying butter or lard to sunburn

---

**Drug Spotlight 11.1** *Abreva® (docosanol 10%)*

| | |
|---|---|
| Define | A nonprescription antiviral topical medication |
| Use | Used to treat cold sores caused by the herpes simplex virus (HSV-1) on the face or lips |
| Action | Approved by the FDA to shorten healing time and duration of symptoms; works by blocking the HSV-1 virus from spreading to healthy cells |
| Application | Applied at first sign (tingle) of a cold sore; used up to five times a day |
| Side effects | Side effects including headaches and nasal congestion |

FDA, Food and Drug Administration

**FIGURE 11-2:** Burn degrees. (A) Burning of the top layer of skin is called a first-degree burn; it commonly causes red skin and swelling. (B) A burn that causes a blister is a second-degree burn; the blisters may open and ooze a clear fluid. This burn is often very painful. (C) A burn that removes the skin and tissue beyond it is a third-degree burn; the area looks brown, even charred. The patient may or may not complain of pain because the nerves have been destroyed in this area. Usually, if pain is present, it is caused by a mixture of second- and third-degree burns.

causes more damage and should not be used. Pharmacological treatment of sunburn includes lidocaine-containing medications such as Solarcaine.

A burn is classified as second degree if a blister forms over the burn, and the burn turns yellow. Cover second-degree burns with a sterile dressing, and administer an antibiotic such as silver sulfadiazine (Silvadene) to the burn as prescribed. The dressing can help absorb exudate if the blister should break. Silvadene helps to prevent infection that could result because the natural barrier against microorganisms has been severely damaged.

A third-degree burn is the most severe and affects all layers of skin, subcutaneous tissue, and possibly even muscle and bone. The patient with such a burn has lost much skin integrity and is at great risk for infection and fluid loss. Immediate treatment includes maintaining the patient's airway (if burns are around face and neck) and administering oxygen and intravenous fluids as needed. Collagenase (Santyl), which débrides (or removes) tissue, is sometimes prescribed to eliminate the dead tissue. However, it also removes healthy tissue and must be applied only to the wound as ordered. An antimicrobial nonstick dressing may be ordered. Other drugs may be ordered to absorb exudates (DuoDERM) or to stimulate formation of healthy new granulation tissue (e.g., becaplermin [Regranex]). Systemic medications may include analgesics, anti-inflammatory agents, and antibiotics.

## Atopic dermatitis

Atopic dermatitis is also called **eczema.** It is an allergic disorder usually associated with other atopic diseases, such as asthma or allergic rhinitis. It causes cutaneous inflammation that is evidenced by extremely dry patches of itchy skin. Initial methods of treatment include avoiding allergens, removing irritants, and maintaining hydration. Agents that may be needed include topical corticosteroids, such as hydrocortisone acetate 1.0% (Cortef), or topical immunomodulators, such as tacrolimus (Protopic) or pimecrolimus (Elidel). Corticosteroids decrease inflammation to reduce the damage it causes. Immunomodulators (immune response modifiers) used for atopic dermatitis are topical preparations that temporarily modify the skin's immune reaction. They do not affect the immune system of the entire body. Oral antihistamines such as diphenhydramine (Benadryl) may relieve itching but can cause mood changes, bone defects, or hematological problems if they are used for prolonged periods.

## Psoriasis

**Psoriasis** is a chronic inflammatory skin disease in which, for unknown reasons, the life cycle of skin cells is shortened (Fig. 11-3). Some investigators believe that the disease has a genetic factor, and others believe that environmental triggers exist. The normal life span of the skin cell is somewhere between 30 and 50 days. With psoriasis, the skin cell matures in 3 to 4 days. The dead skin cells in both healthy and psoriatic skin rise to the surface to be shed. Dead cells in this instance cannot be shed quickly enough, thus causing a buildup of skin cells on the surface. The dead cells take on a flaky white appearance atop a reddened (erythematous) plaque. Treatment of psoriasis may include topical corticosteroids, low-dose antihistamines, salicylic acid, or phototherapy. Specific antipsoriatic agents include the cream anthralin (Psoriatec) and calcipotriene (Dovonex, Calcitrene), which is available as both a cream and an ointment. Oral or injectable methotrexate is used for severe disease unresponsive to other therapy.

Many countries, including Argentina, France, and Iceland, have spas that claim to have healing hot springs containing varying combinations of algae, thermal mud, mineral- and salt-rich water, and other

**FIGURE 11-3:** Psoriasis. *(Reprinted from Barankin, B, and Freiman, A: Derm Notes: Clinical Dermatology Pocket Guide. F.A. Davis, Philadelphia, 2006; p 133.)*

natural substances that cure both psoriasis and dermatitis. Use of UV light has also shown some promise of improvement in psoriatic symptoms.

### Skin cancer and medications

Skin cancer can occur when the skin's tissue is damaged. For example, if a **nevus** (mole) or discolored skin area changes in color, grows, or develops irregular borders, a physician should be notified because this could be a sign of cancer, and a biopsy might be ordered. The three major types of skin cancer are basal cell carcinoma, squamous cell carcinoma, and malignant melanoma. Basal cell carcinoma is the most common form of skin cancer and rarely **metastasizes** (spreads) (Fig. 11-4). Treatment may require surgical excision, but topical preparations for superficial basal cell carcinomas such as fluorouracil, which affects the rapidly dividing cancer cells, or imiquimod (a topical immunomodulator that stimulates the immune system) may be used. Liquid nitrogen cryotherapy is also an option.

Squamous cell carcinoma arises from malignant keratinocytes (the most common type of skin cells that produce keratin) (Fig. 11-5). This form of skin cancer can metastasize. Surgical removal is the treatment of choice, and radiation therapy may be needed. The third type of skin cancer is malignant melanoma, and its incidence is quickly rising (Fig. 11-6). This unpredictable cancer spreads through the lymphatic system and blood. Treatment includes surgery, radiation, and chemotherapy. The medications used in treatment of these more invasive types of cancer are covered in Chapter 17, Immunologic System Medications.

**FIGURE 11-4:** Basal cell carcinoma. *(Reprinted from Barankin, B, and Freiman, A: Derm Notes: Clinical Dermatology Pocket Guide. F.A. Davis, Philadelphia, 2006; p 70.)*

**FIGURE 11-5:** Squamous cell carcinoma. *(Reprinted from Barankin, B, and Freiman, A: Derm Notes: Clinical Dermatology Pocket Guide. F.A. Davis, Philadelphia, 2006; p 150.)*

**FIGURE 11-6:** Melanoma. *(Reprinted from Barankin, B, and Freiman, A: Derm Notes: Clinical Dermatology Pocket Guide. F.A. Davis, Philadelphia, 2006; p 116.)*

●●● S U M M A R Y

The skin is the major defense organ of the body. Any injury, infection, or disease that alters the skin's physiology can compromise the health of the individual. Skin infections are caused by bacteria, parasites, viruses, and fungi. Inflammatory conditions such as burns, atopic dermatitis, and psoriasis can cause pain, itching, and self-consciousness about body image, and some conditions can be life-threatening. Each of these skin conditions requires a specific type of medication for successful treatment. In addition, skin cancer can range from the common basal cell carcinoma to the much more serious squamous cell carcinoma and malignant melanoma`. Skin cancer has a good prognosis if found at an early stage. Therefore, thorough skin assessment can detect problems early on, and an understanding of treatments and available medications is essential for true patient advocacy.

## Activities

To make sure that you have learned the key points covered in this chapter, complete the following activities.

### True or False

Write true if the statement is true. Beside the false statements, write false, and correct the statement to make it true.

Antifungals are used to treat impetigo. _____

Pediculicides kill nits and lice. _____

Vitamin A is used to treat acne. _____

Thrush is a bacterial infection. _____

Oral contraceptives drugs can treat acne. _____

Malignant melanoma is easily treatable with topical creams. _____

The topical antibiotic used for burns is called Silvadene. _____

A nevus is a mole. _____

Rosacea is a type of skin cancer. _____

Psoriasis occurs when a shortened life cycle of skin occurs. _____

### Multiple Choice

Choose the best answer for each question.

**1. HPV is an example of a ___B___.**
   A. Bacterial infection
   B. Viral infection
   C. Parasitic infection
   D. Fungal infection

**2. A comedo is ___C___.**
   A. A louse egg
   B. A nodule
   C. A form of acne
   D. Earwax

**3. Rosacea includes skin irritations called ___B___.**
   A. Comedos
   B. Papules
   C. Verruca
   D. Nevus

**4. An example of a pediculicide is _____.**

A. Compound W

B. Nystatin

C. Rid-X

D. Decadron

**5. Thrush is caused by _____.**

A. HSV-1

B. HSV-2

C. *Candida albicans*

D. *Sarcoptes scabiei*

**6. Thrush is treated with what medication?**

A. Nystatin

B. Ampicillin

C. Acyclovir

D. Any of the above

**7. Which of the following is NOT a type of skin cancer?**

A. Basal cell carcinoma

B. Squamous cell carcinoma

C. Small cell barceloma

D. Melanoma

**8. Atopic dermatitis is also called _____.**

A. Eczema

B. Psoriasis

C. Basal cell carcinoma

D. None of the above

**9. The layer of skin involved in a second degree burn is the _____.**

A. Dermis

B. Epidermis

C. Hypodermis

D. A and B

E. All of the above

F. None of the above

**10. Scabies is caused by this parasite.**

A. Itch mite

B. Body lice

C. Head lice

D. Pubic lice

## Application Exercises

Respond to the following situations on a separate sheet.

1. Harold has been told that his cold sores are caused by herpes. He is very upset and states that he is not promiscuous. What would you say to him?

2. Harold is given Abreva for cold sore treatment. What will you teach him about its use?

3. Cheryl suffers from psoriasis and is given topical corticosteroids. She is very upset and scared to use steroids. How would you explain what steroids are and why she is being asked to use them for her condition?

4. Bill has acne. He asks why he is being placed on an oral antibiotic when it is a skin problem. How would you answer his question?

5. Brenda has sustained a second-degree burn to her hands. She asks why she has to have her hands scrubbed as part of her treatment because it hurts so badly. What would you say?

# Essentials Review

For further study and practice with drug classifications learned in this chapter, complete the following table to the best of your ability. Use resources such as the *PDR,* the Internet, or printed drug guides for help.

| Medication | Classification | Purpose | Side Effects | Contraindications and Precautions | Examples | Patient Education |
|---|---|---|---|---|---|---|
| Lindane | | | | | | |
| Resorcinol | | | | | | |
| Topicort | | | | | | |
| Elidel | | | | | | |

# Musculoskeletal System Medications

*T*he musculoskeletal system comprises muscles, bones, and joints. The skeleton provides the scaffolding for the body, and the muscles hold the bones in place and allow the body to move and interact with the environment. When the musculoskeletal system or any part of it malfunctions, it affects the ability to move. This chapter addresses the medications used to treat conditions that affect muscles, joints, and bones. Medications are used to prevent or treat disease or to decrease symptoms associated with disease that cannot be prevented or cured.

## LEARNING OUTCOMES

At the end of this chapter, the student will be able to:

12.1 Define all key terms.

12.2 Identify the key features of the musculoskeletal system.

12.3 Discuss the importance of healthy endocrine and nervous systems to proper musculoskeletal functioning.

12.4 Recall at least five muscular system disorders and one appropriate treatment for each.

12.5 Discuss at least four bone or joint disorders and one appropriate treatment for each.

---

### KEY TERMS

| | | |
|---|---|---|
| Antispasmodic | Dystonia | Osteoporosis |
| Bisphosphonates | Gout | Rheumatoid arthritis |
| Calcitonin | Hypocalcemia | |
| Disease-modifying antirheumatic drugs (DMARDs) | Osteoarthritis | |
| | Osteomalacia | |

---

# ■ THE MUSCULOSKELETAL SYSTEM

The musculoskeletal system consists of muscles, tendons, and ligaments that attach to the bones and joints (Fig. 12-1), and that rely on the nervous and endocrine systems to function properly. Coordinated and strong movement require healthy nerve signals, healthy muscle tissue, and adequate endocrine function. The nervous system provides the signals that make the muscles contract or relax and thus allow the body to perform tasks such as picking up a spoon and bringing it to the mouth. Even if the signals occur at the appropriate time, a muscle that is not healthy cannot perform its functions. In addition, the skeleton not only gives the body structure, it also stores minerals that help muscles move.

The endocrine system must be healthy to control the deposit of these minerals. The thyroid gland produces calcitonin, which allows calcium to remain in the bone and not move into the blood. Conversely, the parathyroid gland secretes parathyroid hormone, which increases the amount of calcium

(A) Muscles          (B) Bones

**FIGURE 12-1:** The musculoskeletal system is made up of (A) muscles and (B) bones that form the skeleton. The musculoskeletal system gives the body its structure and is the force behind movement.

in the blood and leads to a loss of calcium in the bones. Therefore, if these glands do not function appropriately, abnormal calcium levels may lead to bone abnormalities. Calcium also assists in muscle contraction and nerve impulses, so abnormalities can lead to altered muscle functioning. Other minerals (magnesium and potassium) stored in the bones also affect musculoskeletal functioning (see the Master the Essentials table for descriptions of the most common musculoskeletal system drugs).

## Master the Essentials: Musculoskeletal Medications

This table shows the various classes of musculoskeletal medications and key side effects, contraindications and precautions, interactions, and examples of each class.

| Class | Side Effects | Contraindications and Precautions | Interactions | Examples |
|---|---|---|---|---|
| Antigout drugs | Acute gouty attacks, headache, GI symptoms | Hypersensitivity, uric acid kidney stones, blood dyscrasias, active peptic ulcer | Antibiotics, antineoplastics, warfarin, salicylates, oral antidiabetics | Allopurinol (Zyloprim), colchicine (Colcrys) |
| Anti-inflammatory drugs (NSAIDs) | Albuminuria, hematuria, bronchospasm, constipation, dizziness, epigastric pain, increased bleeding time, hypersensitivity reactions, GERD, GI ulcers and bleeding, headache, tinnitus and hearing loss, vision disturbances | Anemia, asthma, children with viral infections (aspirin), clotting disorders, disorders of the CV and GI systems, GERD, lactation, liver and kidney failure, pregnancy, sulfonamide hypersensitivity, thyroid disorders | Alcohol, anticoagulants, corticosteroids and other steroids, oral hypoglycemics | Aspirin (Ecotrin, Bayer, Buffer), diclofenac with misoprostol (Voltaren, Cataflam), ibuprofen (Motrin, Advil), naproxen (Naprosyn, Aleve) |
| Bisphosphonates | Headache, abdominal pain, bone pain | Hypersensitivity, hypocalcemia, esophageal stricture or achalasia | Calcium supplements, antacids, ranitidine, aspirin | Teriparatide acetate (Forteo) |
| Calcitonin | Rhinitis, nasal irritation (nasal spray); hypertension, dizziness, injection site reactions, nausea, vomiting | Clinical allergy to drug, pregnancy, breastfeeding | None reported | Calcium carbonate (Tums, Os-Cal-D), calcitonin salmon (Miacalcin) |
| Cholinesterase inhibitors | Bradycardia, hypotension, convulsions, rash, increased saliva, weakness, muscle cramps | Hypersensitivity, peritonitis, mechanical intestinal or urinary obstruction | Succinylcholine, aminoglycosides, anesthetics, antiarrhythmics, corticosteroids, magnesium | Neostigmine (Prostigmin) |
| COX-2 inhibitors | Headache, insomnia, rash, abdominal pain, diarrhea, dyspepsia, upper respiratory infection | Hypersensitivity to sulfonamides | Fluconazole, rifampin, theophylline, ACE inhibitors | Celecoxib (Celebrex) |

*Continued*

## Master the Essentials: Musculoskeletal Medications—cont'd

| Class | Side Effects | Contraindications and Precautions | Interactions | Examples |
|---|---|---|---|---|
| DMARDs | Hepatotoxicity, bone marrow suppression, GI disturbances, blood dyscrasias, pruritus, rashes | Hepatic or renal impairment, pregnancy, breastfeeding, active infection, immunosuppression, known hypersensitivity, lupus, pulmonary fibrosis | Vaccines, NSAIDs, probenecid, corticosteroids | Auranofin (Ridaura), azathioprine (Imuran), gold sodium thiomalate (Mycochrysine), methotrexate (Rheumatrex) |
| Muscle relaxants and antispasmodics | Anxiety, ataxia, blurred vision, confusion, decreased blood pressure and respirations, diarrhea, dizziness, drowsiness, dry mouth, headache, slurred speech, tremor, urinary incontinence, weakness | Asthma, lactation, muscular dystrophy, myasthenia gravis, pregnancy | Alcohol, analgesics, antihistamines, psychotropics | Baclofen (Lioresal), cyclobenzaprine (Flexeril), dantrolene (Dantrium), metaxalone (Skelaxin) |

ACE, angiotensin-converting enzyme; COX, cyclooxygenase; CV, cardiovascular; DMARDs, disease-modifying antirheumatic drugs; GERD, gastroesophageal reflux disorder; GI, gastrointestinal; NSAIDs, nonsteroidal anti-inflammatory drugs

Medications used for musculoskeletal disorders can be placed into two categories: those to treat muscular disorders and those to treat bone disorders. Disorders include conditions causing impaired movement, pain, and damage to muscles, bones, and/or joints.

## ■ MEDICATIONS USED TO TREAT MUSCULAR DISORDERS

Muscle disorders comprise a range of ailments. Some originate in the brain (e.g., cerebral palsy, stroke, and multiple sclerosis), and some arise in the muscle tissue itself. Muscle spasms can develop from these disorders or from the use of psychotropic drugs. Certain conditions (e.g., injury to a muscle in the back, muscular dystrophy) cause patients' muscles to move in uncoordinated, or spastic, ways. Other patients have **dystonia,** which is abnormal tension in one area of the body, such as the limbs, neck, face, eyes, or spine. Medications used to treat some of the muscular problems found in these disorders include muscle relaxants such as Flexeril (cyclobenzaprine) and **antispasmodics** such as Skelaxin (metaxalone); these dugs relax muscles and relieve muscle spasms. Both types of medications work with the central nervous system (CNS) to inhibit the neurological activity that causes the spasms or rigidity. Sometimes the antispasmodics or muscle relaxants are classified as benzodiazepines (Valium [diazepam]) or have CNS effects to maximize effectiveness. One of the newer drugs on the market, Cymbalta (duloxetine), which is used for chronic low back pain, is an antidepressant. This drug may decrease the stress felt with chronic pain and help patients live more productive, mobile lives.

### Virtual Field Trip

Using the Internet, locate information to create a patient education plan for someone with chronic back pain.

Other antispasmodics focus on the muscle itself. Botulinum toxin type A (Botox and Botox Cosmetic [onabotulinumtoxin A]) is a toxic substance derived from the bacterium *Clostridium botulinum,* which, in high doses, causes food poisoning (botulism). However, researchers have found that in lower doses it acts as an effective muscle relaxant by blocking acetylcholine release and thus paralyzing the muscle. The most common use of Botox Cosmetic is to reduce wrinkles associated with aging. Botox is used to treat chronic migraines, limb spasticity, abnormal head position and neck pain (cervical dystonia), severe underarm sweating, and certain eye muscle problems. In some situations, once the muscle is paralyzed, the patient can perform strengthening exercises to promote strength in other muscles to correct, for example, abnormal head position. This treatment reaches maximum effectiveness within 6 weeks and must be repeated every 3 to 6 months. Because botulinum toxin causes pain, it is usually administered with a local anesthetic.

Other muscle disorders that require medication include myasthenia gravis and fibromyalgia. Myasthenia gravis is a progressive, autoimmune disease of skeletal muscle fatigue and weakness that is caused by loss of acetylcholine receptors, basically a breakdown in communication between the nerves and the muscles. It can be debilitating. One type of medication for this disease consists of cholinesterase inhibitors, such as neostigmine, which block cholinesterase and therefore facilitate acetylcholine accumulation. Although the disease has no cure, treatment can help reduce symptoms to allow the individual to function more independently.

Fibromyalgia is a disorder of chronic pain in muscles and the soft tissue surrounding joints. This rheumatological illness is difficult to manage. Treatment includes decreasing the contributory factors (e.g., lack of exercise, poor coping response to stress), physical therapy, antidepressants, anti-inflammatory medications, trigger point injections, and narcotic analgesics.

# ■ THE SKELETAL SYSTEM

The skeleton gives the human body structure. It is composed of 206 bones. The human skeleton is a repository for minerals such as calcium. Calcium is needed for nerves, bones, and muscles to function properly. If not enough calcium is stored in bones, the bones can break. If too much calcium is stored, not enough is available for the bloodstream to deliver to the muscles.

The parathyroid and thyroid glands in the endocrine system ensure proper amounts of circulated and stored calcium. The parathyroid glands secrete parathyroid hormone, which pulls calcium from bones into the bloodstream. The thyroid gland secretes **calcitonin,** which deposits calcium into the bones (Fig. 12-2). Both glands work together to keep calcium levels in balance. If either gland fails, musculoskeletal disorders can result.

## Abnormal calcium levels and osteoporosis

When calcium levels are low, supplements may be needed to correct the imbalance. Calcium supplements are prescribed for **hypocalcemia,** or low blood calcium. Vitamin D may be added to facilitate calcium

### Drug Spotlight 12.1 *Lyrica (pregabalin)*

| | |
|---|---|
| Define | Prescription oral antiepileptic drug |
| Use | Used for the treatment of fibromyalgia, shingles pain, and diabetic neuropathy pain |
| Action | Interrupts pain signals from the brain |
| Side effects | • May cause suicidal thoughts in a few patients<br>• Risk of hypersensitivity reaction in patients taking ACE inhibitors<br>• May cause edema of hands, feet, and legs; dizziness or sleepiness |
| Special considerations | Avoid abruptly stopping the medication unless discussed with the prescriber because symptoms may worsen |

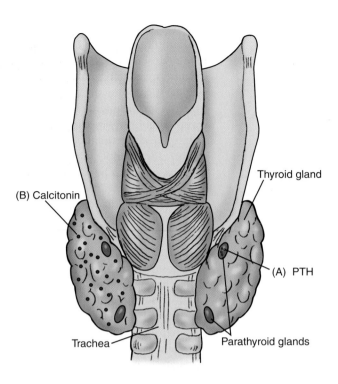

**FIGURE 12-2:** Thyroid and parathyroid glands. Parathyroid hormone (PTH) and calcitonin help keep calcium in the body in balance. (A) The parathyroid glands secrete PTH, which pulls calcium from the bones into the bloodstream. (B) The thyroid gland secretes calcitonin, which puts calcium into the bones.

usage. Vitamin D assists in the absorption of calcium from the stomach and helps to maintain adequate serum calcium levels for proper bone development. Risk factors for hypocalcemia include smoking, lack of exercise, high alcohol consumption, anorexia nervosa, estrogen or testosterone deficiency, poor nutrition, and obesity. Patients with hypocalcemia may be given calcitonin (Miacalcin), which is available as a nasal spray or in an injectable form. Calcitonin is naturally produced by the thyroid gland to deposit calcium into bones. Calcitonin can come from humans or fish such as salmon.

When there is a lack of calcium, the bones can become soft, brittle, and deformed. This condition is known as **osteomalacia** in adults or rickets in children. **Osteoporosis** is a common bone disease that also results from a lack of calcium in the body; this disease creates holes in the bones and gives bone a sponge-like appearance. In all cases, the bones are not firm, and they break easily, even under little stress or pressure. Sometimes calcium and vitamin D are used to prevent bone breaks, as is the case with osteoporosis.

Some medications, such as estrogen (or hormone) replacement therapy (ERT), inhibit bone resorption of calcium and can reduce the extent of osteoporosis. However, this type of treatment has side effects, such as breast and uterine cancer and blood clots. For this reason, these drugs are used with caution. If a patient prefers not to take ERT, she may choose to take a **bisphosphonate,** which is a similar medication without the side effects. These drugs are similar to bisphosphate salts, which are found naturally in the body. An example of a bisphosphonate is alendronate sodium (Fosamax).

*CRITICAL THINKING*

Why would a woman choose to take ERT? Why would she choose not to take it?

Although too little bone calcium can cause fractures, too much bone calcium is a problem as well. Paget's disease is a chronic disease that debilitates patients by enlarging the bone. A patient with Paget's disease resorbs bone excessively, but the new bone is weak and fragile. The bones are deformed (e.g., bowing of the lower legs), leading to pain and fractures. Paget's disease can be diagnosed by a blood test. X-ray studies show irregular bones. Treatment for Paget's disease consists of calcitonin and bisphosphonates, which encourage strong bone formation; supplemental calcium and vitamin D may also be taken as needed.

# Medications for bone and joint inflammation

Arthritis and gout can cause inflammation of the bones and joints (Table 12.1). Arthritis, as indicated in Table 12.1, can be one of two types: osteoarthritis or rheumatoid. In **osteoarthritis,** erosion of bone occurs where the bones meet at the joint. Those affected are mainly middle-aged or older persons and also those who are either extremely sedentary or extremely active.

**Rheumatoid arthritis** is slightly different in that it is an autoimmune condition, in which the joints are affected by inflammation caused by a negative reaction from the immune system. Rheumatoid arthritis usually affects women 30 to 50 years old or children. Nonsteroidal anti-inflammatory drugs (NSAIDs), such as Advil, Motrin, and Aleve, are the most common type of medications used to treat osteoarthritis and rheumatoid arthritis.

**Gout** is a form of arthritis characterized by a sudden, severe attack of pain, redness, and joint tenderness, most commonly at the joint of the big toe and foot. Before middle age, gout primarily affects men, but after women reach menopause, the numbers of men and women affected by gout start to equalize. Risk factors include excessive alcohol use, hypertension, diabetes, hyperlipidemia, and arteriosclerosis. In addition, certain medications and family history are risk factors. Gout is caused by a buildup of uric acid in the joints. Uric acid is a natural by-product of food metabolism and is excreted via the kidneys. In this instance, too much uric acid is produced, or not enough is excreted by the kidneys. Medications used for treating gout are often not administered until the acute attack is over. If medications are given during a gout attack, uric acid may migrate to additional joints. Symptoms of a gout attack are treated first with NSAIDs. High doses may be prescribed to halt an acute attack, and lower doses may be used to prevent future attacks. For patients unable to take NSAIDs, Colcrys (colchicine) is used to relieve the pain. In addition, patients may be given glucocorticoids to control pain and inflammation. When the acute attack has ended, patients start taking antigout medication such as Zyloprim (allopurinol) or Uloric (febuxostat) to lower the uric acid level in the body.

## NSAIDs

NSAIDs reduce inflammation, which is helpful to the patient with gout, osteoarthritis, or rheumatoid arthritis. Some of the concerns regarding NSAIDs are increased gastrointestinal bleeding and renal and cardiac damage caused by long-term use. Thus, these medications should be taken only as ordered, and long-term use should be monitored closely. Aspirin and other analgesics are used for pain. Topical medications containing medication such as menthol, salicylate, and trolamine are usually creams or gels that are rubbed into muscles and joints. Examples are Absorbine, Bengay, Icy Hot, and capsaicin. Stronger pain relief can be obtained by combining analgesics and antidepressants.

## Cyclooxygenase-2 inhibitors

Cyclooxygenase-2 (COX-2) inhibitors (celecoxib [Celebrex]), which technically belong to the larger group of NSAIDs, decrease the production of prostaglandins that cause pain and inflammation. Generally, NSAIDs block the production of both COX-1 and COX-2 enzymes. COX-2 inhibitors block only the production of the COX-2 enzyme and allow the COX-1 enzyme to continue to be produced. COX-1 enzymes are present in many tissues in the body, such as the stomach, where they

## TABLE 12.1  Types of Arthritis

| Type | Cause | Age Affected |
| --- | --- | --- |
| Osteoarthritis | Degeneration (erosion) of bones where they meet, or articulate, at the joints | Strikes middle-aged or older people; extremely sedentary and extremely active people are at increased risk |
| Rheumatoid arthritis | Autoimmune reaction: the body's immune system attacks the joints and causes inflammation | Can affect children, but mostly affects women 30 to 50 years old at symptom onset |

## Drug Spotlight 12.2 *Capsaicin*

| | |
|---|---|
| Define | Topical analgesic; active ingredient comes from the substances that make hot peppers hot, such as chili |
| Use | Used for pain relief from disorders such as diabetic neuropathy, cluster headaches, osteoarthritis, rheumatoid arthritis, shingles, and psoriasis |
| Action | Effective by activating the nerve signals and then decreasing them; patient may have initial increase in pain, followed by relief |
| Application | May be used up to four times a day |
| Side effects | Side effects: rash of hypersensitivity reaction |
| Special considerations and instructions | Education: wash hands well after use to avoid transference to eyes, mouth, or other mucous membranes; do not apply to areas of broken skin |

provide protection to the stomach and intestines. By allowing this enzyme to continue production, the risk of ulceration and bleeding with prolonged use is reduced. COX-2 inhibitors cannot be used by patients who are allergic to sulfa drugs. These medications can also increase the risk of heart problems in certain patients.

### Virtual Field Trip

Using the Internet, find information about Celebrex published within the last 2 years, and write a report about the safety of this drug.

### Disease-modifying antirheumatic drugs (DMARDs)

If anti-inflammatory drugs do not reduce the inflammation adequately, **disease-modifying antirheumatic drugs (DMARDs)** may be used in patients with rheumatoid arthritis. These medications suppress the autoimmune response, but in doing so they suppress immunity systemically. Although not able to cure the disease, these drugs may be able to slow the continual joint destruction. The goal of treatment is not cure but continued joint mobility. One example of a DMARD is Solganal (gold aurothioglucose). Given by injection or sometimes orally, it prevents joint damage and disability. Gold tends to work best in the early stages of rheumatoid arthritis, although it may also help with other types. Gold is used infrequently because other DMARDs, such as Rheumatrex (methotrexate), Neoral (cyclosporine), and Azulfidine (sulfasalazine), are more effective.

### Corticosteroids

Glucocorticosteroids such as Decadron (dexamethasone) and Medrol (methylprednisolone) are medications manufactured to mimic cortisol, which is a hormone produced in the adrenal gland. Corticosteroids reduce inflammation by suppressing the production of materials that trigger allergic and inflammatory responses, but they do not cure inflammatory diseases such as arthritis and gout. Because corticosteroids reduce the body's ability to fight infection, they are used only for short-term therapy during acute symptomatic episodes.

# ◼ MEDICATIONS TO TREAT PHANTOM LIMB PAIN

Patients feel that amputated limbs, as a result of surgery or trauma, often ache as if the limb were still intact because the pain impulse originating in the brain and spinal cord does not recognize that the limb is no longer there. Although some patients report that the pain fades over time, others experience a lifetime of pain management issues. One type of medication that may be effective in managing this chronic pain consists of tricyclic antidepressants such as Elavil (amitriptyline) and Pamelor (nortriptyline). Tricyclic antidepressants alter the chemical messengers that relay pain signals, and they also benefit by helping the patient with sleep. Anticonvulsants and narcotics are two other classifications of drugs that may help. Anticonvulsants such as Tegretol (carbamazepine) quiet damaged nerves to prevent or slow pain signals. Narcotics such as Roxanol (morphine) work by dulling the pain perception center of the brain.

 *CRITICAL THINKING*

Why is it important to know why a patient is taking a medication?

## ●●● SUMMARY

The musculoskeletal system must function well to achieve proper motion and electrolyte storage in the body. Muscles can malfunction if they are too weak or too tight. Bones can weaken from a lack or excess of calcium. Medications for the muscular system act in the brain or in muscle, depending on where the problem is located. Diseases can weaken or inflame bones, or they can retain or eliminate too much calcium. Many drugs are available to help heal malfunctions in the musculoskeletal system. Assisting the patient to maintain independent functioning should be one of the goals of every health-care worker. With independence, patients have dignity and a feeling of well-being.

# Activities

To make sure that you have learned the key points covered in this chapter, complete the following activities.

## True or False

Write true if the statement is true. Beside the false statements, write false, and correct the statement to make it true.

Gout is a disease caused by the buildup of calcium in the joints. _____

Myasthenia gravis is a progressive autoimmune disease affecting the muscles. _____

Capsaicin is a drug made from hot peppers. _____

NSAIDs are used for phantom limb pain. _____

Osteoporosis can lead to increased risk of fractures. _____

Fibromyalgia is an acute disorder of the bones. _____

Lyrica is a drug used to treat osteoarthritis. _____

The endocrine system is very important to maintaining proper levels of calcium in the bones. _____

Side effects of estrogen replacement therapy (ERT) can include breast and uterine cancer. _____

Examples of topical NSAIDs for gout, osteoarthritis, and rheumatoid arthritis include Icy Hot, Bengay, capsaicin, and Absorbine. _____

## Multiple Choice

Choose the best answer for each question.

1. **Osteomalacia is a _____.**
   A. Rheumatologic disease
   B. Gout
   C. Joint degeneration
   D. Calcium disorder

2. **Which is a buildup of uric acid in the joints?**
   A. Fibromyalgia
   B. Gout
   C. Paget's disease
   D. Myasthenia gravis

3. **Which is an example of DMARDs?**
   A. Salicylate
   B. Gold salts
   C. Cyclosporine
   D. NSAIDs
   E. B and C

4. **Which is used to treat dystonia?**

   A. Muscle relaxant

   B. Antispasmodic

   C. Calcitonin

   D. Parathyroid hormone

   E. A and B

5. **Which disorder is characterized by chronic pain in muscles and soft tissue surrounding joints?**

   A. Paget's disease

   B. Myasthenia gravis

   C. Gout

   D. Fibromyalgia

6. **Examples of corticosteroids include _____.**

   A. Decadron

   B. Rheumatrex

   C. Celebrex

   D. Morphine

7. **Examples of DMARDs include _____.**

   A. Decadron

   B. Rheumatrex

   C. Celebrex

   D. Morphine

8. **Examples of narcotics include _____.**

   A. Decadron

   B. Rheumatrex

   C. Celebrex

   D. Morphine

9. **Examples of COX-2 inhibitors include _____.**

   A. Decadron

   B. Rheumatrex

   C. Celebrex

   D. Morphine

10. **Which endocrine gland produces calcitonin?**

    A. Parathyroid

    B. Thyroid

    C. Adrenal

    D. Pancreas

Respond to the following situations on a separate sheet.

1. Shelly is an army veteran who lost one of her legs in the Iraq War. She asks how she can feel pain in a foot that is no longer there. What would you say?

2. Harold has been diagnosed with Paget's disease. He does not understand why he is being told to make sure he eats enough calcium when his bones are already big. What would you tell him?

3. Joette is entering menopause. Why would she refuse estrogen replacement therapy?

4. Ruth has rheumatoid arthritis. She wants to know why the medications she is taking are not making the disease go away. What would you tell her about the goals of treatment for arthritis?

5. Vicki is taking NSAIDs for osteoarthritis. She has developed stomach pains. Should she be told to stop taking this medication? Why or why not?

# Essentials Review

For further study and practice with drug classifications learned in this chapter, complete the following table to the best of your ability. Use resources such as the *PDR,* the Internet, or printed drug guides for help.

| Example | Generic Name | Classification | Purpose | Side Effects | Contraindications and Precautions | Examples | Patient Education |
|---------|--------------|----------------|---------|--------------|-----------------------------------|----------|-------------------|
| Flexeril |  |  |  |  |  |  |  |
| Capsaicin |  |  |  |  |  |  |  |
| Azulfidine |  |  |  |  |  |  |  |
| Elavil |  |  |  |  |  |  |  |

# Nervous System Medications

*The most complex system in the body is the nervous system. This system starts with the brain, which houses billions of neurons and innumerable internal connections. The brain is attached to the central nervous and peripheral nervous systems. The nervous system processes all incoming information before acting on it; it controls everything we do from breathing to walking. Nervous system medications, as described in this chapter, are used to treat pain, anxiety, depression, mania, insomnia, convulsions, and schizophrenia.*

## LEARNING OUTCOMES

At the end of this chapter, the student will be able to:

| | |
|---|---|
| 13.1 | Define all key terms. |
| 13.2 | Identify the two major branches of the nervous system. |
| 13.3 | Identify four categories of medications used to treat pain and fever. |
| 13.4 | Recall at least one category of medication used to treat anxiety, insomnia, sedation, and seizures. |
| 13.5 | Identify at least one category of medication used to treat behavioral, emotional, or mood disorders. |
| 13.6 | Identify one medication commonly used to stabilize mood in bipolar disorder. |
| 13.7 | Discuss medications used to treat psychosis, and identify other disorders for which these medications may be prescribed. |
| 13.8 | Recall at least one category of drug used to treat the dementia and two categories of drugs used to treat Parkinson's disease. |
| 13.9 | Compare and contrast the actions of local and general anesthetics. |
| 13.10 | Discuss how alcohol can influence medication use and its effect on the body. |

## KEY TERMS

Adrenergic (Sympa-
   thomimetics)
Analgesic
Anxiolytic
Aura
Autonomic nervous
   system
Blood-brain barrier
Central nervous system
   (CNS)
Cholinergic (Parasympa-
   thomimetic)

Drug holiday
Gamma-aminobutyric
   acid (GABA)
Hydantoins
Monoamine oxidase
   inhibitors (MAOIs)
Narcotic
Neuroleptic
Neurotransmitters
Parasympathetic
Peripheral nervous
   system (PNS)

Psychotropic
Selective serotonin reup-
   take inhibitors (SSRIs)
Somatic nervous system
Status epilepticus
Sympathetic nervous
   system
Synapse

# THE NERVOUS SYSTEM

The nervous system is divided into the **central nervous system (CNS)** and the peripheral nervous system (PNS), which also includes the autonomic nervous system. The CNS includes the brain and spinal cord, which contain billions of neurons. Neurons make up nerves, which make communication and interaction possible between the brain and every part of the body. The brain processes both internal and external information and tells the body how to respond. For example, if the brain receives a signal via nerves that you are cold, it signals your body via nerves to shiver to raise its temperature. Additionally, if your body is not receiving enough glucose because you skipped lunch, nerves send a signal to the brain to stimulate a headache and remind you to eat.

Nervous system medications are used to treat pain, anxiety, depression, mania, insomnia, convulsions, and schizophrenia. Any medication that affects the mind, emotions, or behaviors is known as a **psychotropic.** Nervous system medications act on the CNS and the PNS (discussed in the next section) (Fig. 13-1). Because the PNS extends throughout the body, these drugs can affect other body systems. For example, a drug meant to ease uterine pain may also relieve leg pain.

Most of these drugs act at the **synapse** (gap) between nerves and can adjust the transmission of messages by **neurotransmitters,** which are chemicals that facilitate the movement of messages across the synapses. Medications work by either exciting the CNS or depressing it. Because these drugs are powerful enough to cross the **blood-brain barrier,** which is the barrier in the brain that prevents toxic substances and some medications from entering the brain, they frequently have serious side effects (see the Master the Essentials table for descriptions of the most common nervous system drugs).

### The peripheral nervous system

The **peripheral nervous system** consists of the **somatic** (voluntary) and **autonomic** (involuntary) nervous systems. The somatic nervous system consists of those muscles over which we have conscious control (e.g., for lifting your arm to scratch your nose). The autonomic nervous system, conversely, controls our internal organs. For example, if you are watching a scary movie, and a monster jumps out from behind a door, your heart begins to race, your stomach may hurt, your pupils dilate, and/or your mouth gets dry, but you do not voluntarily cause these changes; they occur involuntarily based on a stimulus sent to your brain. Medications described in this section include those that affect the autonomic system.

### The autonomic nervous system

The **autonomic nervous system** is broken down further and consists of two parts: the **sympathetic nervous system,** which controls the body's "fight or flight" response, and the **parasympathetic** nervous system, which helps the body to rest and relax (see Fig. 13-1). Acetylcholine and norepinephrine are the

Central nervous
system

Peripheral nervous
system

**Autonomic nervous
system**

Parasympathetic
system

Sympathetic
system

**FIGURE 13-1:** Central and peripheral nervous systems. The brain and the spinal cord make up the central nervous system. The PNS contains nerves outside the brain and spinal cord that lead to the arms, legs, hands, and feet. The autonomic nervous system is part of the PNS.

two main neurotransmitters that affect the autonomic nervous system. A nerve cell that releases acetylcholine is referred to as **cholinergic,** which relaxes the body. One that releases epinephrine or nor-epinephrine is considered **adrenergic,** which excites the body. These cholinergic and adrenergic substances are naturally occurring in the body, but the substances must be provided artificially when the body's reaction is not appropriate to counteract disease states. The next section describes in more detail when cholinergic and adrenergic drugs are used and why.

## Master the Essentials: Nervous System Medications

This table shows the various classes of nervous system medications and key side effects, contraindications and precautions, and interactions for each class.

| Class | Side Effects | Contraindications and Precautions | Interactions | Example |
|---|---|---|---|---|
| Adrenergics | Chest pain, fast heart rate, headache, increase blood glucose, nervousness, tissue death, tremors | Brain damage, CV and heart problems, glaucoma, hyperthyroidism | Adrenergic blockers, CNS drugs | Norepinephrine (Levophed), epinephrine |
| Adrenergic blockers | Confusion, decreased blood pressure, blood glucose, energy, heart rate | Asthma, atrioventricular block (heart block), chronic heart failure, diabetes, low blood pressure | Alcohol, digitalis, epinephrine, insulin, MAO inhibitors (drugs that inhibit the actions of MAO), theophylline, TCAs | Alfuzosin (Uroxatral), doxazosin (Cardura), prazosin (Minipress) tamsulosin (Flomax), terazosin (Hytrin), acebutolol (Sectral) atenolol (Tenormin), bisoprolol (Zebeta), metoprolol (Lopressor), nadolol (Corgard), nebivolol (Bystolic), propranolol (Inderal LA) |
| Cholinergics | Bronchospasm; decreased heart rate, respirations, blood pressure; increased salivation, tears, and sweating; muscle cramps and weakness | Asthma, benign prostatic hypertrophy, cardiac disease, GI disorders, hyperthyroidism | Quinidine, procainamide | Pilocarpine (Pilopine), donepezil (Aricept) |
| Anticholinergics | Blurred vision, confusion, decreased GI motility, dilation of pupils, drying of secretions, fever, flushing, headache, increased heart rate | Asthma, cardiac arrhythmias, COPD, GI or GU obstruction, glaucoma, hypertension | Digoxin, nitroglycerin, TCAs | Atropine (Atropen) |
| Salicylates | Coma, depression, dizziness, headache, drowsiness, increased bleeding time, bruising, GI bleeding, liver and kidney disorders, tinnitus, rash | Asthma, bleeding disorders, lactation, pregnancy, vitamin K deficiency | Alcohol, antacids, anticoagulants, heparin, NSAIDs, insulin | Salicylic acid (aspirin) |
| Acetaminophen | Rash, urticaria (high dosages can cause liver failure) | Alcohol abuse, hypersensitivity, liver disease, malnutrition | Alcohol, oral contraceptives, phenytoin, loop diuretics | Acetaminophen (Tylenol) |

## Master the Essentials: Nervous System Medications—cont'd

| Class | Side Effects | Contraindications and Precautions | Interactions | Example |
|---|---|---|---|---|
| NSAIDs | Blurred vision, constipation, dizziness, drowsiness, dyspepsia, edema, GI bleeding, headache, hepatitis, irregular heart rate, kidney disorders, prolonged bleeding, psychic disturbances, rash, tinnitus | Active GI bleeding, CV disease, hypersensitivity, liver disease, pregnancy, renal disease, ulcer | Corticosteroids, salicylates, cyclosporine, anticoagulants, beta blockers, digoxin | Ibuprofen (Advil, Motrin) |
| Narcotics | Decreased blood pressure, heart rate, and respirations; agitation, blurred vision, confusion, constipation, flushing, headache, oversedation, rash, restlessness, seizures, urinary retention | Lactation and pregnancy, patients with head injury, CNS depression, COPD, hypothyroidism, liver or kidney disease; used with caution in addicted patients, children, elderly patients, hypersensitive patients, suicidal patients | Alcohol, antiemetics, antihistamines, antihypertensives, antiarrhythmics, muscle relaxers, psychotropics, sedative-hypnotics | Morphine, Demerol, fentanyl |
| Non-narcotic benzodiazepine hypnotics | Outgoing or aggressive behavior, confusion, agitation, hallucinations, worsening of depression, suicidal thoughts or actions, memory loss, anxiety, sleep activity | Hypersensitivity to ingredients, pregnancy, lactation, children | Alcohol, paroxetine, lorazepam, olanzapine | Zolpidem (Ambien), eszopiclone (Lunesta) |
| Antiseizure Medications | Multiple side effects different for each medication | Dilantin: hypersensitivity, caution in pregnancy, impaired liver function;   Luminal: blood disorder porphyria, patients taking GHB;   Zarontin: hypersensitivity to succinimides;   Sabril: none;   Lamictal: hypersensitivity;   Gabitril: hypersensitivity;   Topamax: hypersensitivity, glaucoma; | Alcohol, salicylates, succinimides, sulfonamides, valproic acid, oral contraceptives, rifampin and many more than possible to list | Phenytoin (Dilantin), phenobarbital (Luminal), ethosuximide (Zarontin), vigabatrin (Sabril), lamotrigine (Lamictal), tiagabine (Gabitril), topiramate (Topamax), carbamazepine (Tegretol), diazepam (Valium) |

*Continued*

## Master the Essentials: Nervous System Medications—cont'd

| Class | Side Effects | Contraindications and Precautions | Interactions | Example |
|-------|--------------|-----------------------------------|--------------|---------|
| | | Tegretol: history of bone marrow depression, hypersensitivity; Valium: hypersensitivity, children under 6 months old, myasthenia gravis, severe respiratory or hepatic insufficiency, sleep apnea, acute narrow-angle glaucoma | | |
| Anxiolytics | Agitation, amnesia, bizarre behaviors, confusion, decreased white blood cell count, depression, drowsiness, hallucinations, headache, lack of coordination, lethargy, oversedation, sensitivity to light, tremors | Not used in children, decreased vital signs, depression, lactation, pregnancy, suicidal ideation; observe for addiction and for evidence that the patient is considering suicide | Alcohol, antiemetics, antihistamines, analgesics, CNS depressants, digoxin, grapefruit juice, muscle relaxants, phenytoin, psychotropics | Alprazolam (Xanax), diazepam (Valium), lorazepam (Ativan) |
| Barbiturates | Lethargy, dizziness, irritability, constipation, vessel swelling, confusion, decreased respirations and heart rate, bone softening, coma, fatal overdose, unsteady balance, liver inflammation, bone marrow suppression, vision disorders, anorexia, inflammation of the gums | Pregnancy, hypersensitivity, hepatitis, cardiac and renal disease, hemolytic disorders, decreased heart rate | Alcohol, analgesics, antacids, antineoplastics, CNS depressants, corticosteroids, folic acid, grapefruit juice, MAO inhibitors, oral anticoagulants, oral contraceptives, theophylline, sedatives | Seconal, Nembutal |
| CNS Stimulants | Nervousness, insomnia, irritability, seizures or psychosis; increased heart rate, blood pressure, and irregularity of heart rhythm; dizziness, headache, blurred vision, GI disorders, dependence | Nervousness, insomnia, irritability, seizures, or psychosis; increased heart rate, blood pressure, and irregularity of heart rhythm; dizziness, headache, blurred vision, GI disorders, dependence | Antacids, anticoagulants, anticonvulsants, clonidine, TCAs | Methylphenidate (Ritalin), amphetamine/ dextroamphetamine (Adderall), phentermine (Zantryl) |

## Master the Essentials: Nervous System Medications—cont'd

| Class | Side Effects | Contraindications and Precautions | Interactions | Example |
|---|---|---|---|---|
| MAO Inhibitors | Nervousness, headache, stiff neck, increased heart rate and blood pressure, diarrhea, blurred vision | Known hypersensitivity, heart disease, hepatic or renal impairment, headaches, cerebrovascular disease, pregnancy, lactation | Adrenergics, diuretics, antidepressants, CNS depressants, insulin, levodopa, foods containing tyramine, herbs such as St. John's wort | Selegiline (Eldepryl) |
| TCAs | Dry mouth, increased appetite, weight gain, blurred vision, drowsiness, dizziness, constipation, urinary retention, postural hypotension, irregular heart rhythms, headache | Pregnancy and lactation; cardiac, kidney, liver, and GI disorders; glaucoma; obesity; seizures | Alcohol, CNS drugs, MAO inhibitors | Amitriptyline (Elavil) |
| SSRIs | Sexual dysfunction, anorexia, diarrhea, sweating, insomnia, anxiety, nervousness, tremor, fatigue, dizziness, drowsiness, headache | Pregnancy and lactation; patients with thoughts of suicide, diabetes, bipolar disorders, eating disorders | CNS drugs, MAO inhibitors, anticoagulants, beta blockers, antiarrhythmics | Fluoxetine (Prozac), sertraline (Zoloft), paroxetine (Paxil), citalopram (Celexa) |
| Lithium | GI distress, hypotension, cardiac irregularities, polyuria, tremors, thyroid problems | Seizure disorders; Parkinson's disease; CV, kidney, and thyroid diseases; dehydration, pregnancy, lactation | NSAIDs, diuretics, ACE inhibitors, sodium salts | Lithium citrate |
| Antipsychotics | ECG changes, hypotension, agitation, dizziness, sedation, drowsiness, dystonia, headache, constipation, dry mouth, photosensitivity, nausea | Known hypersensitivity, cardiac arrhythmias, seizure disorder, thyroid disease, renal or hepatic impairment | Anticholinergics, CNS depressants, alcohol, beta blockers, caffeine, antidepressants, lithium | Clozapine (Clopine), thioridazine (Mellaril), chlorpromazine (Thorazine) |
| Antiparkinsonian drugs | Involuntary movements, loss of appetite, anxiety, confusion, depression, psychosis, decreased blood pressure, dizziness, fainting | Pregnancy and lactation, asthma and emphysema, cardiac disease, decreased blood pressure, peptic ulcer, diabetes, glaucoma | Benzodiazepines, pyridoxine, phenothiazines, haloperidol, antihypertensives, phenytoin, vitamin $B_6$, MAO inhibitors | Ropinirole (Requip), selegiline (Eldepryl), bromocriptine (Parlodel), benztropine (Cogentin), carbidopa/levodopa (Sinemet), biperiden (Akineton) |

*Continued*

## Master the Essentials: Nervous System Medications—cont'd

| Class | Side Effects | Contraindications and Precautions | Interactions | Example |
|---|---|---|---|---|
| Local anesthetics | Heart block, hypotension, bradycardia, arrhythmias, restlessness, anxiety, dizziness, headache, nausea, vomiting | Known hypersensitivity, severe hypertension, shock, hematologic disorders, psychosis | Sedatives, sulfonamides | Lidocaine/ prilocaine (EMLA cream), benzocaine/ butamben/ tetracaine (Exactacain), benzocaine (Americaine otic), lidocaine (Xylocaine), tetracaine (Tetcaine ophthalmic) |
| General anesthetics | Cardiopulmonary depression, confusion, sedation, nausea, vomiting, hypothermia, malignant hyperthermia | Known hypersensitivity, hepatic disorder, malignant hyperthermia, pregnancy, lactation | CNS depressants, neuromuscular blockers, catecholamines | Midazolam (Versed), propofol (Diprivan), ketamine (Ketalar), desflurane (Suprane), isoflurane (Forane), sevoflurane (Ultane), nitrous oxide |

ACE, angiotensin-converting enzyme; CNS, central nervous system; COPD, chronic obstructive pulmonary disease; CV, cardiovascular; ECG, electrocardiogram; GI, gastrointestinal; GU, genitourinary; MAO, monoamine oxidase; NSAIDs, nonsteroidal anti-inflammatory drugs; SSRIs, selective serotonin reuptake inhibitors; TCAs, tricyclic antidepressants.

## The autonomic nervous system and medications

Autonomic drugs stimulate the sympathetic nervous system when the body needs to be excited. These drugs are also called **sympathomimetics** or adrenergic agonists. Drugs that stimulate the parasympathetic nervous system calm the nervous system. They are also called **parasympathomimetics** or **cholinergic agonists.**

### Sympathomimetics (Adrenergic)

Adrenergic drugs are called sympathomimetics because they mimic the sympathetic nervous system and stimulate the fight or flight impulse. They work to stimulate the heart, increase blood flow to the skeletal muscles, and constrict peripheral blood vessels, which then dilate certain parts of the body, such as the bronchi for patients with asthma and pupils for patients who may be having an eye procedure. They are also used to restore heart rhythm during cardiac arrest and to increase blood pressure with drugs such as Levophed (norepinephrine) in cases of shock. They constrict capillaries if the patient is bleeding, such as during a nosebleed. Adrenergic medications can dilate the bronchioles of the patient with asthma or the pupils of patients having eye procedures. The major contraindication for adrenergic drugs is hypersensitivity to the drug. These drugs should be used cautiously in patients with hypertension, myocardial infarction, atrial fibrillation, or hypovolemia, in children, and in women who are pregnant or breastfeeding.

### Adrenergic blockers

As the name suggests, adrenergic blockers block the action of adrenergics (drugs that stimulate the sympathetic nervous system) and thus have a parasympathetic effect. As discussed earlier, the parasympathetic effect calms the nervous system. Adrenergic blockers are useful for treating cardiac arrhythmias (heart rhythm problems), high blood pressure, migraine headaches, and chest pain because they slow the heart rate, relax the blood vessels, and allow blood to flow more freely, thus decreasing the workload on the heart.

Adrenergic blockers are broken down into two groups, based on the muscles they affect. Alpha blockers such as alfuzosin (Uroxatral), doxazosin (Cardura), prazosin (Minipress), tamsulosin (Flomax), and terazosin (Hytrin) affect vascular smooth muscle and are used to alleviate hypertension and benign prostatic hypertrophy (this condition, which affects the male reproductive and urinary systems, is discussed in Chapter 20). Beta blockers work by blocking the effects of the hormone epinephrine. This action affects the heart and blood vessels and causes the heart to beat more slowly and with less force, thereby reducing blood pressure. Beta blockers such as acebutolol (Sectral), atenolol (Tenormin), bisoprolol (Zebeta), metoprolol (Lopressor), nadolol (Corgard), nebivolol (Bystolic), and propranolol (Inderal LA) are used for hypertension, migraine headaches, and glaucoma.

### Parasympathomimetics (Cholinergics)

Parasympathomimetics (cholinergics) are so named because they mimic the action of the parasympathetic system; cholinergics release acetylcholine, which relaxes the body's fight or flight mechanism. Cholinergics are rarely used because they severely slow body system activity (including the heart rate) and constrict respiratory passages. Nerve gases are an example of this class. One of the few cholinergic drugs still used is pilocarpine (Pilopine) for the treatment of open-angle glaucoma. This drug increases the drainage of fluid (aqueous humor) out of the eye to reduce ocular pressure. The drug must be stopped several weeks before surgical procedures because of an increased risk of intraoperative breathing problems.

### Anticholinergics or cholinergic blockers

Anticholinergics or cholinergic blockers inhibit the parasympathetic branch of the autonomic nervous system and thus promote fight or flight symptoms. These drugs dry secretions, including those in the respiratory tract, and are used for asthma and motion sickness. They are also used for preoperative relaxation, for neuromuscular blocking of spasms, as antidotes to insect stings, and in cholinergic crises. A cholinergic crisis manifests with extreme muscular weakness and respiratory depression caused by surplus acetylcholine. This crisis is most commonly seen in patients with myasthenia gravis who are overmedicated with anticholinesterase drugs. In an emergency, atropine (Atropen) can be used to treat a slow heart rate, heart block, or bronchospasm.

## ■ MEDICATIONS TO CONTROL PAIN AND FEVER

Pain is an unpleasant sensory and emotional experience arising from actual or potential tissue damage. The perception of pain varies greatly among patients, but it is important to treat each person's pain based on his or her description of it. Pain management is based on a thorough patient assessment that includes the location and intensity of pain.

**Analgesics** reduce pain without eliminating feeling or sensation, as occurs with anesthetics. Choices include salicylates, acetaminophen, nonsteroidal anti-inflammatory drugs (NSAIDs), and narcotics. Some of these drugs are also antipyretic, which means they reduce fever.

### Salicylates

Salicylates, such as aspirin (acetylsalicylic acid), relieve mild to moderate pain and reduce inflammation and fever. Salicylates are also used to decrease inflammation in blood vessels, to improve cardiovascular flow. Aspirin has the disadvantage of causing gastrointestinal (GI) distress, and it should not be used in children with viral infections because of the danger of Reye's syndrome.

Methylsalicylate is a topical anti-inflammatory medication used to irritate the surface of the skin. This irritation increases blood flow to the area where it was applied and thus decreases pain. An example of this class is Bengay.

*CRITICAL THINKING*

Based on what you learned in previous chapters and your understanding of how different routes of medication adminstration affect absorption, why would powders (aspirin in a powder form that you place on your tongue) work more rapidly than aspirin tablets?

### Acetaminophen

Acetaminophen (Tylenol) decreases pain and fever, but it has no anti-inflammatory effect. Acetaminophen is often an ingredient in combination products used to relieve pain or in products used for cold and flu symptoms such as Alka-Seltzer Plus cold medications. Because it typically does not produce severe side effects, acetaminophen is frequently combined with narcotics such as oxycodone with acetaminophen (Percocet) to treat moderate to severe pain.

### Nonsteroidal anti-inflammatory drugs (NSAIDs)

NSAIDs, in the context of pain and fever relief, refer to medications such as ibuprofen (Motrin or Advil). These drugs reduce pain and swelling caused by inflammation. Fever is also reduced using this type of drug. As with acetaminophen, NSAIDs can be combined with narcotics to relieve moderate to severe pain. An example is oxycodone with ibuprofen (Combunox).

### Narcotics

**Narcotics** are strong painkillers that suppress the CNS. They are an excellent choice when pain cannot be relieved by milder drugs. The active ingredient in most narcotics is opium, which is extracted from the poppy plant. However, a patient taking narcotic medication to relieve pain must be closely monitored because an excess amount of a narcotic medication can slow respirations to dangerous levels. It can also decrease blood pressure significantly as a result of peripheral vasodilation. Further drops in blood pressure occurring with changes in position lead to the risk of falls.

Opioid analgesics such as morphine, codeine, and fentanyl are the strongest. They are not routinely prescribed because of their addiction potential and the possibility of severe side effects, particularly in large doses. Because narcotics produce euphoria, or happy feelings, they can also cause physiological or psychological dependence. For this reason, patients must use caution with certain activities, such as driving. In addition, limited amounts of medications are ordered, to force close supervision and reassessment of these patients. However, if a patient has pain that does not respond to other medications, he or she should not be denied adequate pain relief out of concern for addiction or dependence. Narcotics are rarely addictive in patients who take them for relief of acute pain for a short period of time. Narcotics can also be used for general anesthesia during surgery.

Sometimes combining analgesics with alternative methods of pain relief, such as meditation, can reduce pain effectively.

---

### A CLOSER LOOK: Headaches

The two main types of headaches are tension headaches and migraine headaches. Tension headaches occur when the head and neck become tight because of tension and stress. This causes a steady throbbing pain. These headaches can usually be treated with NSAIDs or mild narcotics.

Migraine headaches are more painful. They are usually preceded by a sensory cue known as an **aura**. The aura may include seeing flashing lights, smelling bizarre odors, tasting food in an empty mouth, and hearing sounds that do not exist. The pain is often localized behind the eye, and patients frequently have nausea and vomiting. Patients with migraines need special medications, such as sumatriptan (Imitrex), to prevent or stop the pain. Other patients may be treated with tricyclic antidepressants or a beta-adrenergic blocker such as propranolol to prevent or decrease the frequency of migraine headaches.

---

### A CLOSER LOOK: Headaches—cont'd

**Migraine Triggers**

| Environmental | Food |
|---|---|
| **Environmental** | **Food** |
| Changes in barometric pressure and weather | Alcohol |
| Bright colors | Aged cheese |
| Unusual odors | Aspartame (NutraSweet) |
| Sun glare | Caffeine |
| Tobacco smoke | Chocolate |
| **Emotional and hormonal** | Monosodium glutamate (MSG) |
| Stress and anxiety | **Medications** |
| Pregnancy | Tagamet |
| Menstruation | Nifedipine |
| Decreased blood glucose | Theophylline |
| Physical or sexual stress | |

---

### CRITICAL THINKING

What methods, other than drugs, can be used to decrease pain?

---

## MEDICATIONS TO TREAT ANXIETY, INSOMNIA, SEDATION, AND SEIZURES

The limbic system of the brain is integral to such emotions as love, fear, and anger, as well as being important to our memory and level of alertness. The connections in this part of the brain allow the limbic system to control and mediate these emotions. If the structures in this system are not operating optimally, difficulty with anxiety, sleeplessness, alertness, or seizures may occur. Medications help to relieve anxiety, promote sleep, increase alertness, or help stop seizures.

### Anxiolytic medications

Anxiety is apprehension, tension, or uneasiness that originates from anticipating danger, or an inappropriate fear, the source of which is often unknown or unrecognized. Some fears are exaggerations of normal anxieties (heights, animals), and others are based on previous experiences (e.g., being trapped in an elevator). Anxiolytic medications reduce the intensity of these fears, dangers, and/or tension that a patient may be experiencing. The following is a list of phobias (fears). Use a medical dictionary to define them on a separate sheet.

- Acrophobia
- Agoraphobia
- Ailurophobia
- Arachnophobia
- Claustrophobia
- Mysophobia
- Xenophobia
- Zoophobia

Types of anxiety disorders include generalized anxiety disorder and panic disorder. As mentioned earlier, **anxiolytic** medications reduce anxiety. They can be taken routinely or only when the patient feels increasing anxiety. These drugs work in the limbic system of the brain by depressing the subcortical levels of the CNS and have a calming effect. This effect can range from mild sedation to coma, depending on the medication and dose used. CNS depressants comprise a type of anxiolytic used to treat anxiety and restlessness. Benzodiazepines, another type of anxiolytic, such as lorazepam (Ativan), diazepam (Valium), and alprazolam (Xanax), are used for anxiety, seizures, alcohol withdrawal symptoms, and muscle relaxation. They can also be used to reduce anxiety before general anesthesia.

### Insomnia and medications

Insomnia (trouble sleeping) is a common complaint from patients. Sometimes barbiturates are used to induce sleep by depressing the CNS (slowing heart rate, respirations). They are also used to help the patient relax before a minor procedure or general surgery. Other newer non-narcotic benzodiazepine hypnotics such as zolpidem (Ambien) and eszopiclone (Lunesta) help to promote sleep with fewer side effects. Both types of medications target the same portion of the brain, but the newer non-narcotic medications are able to target just the areas promoting sleep without depressing the entire CNS. These medications are therefore becoming the preferred sleep aids, but they continue to pose a possible addiction risk. Therefore, they should be used on a limited basis.

### Barbiturates and antiseizure medications

Barbiturates are also used to control seizures. Barbiturates that are **hydantoins,** such as phenytoin (Dilantin), delay sodium from crossing the neural membranes. This effect decreases the potential for too much electrical activity and calms the cell. Hydantoins are the drug of choice for tonic-clonic (grand mal) and partial seizures. Other barbiturates such as phenobarbital (Luminal) are used for tonic-clonic and febrile seizures in children. Succinimides such as ethosuximide (Zarontin) comprise a class of antiseizure drugs that delay the movement of calcium over the neurons. Like hydantoins, they relax nerve cells. The succinimides are the drugs of choice for absence (petit mal) seizures.

Although the reason that traditional antiseizure medications decrease seizure activity is poorly understood, once **gamma-aminobutyric acid (GABA)** was discovered to be a naturally occurring neurotransmitter inhibitor, research began to stimulate the production of GABA production. In other words, GABA inhibits abnormal electrical activity in the brain, and an increased presence of this amino acid decreases seizure activity (see Fig. 13-2). An example of this category of drug is vigabatrin (Sabril). Benzodiazepines such as diazepam (Valium) can also intensify the effect of GABA transmitters in the brain and allow more GABA to reach the receptors in the brain to trigger the actions needed to suppress abnormal electrical activity.

Other medications that work as anticonvulsants are lamotrigine (Lamictal), tiagabine (Gabitril), topiramate (Topamax), and carbamazepine (Tegretol). Some drugs such as diazepam (Valium) that are used to decrease seizures also help manage the symptoms of alcohol withdrawal by reducing associated anxiety symptoms.

---

### A CLOSER LOOK: Seizures

Abnormal electrical activity in the brain can cause seizures. A patient may have a diagnostic test called electroencephalography (EEG) to detect seizure activity. Seizures may be mild (petit mal) or severe (grand mal). The most severe seizure is called **status epilepticus.** In this instance, the patient is having a tonic-clonic (grand mal) seizure that lasts for longer than 30 minutes and cannot regain consciousness. Because the patient is not breathing during this episode, there is a high risk of brain damage and death without immediate medical intervention, usually with IV benzodiazepines such as Valium.

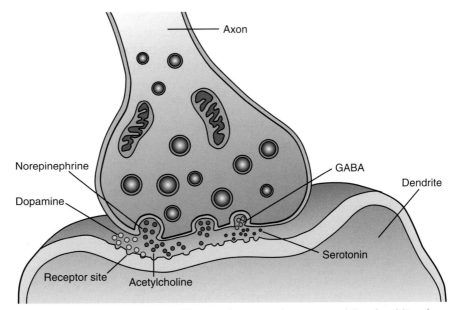

**FIGURE 13-2:** Nerve synapse. The gap between the axon and the dendrite of a nerve is called the synapse. Neurotransmitters such as gamma-aminobutyric acid (GABA), serotonin, dopamine, norepinephrine, and acetylcholine help transmit the electrical impulse from the axon to the dendrite. The neurotransmitters fit into receptors on the dendrites. Some psychotropic drugs act by inhibiting the work of the neurotransmitters, thereby slowing the electrical impulses; others act by stimulating neurotransmitters, thereby promoting electrical impulses.

# MEDICATIONS TO TREAT BEHAVIORAL, EMOTIONAL, AND MOOD DISORDERS

Behavioral and emotional disorders are becoming more common in the United States. Mood disorders are characterized by extreme emotions from very elevated, which is referred to as mania, to very low, such as depression. Some patients bounce between mania and depression, a condition called bipolar disorder. Several categories of drugs, including antidepressants, mood stabilizer drugs, and antipsychotics, can be used to help patients with these disorders. These drugs are discussed later in this chapter.

## Central nervous system stimulants

Attention deficit disorder (ADD) and attention deficit hyperactivity disorder (ADHD) are common in both children and adults. These disorders stem from the ineffectiveness of the impulse control center of the frontal cortex of the brain.

It may seem counterintuitive to give a distracted, unfocused, overactive patient a stimulant, but CNS stimulants such as amphetamine/dextroamphetamine (Adderall), pemoline (Cylert), and methylphenidate (Ritalin) have the opposite effect in these patients in that they calm them and increase their ability to focus. An alternate way to view this disorder is to understand that the patient is being bombarded by a multitude of stimuli and is unable to focus on any one of them. The CNS stimulants help these patients to focus on only a few of the stimuli and not be distracted by the others and therefore allow patients to become more successful in their daily activities. People who do not have ADD or ADHD but who take the medication anyway find that it acts as a CNS stimulant.

Sometimes an amphetamine, a type of CNS stimulant, such as phentermine (Zantryl), is prescribed for obesity. Usually, it is given 30 to 60 minutes before meals to increase metabolism, but only for short periods of time. Diet and exercise regimens should be used concurrently with amphetamine use for weight loss.

*CRITICAL THINKING*

Why should amphetamines not be prescribed routinely for obese patients who are trying to lose weight?

## Antidepressants

Clinical depression is characterized by excesses of sleeping and eating, an inability to concentrate, avoidance of the companionship of other people, decreased interest in sex and activities one usually enjoys, and feelings of despair. Depression is usually a combination of genetic and environmental causes and can be devastating to the patient. When neurotransmitters are depleted, the patient does not think as clearly as usual, and mood becomes depressed. Antidepressants preserve neurotransmitters at the synapse.

Three categories of antidepressant agents are monoamine oxidase (MAO) inhibitors (MAOIs), tricyclic antidepressants (TCAs), and selective serotonin reuptake inhibitors (SSRIs).

■ **Monoamine oxidase inhibitors (MAOIs).** MAOIs inhibit MAO, an enzyme that terminates the action of neurotransmitters at the synapse. Inhibiting or stopping MAO improves the retention of neurotransmitters at the site. An example of an MAOI is selegiline (Eldepryl). Unfortunately, this drug classification requires dietary exclusion of foods containing tyramine (Box 13.1). A patient who eats any of these foods while taking an MAOI can suffer critical hypertension. Because tyramine is common in many foods, these drugs are rarely prescribed today.

*CRITICAL THINKING*

If a patient who is taking an MAOI went to a Super Bowl party, which typical party foods would he or she be unable to eat?

■ **Tricyclic antidepressants (TCAs).** Many medication options for depression exist, and most patients find that the first medication they try is a good fit. Other patients must try numerous medications before they find an antidepressant that works for them and has tolerable side effects. Patients suffering from insomnia are generally prescribed TCAs because of the sedative side effects of these drugs. TCAs are medications with a three-ring (tricyclic) chemical structure that keeps norepinephrine and serotonin at the nerve terminals and thereby helping electrical impulses cross the synapse (see Fig. 13-2). TCAs such as amitriptyline (Elavil) have been used for decades but have many more side effects than the more popular SSRIs. TCAs are still the drugs of choice for severe depression and inpatient treatment of depression.

## BOX 13.1 Foods High in Tyramine

| | |
|---|---|
| Avocados | Papayas |
| Bananas | Paté, beef |
| Beer | Pepperoni |
| Bologna | Raisins |
| Chocolate | Salami |
| Dairy products, aged | Sausage |
| Fava beans | Soy sauce |
| Figs | Wine |
| Herring | Yeast |
| Hot dogs | |

■ **Selective serotonin reuptake inhibitors (SSRIs).** SSRIs such as citalopram (Celexa), fluoxetine (Prozac), paroxetine (Paxil), and sertraline (Zoloft) prevent serotonin from being used up at the synapse. Serotonin is a chemical produced in the brain that acts as a neurotransmitter to help signals transfer from one part of the brain to another. Low serotonin levels have been implicated in depression, and keeping serotonin at the synapse improves mood. Because they have so few side effects compared with MAOIs and TCAs, SSRIs are frequently the first class of drug prescribed for depression. However, each drug within the classification can affect the patient differently. If one drug does not work well for the patient, the prescriber may change the dosage or change to another medication.

### CRITICAL THINKING

Why are antidepressants used to decrease pain?

## MEDICATIONS TO STABILIZE MOOD

Mood stabilizers (antimanic agents) stabilize the extreme mood shifts seen in patients with bipolar disorder. In a very short period of time, patients vacillate between severe depression and a manic state in which they make grandiose plans and possibly act on those plans because they feel invincible. Therapy can decrease the number and intensity of these manic episodes and the frequency of these shifts in mood.

A common drug used to treat bipolar disorder is lithium. Lithium is a salt, so it is important for patients who are taking lithium not to become dehydrated. These patients should avoid using table salt. Lithium has a small therapeutic range. Because lithium toxicity can be fatal, blood lithium assays (levels) must be performed regularly. Signs of toxicity include drowsiness, blurred vision, confusion, sensitivity to light, tremors, muscle weakness, cardiovascular collapse, seizures, and coma.

## MEDICATIONS FOR TREATING PSYCHOSES

Psychoses comprise a class of disorders characterized by abnormal thoughts, disorganized communication, and lack of interaction with the environment. Delusions, hallucinations, paranoia, and bizarre thoughts and behaviors are frequent symptoms of psychoses.

Antipsychotic medications called **neuroleptics,** such as chlorpromazine (Thorazine), clozapine (Clopine), and thioridazine (Mellaril), treat the abnormal actions and behavior of psychoses such as talking and interacting with a situation that only patients can see and hear. Some antipsychotic medications are used for nausea and vomiting, dementia, agitation, and spasms, as well as for psychoses. Be sure you know why the neuroleptic was prescribed.

## MEDICATIONS TO TREAT DEGENERATIVE DISORDERS

Degenerative disorders of the nervous system are characterized by a continuous decline in mental and/or physical functioning, and they have no cure. These disorders may be caused by genetics, environment, or injury to the nervous system, although the cause is often unknown. The goals of treatment are to relieve symptoms and to maintain independence for as long as possible. The following are two of the more common degenerative disorders affecting the nervous system.

### Dementia

Dementia is a progressive, irreversible decline in mental function. Alzheimer's disease is the most frequent cause of dementia, but there are dozens of other less commonly known causes. Currently, few drugs are available to treat dementia, and the ones that do cause only a minor reduction in symptoms of confusion and decreased memory. The goal of drug therapy is to prevent or slow further mental deterioration. Therefore, the best outcome is early diagnosis, so treatment can begin. Although it is unclear how they work, cholinesterase inhibitors are the drugs of choice in treating mild to moderate

Alzheimer's disease. Research shows that this class of drugs prevents the breakdown of cholinesterase in the brain that is responsible for memory and thinking. Aricept (donepezil HCL) is an example of a cholinesterase inhibitor that shows some promise in slowing the progression of this disease.

### CRITICAL THINKING

If a patient is diagnosed with dementia, what precautions may need to be taken in the home?

### Virtual Field Trip

Google the following:
Local support groups for families and patients with Alzheimer's disease
The latest research on Alzheimer's disease, to report on any new medications being researched for use

## Parkinson's disease

Parkinson's disease is a degenerative disorder of the CNS. When neurons that produce the neurotransmitter dopamine die, muscle movements become disorganized. The lack of dopamine and the increase in acetylcholine cause tremors, slow movement, rigid muscles, and balance problems. Antiparkinsonian drugs focus on keeping dopamine and acetylcholine at the nerve synapse and thereby promote the transmission of nerve signals. These drugs are classified as dopaminergic (replacing or increasing dopamine), such as selegiline (Eldepryl), bromocriptine (Parlodel), ropinirole (Requip), and carbidopa/levodopa (Sinemet), or cholinergic agents (those that inhibit the action of acetylcholine), such as biperiden (Akineton).

Because of the blood-brain barrier, it is difficult to ensure that a sufficient amount of dopamine reaches the brain to control the symptoms of this disease effectively. As a result, patients with Parkinson's disease are given a combination of drugs that allow smaller doses of medications to achieve the dopamine levels needed. These patients tend to become acclimatized or tolerant of their medication, and thus the doses must be increased to have the same effect. When the dose cannot be increased or the side effects become intolerable, the doctor will request a **drug holiday,** in which the patient stops taking antiparkinsonian medications for a week or so and then restarts them at a lower dose, to produce the desired effects.

### Virtual Field Trip

Google the following:
The latest research on Parkinson's disease
Local support groups for families and patients with Parkinson's disease

### Drug Spotlight 13.1 *Exelon Patch (rivastigmine transdermal system)*

| | |
|---|---|
| Define | Used in the treatment of mild to moderate dementia of the Alzheimer's type or that associated with Parkinson's disease |
| Use and application | Transdermal patch applied once a day |
| Special considerations | • Dosage titrated to avoid nausea and vomiting associated with higher doses; body weight should be monitored because low body weight may lead to more adverse effects, care with use in patients weighing less than 50 kg |
| Side effects | Most commonly nausea, vomiting, and diarrhea |
| Contraindications | Hypersensitivity to rivastigmine or carbamate |

# ■ LOCAL AND GENERAL ANESTHETIC MEDICATIONS

Anesthesia means loss of sensation. Anesthesia administered locally creates a lack of feeling without a loss of consciousness. For instance, lidocaine is used to numb the skin before stitches are placed to close a wound. General anesthesia causes patients to lose both feeling and consciousness, such as during a surgical procedure.

## Local Anesthesia

Local anesthesia can be applied to a body surface to numb an area before a procedure. The local anesthetic blocks the entry of sodium ions into nerve fibers. Adequate amounts must be applied or injected to keep the area numb throughout the procedure. Local anesthetics come in a variety of forms: cream (lidocaine/prilocaine [EMLA]), aerosol spray (benzocaine/butamben/tetracaine [Exactacain]), otic (benzocaine [Americaine otic]) or ophthalmic drops (tetracaine [Tetcaine ophthalmic]), or an injectable solution such as lidocaine (Xylocaine). Local anesthetics are classified as esters or amides, depending on the structure of their molecules.

Amides, such as lidocaine and novocaine, tend to last longer, so they are more popular. Adverse effects and allergies are rare. The patient must be observed during the procedure to be sure that the anesthetic is still in effect and to monitor any negative reactions. Be sure to document your observations.

Esters, such as procaine and tetracaine, have the potential for severe allergic reactions such as anaphylactic shock because of the release of para-aminobenzoic acid (PABA), a known allergen, during the metabolism process. Because of this, the use of esters is limited to topical preparations, in which exposure to PABA is much less significant than in injections.

## General Anesthesia

General anesthetics can be administered by intravenous (IV) infusion or inhalation. For longer procedures, an IV agent such as midazolam (Versed), propofol (Diprivan), or ketamine (Ketalar) may be used initially, followed by inhalation therapy with medications such as desflurane (Suprane), isoflurane (Forane), or sevoflurane (Ultane). Use of the IV agent allows smaller doses of inhalation therapy medications to be used and thus reduces the risk of severe side effects of these medications.

*CRITICAL THINKING*

Why would an IV anesthetic be given before an inhaled gas is administered by mask?

Inhaled general anesthetics are volatile agents that can depress respiratory and cardiovascular function, so patients must be observed carefully during procedures in which these drugs are used. An example of an inhaled general anesthetic in ambulatory care is nitrous oxide, which is used for dental and brief surgical procedures.

Contraindications to inhalation anesthetics include any known hypersensitivity to specific anesthetic agents or respiratory system disease.

# ■ ALCOHOL

Alcohol, which is a CNS depressant, is rarely prescribed as a medication. However, because it interacts with other medications and can have powerful effects on the body, it is included in this discussion. Alcohol added to medication can cause confusion, peripheral vasodilation, increased heart rate, electrolyte imbalances, decreased motor coordination, unsteady gait, and slurred speech. Prolonged use can permanently damage the CNS and liver.

Signs and symptoms of chronic alcoholism include irritability, tremors, GI disorders, frequent falling accidents, blackouts, memory loss, confusion, neural and muscular weakness, and conjunctivitis. Treatment includes disulfiram (Antabuse), behavior modification, vitamin B injections, and dietary changes (e.g., supplements to replace vitamins lost through poor nutrition).

Patients abusing alcohol should be assessed for respiratory problems, vomiting, convulsions, cerebral swelling, electrolyte imbalances, and tremors when they are withdrawing from alcohol.

 S U M M A R Y

Medications that affect the central and peripheral nervous systems can be used to treat many brain and nervous system disorders, ranging from mild headaches to severe symptoms of Parkinson's disease. Always assess carefully any patient who is taking medications that affect the neurological system. Any drug that crosses the blood-brain barrier has the risk of creating severe side effects and permanent damage.

# Activities

To make sure that you have learned the key points covered in this chapter, complete the following activities.

## True or False

Write true if the statement is true. Beside the false statements, write false, and correct the statement to make it true.

Parasympathomimetics have many therapeutic uses because of relatively few side effects. _____

Some antipsychotic drugs are used to manage alcohol withdrawal. _____

Benzodiazepines are a type of local anesthesia. _____

Salicylates have the side effect of prolonging bleeding time. _____

Barbiturates are use for insomnia. _____

The nervous system is divided into three sections: the central, peripheral, and lateral nervous systems. _____

The somatic nervous system controls voluntary movement such as lifting your hand. _____

The somatic nervous system controls involuntary movements such as the constriction of pupils. _____

The blood-brain barrier restricts very few substances from entering the brain. _____

Hydantoins are used to control seizures. _____

## Multiple Choice

Choose the best answer for each question.

**1. The classification of drugs used to treat depression is _____.**

    A. Benzodiazepine

    B. Antidepressants

    C. CNS stimulants

    D. Narcotic analgesics

**2. The classification of drugs usually used for surgical procedures is _____.**

    A. Benzodiazepines

    B. Anesthetics

    C. Barbiturates

    D. Beta blockers

**3. The disease most commonly associated with a drug holiday is _____.**

    A. Parkinson's disease

    B. Alzheimer's disease

    C. Myasthenia gravis

    D. Fibromyalgia

# ■ THE EYE

It is important to review the anatomy of the eye (Fig. 14-1). The eyes are protected by their placement in the orbits of the skull. Eyelids, eyelashes, and eyebrows protect the eye from irritants and infectious microbes. A hard sclera protects the outer eye. The sclera contains a layer called the choroid, which consists of a network of blood vessels that nourish the majority of the eye with oxygen and nutrients. The iris regulates the amount of light that enters the eye by dilating and constricting the pupil. The pupil is basically a hole in the iris. The outer eye is bathed with tears. The anterior chamber contains a watery **aqueous humor** (fluid). The clear structure that covers the iris, the pupil, and the anterior chamber is the cornea. The cornea is provided with oxygen and nutrients through tears, not blood vessels; thus, it is clear. The dark cavern of the posterior chamber contains a viscous (thick) **vitreous humor.**

Images are projected through the pupil and lens onto the rods (black and white) and cones (color) of the retina. The retina is the light-sensitive tissue located at the back of the eyeball. The inverted images are then sent to the brain via the optic nerve for interpretation.

---

### A CLOSER LOOK: Eye Health

Good eye health requires that patients have their eyes assessed annually. Family practitioners should encourage their patients, particularly older patients, to see an ophthalmologist or optometrist annually. These specialists use a **tonometer** to measure pressure in the eye. If pressure builds in the eye, it is usually because the aqueous humor is not flowing out of the eye correctly. This causes intraocular pressure (IOP) to increase. Pressure on the optic nerve eventually can lead to blindness.

---

**FIGURE 14-1:** Anatomy of the eye.

# EYE MEDICATIONS

The eye is vulnerable to several disorders, irritations, and infections, such as glaucoma, conjunctivitis, macular degeneration, keratitis, chalazion, and cataracts, all of which require medication as part of a treatment plan. Some medications, such as atropine, are also used to facilitate eye examinations (see the Master the Essentials table for descriptions of the most common medications for disorders of the eye).

## Master the Essentials: Eye and Ear Medications

This table shows the various classes of eye and ear medications, the key side effects, contraindications, precautions, interactions, and examples of each class.

| Class | Indications for Use | Side Effects | Contraindications and Precautions | Interactions | Examples |
|---|---|---|---|---|---|
| Ophthalmic alpha blockers | Treatment of eye irritation | Hypertension, somnolence, oral dryness, ocular hyperemia, eye burning or stinging | Hypersensitivity | MAO inhibitors, tricyclic antidepressants, beta blockers, antihypertensives, digoxin | Apraclonidine HCl (Iopidine), brimonidine tartrate (Alphagan P), dipivefrin (Propine), epinephrine (Epifrin, Glaucon) |
| Ophthalmic beta blockers | Treatment of open-angle glaucoma | Headache, depression, arrhythmia, syncope, nausea, keratitis, visual disturbances, bronchospasm | Bronchial asthma, COPD, sinus bradycardia, AV block, heart failure, hypersensitivity | Oral beta blockers calcium antagonists, digoxin, quinidine, phenothiazines | Betaxolol (Betoptic S), levobunolol HCl (Betagan), metipranolol (OptiPranolol), timolol hemihydrate (Betimol ), timolol maleate (Timolol Maleate USP, Istalol), timolol maleate ophthalmic gel (Timoptic-XE) |
| Carbonic anhydrase inhibitors | Treatment of glaucoma | Ocular burning or sting, blurred vision, bitter taste | Hypersensitivity | Salicylates, amphetamines, quinidine, methamine | Acetazolamide (Diamox, Sequels), brinzolamide ophthalmic suspension (Azopt), dorzolamide HCl (Trusopt) |
| Cycloplegic mydriatics | Dilation of pupil in inflammatory conditions or for diagnostic or surgical procedures | Increased IOP, transient burning/stinging, blurred vision, dry mouth, dry skin | Hypersensitivity, children with history of reaction to atropine, pregnancy | None reported | Pilocarpine (Isopto Carpine Solution), homatropine (Isopto Homatropine Solution 2-5%), scopolamine (Scopace) |
| Immunomodulators | Used to increase tear production | Burning, itching, discharge, red eyes, blurred vision, overflow of tears | Active infections, hypersensitivity, contacts | None reported | Cyclosporine (Restasis 0.05% emulsion) |

*Continued*

## Master the Essentials: Eye and Ear Medications—cont'd

| Class | Indications for Use | Side Effects | Contraindications and Precautions | Interactions | Examples |
|---|---|---|---|---|---|
| Miotics | Treatment of glaucoma | Corneal edema, clouding, stinging, burning, tearing, headache | Hypersensitivity, any condition in which pupillary constriction is undesirable | Topical NSAIDs | Carbachol (Isopto Carbachol), pilocarpine HCl (Isopto Carpine, Pilocarpine HCl Ophthalmic Solution USP), pilocarpine HCl gel (Pilopine HS Gel) |
| Ophthalmic antibiotics | Infection | Burning sensation in the eyes, conjunctivitis, hypersensitivity reactions, rash, urticaria | Allergy, fungal or viral diseases in the eye | Cortico-steroids | Gentamicin ophthalmic (Garamycin ophthalmic, Genoptic, Gentasol), tobramycin (Tobrex, Tobralcon), ciprofloxacin (Ciloxan), azithromycin (AzaSite), erythromycin (Eyemycin, Ilotycin, Romycin), bacitracin/polymyxin B (Ocumycin, Polycin-B, Polysporin ophthalmic), neomycin/polymyxin B |
| Ophthalmic corticosteroids | Inflammation and pain resulting from injury or surgery | If used for prolonged period: immunosuppression | Immunosuppression, purulent drainage from infection | None reported | Dexamethasone (AK-Dex, Ocu-Dex), prednisolone ophthalmic (Econopred Plus, Omnipred, Pred Forte, Prednisol) |
| Ophthalmic local anesthetics | Anesthetic before surgery | Stinging, burning | Hypersensitivity, prolonged use | None reported | Tetracaine (Altacaine, Opticaine), proparacaine (Alcaine, Ophthetic) |
| Ophthalmic NSAIDs | Inflammation and pain in eye | Burning, stinging, irritation, corneal edema, risk of increased bleeding | Diabetes mellitus, children, infections, pregnancy, known hypersensitivity, bleeding disorders | None reported | Diclofenac 0.1 % solution (Cambia, Voltaren), ketorolac tromethamine 0.5% solution (Acular), nepafenac 0.1% suspension (Nevanac) |

## Master the Essentials: Eye and Ear Medications—cont'd

| Class | Indications for Use | Side Effects | Contraindications and Precautions | Interactions | Examples |
|---|---|---|---|---|---|
| Osmotic diuretics | Treatment of glaucoma; decreases intraocular pressure | Dizziness, dry mouth, fluid and electrolyte imbalance, headache, tremors, nausea, vomiting, disorientation, confusion | Anuria, dehydration, pulmonary edema, hypersensitivity | Amphetamines, quinidine | Glycerin (Osmoglyn, Ophthalgan Solution) |
| Ophthalmic prostaglandin agonists | Treatment of open-angle glaucoma and ocular hypertension | Ocular hyperemia, decreased visual acuity, eye discomfort | Hypersensitivity, pregnancy | None reported | Bimatoprost (Lumigan), latanoprost (Xalatan Solution), travoprost (Travatan Z) |
| Antivertigo agents | Prevention and treatment of motion sickness | Blurred vision, confusion, extrapyramidal symptoms, restlessness, sedation, hypotension, rash, dry mouth | Benign prostatic hypertrophy, children, glaucoma, hypertension, lactation, pregnancy, seizures, hypersensitivity | Alcohol, CNS depressants, muscle relaxants | Meclizine (Anti-Vert, Bonine), diphenhydramine (Benadryl), dimenhydrinate (Dramamine), scopolamine (Transderm-Scop Transdermal Patch) |
| Otic antibiotics | Treatment of ear infections | Irritation in the ear | Hypersensitivity, eardrum rupture, breastfeeding, pregnancy | Other ear drops | Acetic acid and aluminum acetate otic (Domeboro Otic), ofloxacin otic (Floxin), acetic acid (Vosol) |
| Otic combination drugs | Treatment of ear infections with inflammation | Unusual taste in the mouth | Hypersensitivity to antibiotics or steroids, eardrum rupture, pregnancy, breastfeeding | Other ear drops | Ciprofloxacin and dexamethasone otic (Ciprodex), hydrocortisone, neomycin and polymyxin B otic (Vosol HCl) |
| Cerumenolytics | Softening of earwax (cerumen) | None | Hypersensitivity, ear drainage or discharge, recent ear injury, surgery, dizziness, ruptured eardrum | None noted | Carbamide peroxide solution (Auro, Debrox) |

AV, atrioventricular; CNS, central nervous system; COPD, chronic obstructive pulmonary disease; MAO, monoamine oxidase; NSAIDs, nonsteroidal anti-inflammatory drugs.

## Medications for glaucoma

Glaucoma is a leading cause of blindness. In this disease, an increase in pressure in the eye damages the optic nerve and thus impairs its ability to transmit visual information from the eye to the brain. Glaucoma is actually a group of diseases. Primary open-angle glaucoma, the most common form, occurs when the eye's **Schlemm canal** (drainage tube for aqueous humor) becomes obstructed, thus leading to a gradual increase in pressure. This disease traditionally has no symptoms, and if not diagnosed, it can cause loss of vision. Primary open-angle glaucoma is routinely treated effectively with medications, especially when it is diagnosed early.

Another type of glaucoma is angle-closure, also known as acute or narrow-angle, glaucoma. This type is rarer, and it differs from open-angle glaucoma in that eye pressure usually increases very rapidly. Angle-closure glaucoma occurs when drainage is obstructed, but at a different place in the eye. The iris is usually too small, and it covers up the drainage canals. Symptoms of this type of glaucoma include headaches, eye pain, nausea, multicolored halos around lights at night, and blurred vision. Angle-closure must be corrected surgically.

A third type of glaucoma is called normal-tension glaucoma. As the name implies, the optic nerve is damaged even though the pressure in the eye is not elevated enough to indicate this likelihood. The patient has no symptoms, and diagnosis is made only by examining the optic nerve for damage. Because the cause of this type of glaucoma is still a mystery to physicians, treatment consists of lowering the pressure in the eye as much as possible through medications or surgery.

A few other types of glaucoma fall into an "other" category. These include congenital glaucoma, in which an infant is diagnosed early with increased pressure resulting from a hereditary congenital malformation or abnormal fetal development. Secondary glaucoma is secondary to another disease that causes or contributes to increased eye pressure or is a result of injury or certain medications. Some medications, such as glucocorticoids, antihypertensives, antihistamines, and antidepressants, can predispose a patient to increased **intraocular pressure (IOP)** because of a decrease in aqueous humor flow in the eye. In many cases, this is temporary and subsides with discontinuation of the medication. In a few rare instances, it is permanent. Pigmentary glaucoma results when the pigment granules giving the eye its color break off and lodge in the drainage system.

Medications used to treat glaucoma act by increasing the flow of aqueous humor; they include miotics and prostaglandins. Drugs such as pilocarpine HCl (Isopto Carpine, Pilocarpine HCl Ophthalmic Solution USP), carbachol (Isopto Carbachol), and pilocarpine HCl gel 4% (Pilopine HS Gel) that increase the outflow of aqueous humor are called miotics. They also constrict the pupil. Some of these drugs activate cholinergic receptors, which decrease the IOP. They dilate the meshwork of the Schlemm canals, and allow increased output of aqueous humor. As more aqueous humor is absorbed, the IOP decreases.

Prostaglandins such as bimatoprost (Lumigan), latanoprost (Xalatan), and travoprost (Travatan Z) do not affect pupil diameter but rather dilate the meshwork of in the anterior chambers in the Schlemm canals. However, one side effect of prostaglandins is that they change the pigmentation of the iris and thus the color of the eye.

Other medications decrease IOP by reducing the flow of aqueous humor. These agents include alpha and beta blockers, carbonic anhydrase inhibitors, and osmotic diuretics.

■ Alpha blockers. Alpha blockers such as apraclonidine HCl (Iopidine) and brimonidine tartrate (Alphagan P) dilate blood vessels in the eye and have a mild effect on the cardiovascular and respiratory systems. They treat glaucoma by decreasing the production of and increasing the drainage of aqueous humor.

■ Beta blockers. Beta blockers such as betaxolol HCl (Betoptic S) and timolol maleate (Istalol) also work by decreasing the production of intraocular fluid. In low dosages, beta blockers affect the eye but do not have a systemic effect. If they do enter the cardiovascular system, these drugs can constrict the bronchi, slow the heart rate, and cause hypotension. These systemic effects can be minimized by closing the eyes following application to prevent the drops from entering the tear drainage duct.

■ Carbonic anhydrase inhibitors. Medications such as acetazolamide (Diamox and Sequels) decrease IOP by reducing the production of intraocular fluid. They can be administered topically or systemically, although systemic use is reserved for patients who do not respond to the topical medications.

■ Osmotic diuretics. This class of medications, which include glycerin (Osmoglyn, Ophthalgan Solution), are used for eye surgery to decrease the amount of aqueous humor rapidly.

Although the cause is not clear, glaucoma is more prevalent among patients with hypertension, diabetes, migraines, nearsightedness, and farsightedness and patients of advanced age.

## Medications for eye irritations and infections

For minor eye injury and irritation, the following can be used: local anesthetics such as tetracaine (Pontocaine 0.5% solution) and proparacaine (Ophthaine, Ophthetic 0.5% solution); antimicrobials such as gentamicin, tobramycin, and erythromycin; nonsteroidal anti-inflammatory drugs (NSAIDs) such as ketorolac tromethamine 0.5% solution (Acular) and nepafenac 0.1% suspension (Nevanac); and glucocorticoids such as dexamethasone (Maxidex suspension, Decadron solution and ointment) and hydrocortisone acetate (Hydrocortone). These medications can be administered as drops or salves or by injection. For milder irritations and injuries, the medications, such as eye lubricants, simply soothe the outer eye. For more serious irritations and injuries such as keratitis (an inflammation of the cornea caused by irritation or microbial infection), the medications must penetrate beyond the surface. Ophthalmic glucocorticoids should not be used for long-term treatment because they can suppress the immune response.

Anti-infectives are used for eye infections. Similar to infections elsewhere in the body, t eye infections must be treated swiftly and completely. One of the most common infections of the eye is conjunctivitis (pinkeye), and it is treated with an antibiotic such as gentamicin ophthalmic ointment. Eye infections can spread to other parts of the body, especially if patients rub their eyes with their fingers and then touch another part of the body. Meticulous hand washing is important, and patients should be advised to not rub the infected eye. Another common eye infection is a stye. A stye is a bacterial infection in an oil gland in the eyelid that causes a painful red bump. This is usually treated with topical ophthalmic antibiotics or oral antibiotics such as doxycycline (Vibramycin, Oracea, Adoxa) for persistent or multiple styes.

## Medications for eye examinations

Some drugs are used to make it easier for a health-care professional to examine the eyes. Cycloplegic mydriatics, for example, relax ciliary muscles and dilate the pupils so the examiner can peer into the eye.

Local ophthalmic anesthetic agents are used for removing foreign objects. The blink reflex is impaired, so it is important to inform the patient to wear darkened glasses when going outside until the effect of the medication wears off.

Staining agents are nontoxic, water-soluble dyes used to diagnose corneal epithelial defects caused by infection or injury. They can also be used to find foreign bodies or contact lenses in the eye. The stain colors the object green.

## Miscellaneous eye medications

Immunomodulators such as Restasis work to treat a certain type of chronic dry eye by increasing tear production. The patient must understand that it will take time before the effects of this drug are felt and up to 6 months for maximum benefit. The liquid portion of the medication is castor oil, which provides some immediate moisturizing benefit.

# ■ THE EAR

Otic, or ear, medications can be used to treat inflammation, wax buildup, or infections. To understand ear disorders, you must understand the anatomy of the ear, which is divided into the outer, middle, and inner ear (Fig. 14-2). The outer ear consists of the pinna, which is the visible part of the ear, and the external auditory canal. The pinna protects the middle and inner ear, and it also collects sound and funnels it through the external auditory canal. The external auditory canal contains glands that secrete cerumen (earwax). The purpose of this wax is to protect the inner ear from damage and infections. Thus, a lack of wax can lead to an increased risk of ear infections. Too much earwax can cause a blockage leading to loss of hearing.

The middle ear is separated from the outer ear by the tympanic membrane (eardrum), and it includes the auditory ossicles (malleus, incus, stapes), the middle ear cavity (hollow area containing ossicles), and the eustachian tube. Once sound waves hit the tympanic membrane, three flexible bones called the ossicles convert that sound into mechanical vibrations. The eustachian tube connects the ear and the throat and functions to equalize pressure on both sides of the tympanic membrane.

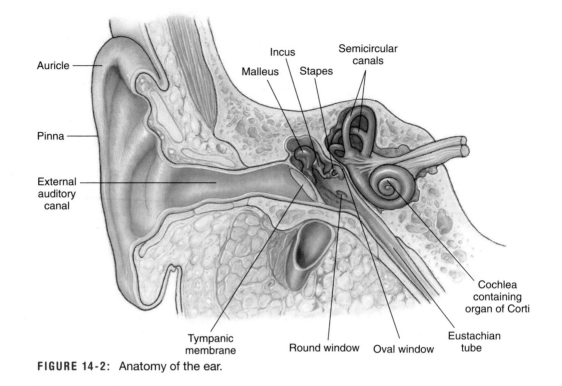

**FIGURE 14-2:** Anatomy of the ear.

The inner ear includes the oval window, round window, cochlea, and semicircular canals. The oval window is located directly behind the stapes and vibrates when that bone strikes it. This sets in motion the fluid-filled tubes, which generate nerve impulses that travel to the brain. The round window serves as a pressure relief valve, bulging outward as pressure rises. The inner ear consists of fluid-filled tubes containing the actual hearing cells of the body. The front portion contains the following: the cochlea, which helps with hearing; the semicircular cells, which help maintain balance; and the vestibule, which also is responsible for balance. Thus, hearing and equilibrium are very closely intertwined in the anatomy of the ear.

## ■ EAR MEDICATIONS

The most common disorders requiring ear medications are infections of some type. Swimmer's ear (otitis externa) is an infection of the outer ear, and otitis media is a middle ear infection. Other common conditions requiring medication are impaction of cerumen (earwax) and motion sickness. Otic medications are usually deposited in the outer ear, or pinna, from where they flow through the auditory canal toward the eardrum. If the eardrums are intact, they provide a barrier that prevents infection from entering the inner ear. Conversely, if the eardrum is ruptured, otic medications should be used only under strict medical supervision.

Several types of medication are used to treat ear disorders. Antibiotics such as acetic acid and aluminum acetate otic (Domeboro Otic), ofloxacin otic (Floxin) and acetic acid (Vosol) can be given directly into the ear to fight infections. In the case of swimmer's ear, they may be combined with a glucocorticoid to reduce associated inflammation. Examples of these combination drops are as follows: ciprofloxacin and dexamethasone otic (Ciprodex); hydrocortisone, neomycin, and polymyxin B otic (Cortisporin); and hydrocortisone and acetic acid (Vosol HC). Systemic antibiotics, such as amoxicillin (Amoxil, Trimox), amoxicillin and clavulanate potassium (Augmentin), sulfamethoxazole and trimethoprim (Bactrim, Septra), cefaclor (Ceclor), erythromycin and sulfisoxazole (Pediazole), are needed for middle or inner ear infections.

Pain medications such as antipyrine and benzocaine (A/B otic, Aurodex, and Auroguard) may also be prescribed for the pain that accompanies trauma or infection (see the Master the Essentials table for descriptions of the most common medications for disorders of the ear).

**Drug Spotlight 14.1** *Transderm Scop (transdermal scopolamine)*

| | |
|---|---|
| Define | Transdermal circular patch applied to skin behind ear |
| Use | Used in adults for prevention of nausea and vomiting associated with motion sickness and recovery from anesthesia and surgery |
| Application | Should be applied at least 4 hours before anticipated event producing nausea and vomiting |
| Effectiveness | Patch delivers drug for up to 3 days; for surgery, remove after 24 hours; for longer travel; remove after 3 days and place a new patch behind the other ear |
| Side effects | Dry mouth, dizziness |
| Contraindications and withdrawal symptoms | Drug withdrawal symptoms noted after patch removal: dizziness, nausea, vomiting, headache; usually occurs 24 hours after patch removal |

As was discussed earlier, earwax is a normal product of a healthy ear. Mineral oil, **cerumen** (earwax) softeners (cerumenolytics), and hydrogen peroxide can be used to decrease the amount of earwax if problems are occurring. Although earwax can protect the ear from infection, a buildup of earwax can decrease hearing, cause pain, and sometimes trap and promote growth of bacteria.

In addition to hearing, the ear is also responsible for balance. Motion sickness is caused by the ear's inability to determine the body's position relative to its motion. It can be treated with tablets or transdermal patches that are placed behind the ear (see Drug Spotlight 14.1). Medications such as Dramamine or Bonine should be taken 20 to 60 minutes before travel.

Drugs such as meclizine (Antivert), which is an anticholinergic, are given for dizziness, or **vertigo,** and the nausea that sometimes accompanies it.

## MEDICATIONS AND OTOTOXICITY

As discussed in Chapter 2, many drugs can cause **ototoxicity** (damage to ears). Commonly, this is occurs with certain antibiotics such as gentamicin. Symptoms of ear damage include **tinnitus** (ringing in the ears), hearing loss, and severe headache, ataxia, and balance disturbances.

## SUMMARY

The eyes and ears provide critical sensory information to the brain. Conditions, disease, infections, and other irritants can disrupt sensory communication and cause pain and discomfort not only at the source but also systemically. The eye is made up of many interconnected structures working together to provide clear vision. Glaucoma is a term for a group of diseases that cause increased pressure in the eye that, if untreated, will lead to blindness. The basis of treatment for all types of glaucoma is the reduction of aqueous humor in the eye to decrease IOP. This is accomplished through the use of various eye drops, although sometimes surgical intervention is required. Eye infections such as conjunctivitis and styes vary from minor to serious and must be treated with appropriate antibiotics. Other medications such as miotics and anesthetics are administered to the eye to assist in ophthalmic examinations.

The ear is made up of three major parts: the outer, inner, and middle ear. These parts work together to provide hearing and balance to each individual. When these pieces do not fit together and function well, hearing and balance are adversely affected. Otic medications are given to treat infections and motion sickness.

Good eye and ear health is fundamental to retaining our ability to see and hear. Patients should be encouraged to be alert to changes in their vision and hearing. They should also have a thorough assessment of these organs regularly because some diseases, such as glaucoma, can be symptom free until quite advanced. Early detection and treatment may save the individual's eyesight or hearing for many years to come.

## Activities

To make sure that you have learned the key points covered in this chapter, complete the following activities.

### True or False

Write true if the statement is true. Beside the false statements, write false, and correct the statement to make it true.

Half-angle is a type of glaucoma. _____

Pinkeye is an injury occurring from surgery. _____

Aqueous humor is located behind the eardrum. _____

The Schlemm canal is located in the eye. _____

Mydriatics are used to examine the inner eye. _____

The stapes is located in the inner ear. _____

Cerumen is another name for earwax. _____

Glaucoma can occur suddenly or gradually over time. _____

IOP stands for in other places. _____

The pinna functions by funneling sound through the outer ear canal. _____

### Multiple Choice

Choose the best answer for each question.

**1. Which physician is an ear specialist?**

A. Audiologist

B. Ophthalmologist

C. Optician

D. Dermatologist

**2. Which of the following are used to treat edema in the eye?**

A. Cerumenolytics

B. Glucocorticoids

C. Mydriatics

D. Miotics

**3. Which drug is used to treat glaucoma?**

A. Cerumenolytics

B. Glucocorticoids

C. Mydriatics

D. Miotics

**4. What class of drugs is used to treat pinkeye?**

   A. Miotics

   B. Antibiotics

   C. Diuretics

   D. Corticosteroids

**5. Scopolamine is given via which route?**

   A. Oral

   B. Injection

   C. Transdermal

   D. Rectal

**6. A stye is caused by _____.**

   A. Bacteria

   B. Fungus

   C. Parasite

   D. Virus

**7. The part of the eye covering the outer eye is called the _____.**

   A. Iris

   B. Cornea

   C. Eyelid

   D. Sclera

**8. Signs of ototoxicity include _____.**

   A. Tinnitus

   B. Severe headache

   C. Ataxia

   D. All of the above

**9. The category of ophthalmic medication that may alter the color of the iris and change the patient's eye color is called _____.**

   A. Glucocorticoids

   B. Prostaglandins

   C. Antibiotics

   D. Beta blockers

**10. Motion sickness medication should be taken _____.**

   A. 1 hour before travel

   B. 1 day before travel

   C. 20 to 60 minutes before travel

   D. At time of travel

# THE ENDOCRINE SYSTEM

The endocrine system uses chemicals known as hormones, acting as messengers, to various parts of the body to trigger a reaction. Several components make up this system (Fig. 15-1), which is controlled by the hypothalamus. The hypothalamus gland, located in the brain, secretes chemicals called releasing factors that trigger the release of several hormones from the pituitary gland. The pituitary gland, also located in the brain, is known as the master gland because it secretes most of the body's hormones. The pituitary gland secretes follicle-stimulating hormone (FSH) and luteinizing hormone (LH), which are important to female reproduction, and **antidiuretic hormone (ADH),** which helps prevent loss of water by the kidneys. In addition, the pituitary gland secretes **thyroid-stimulating hormone (TSH),** which

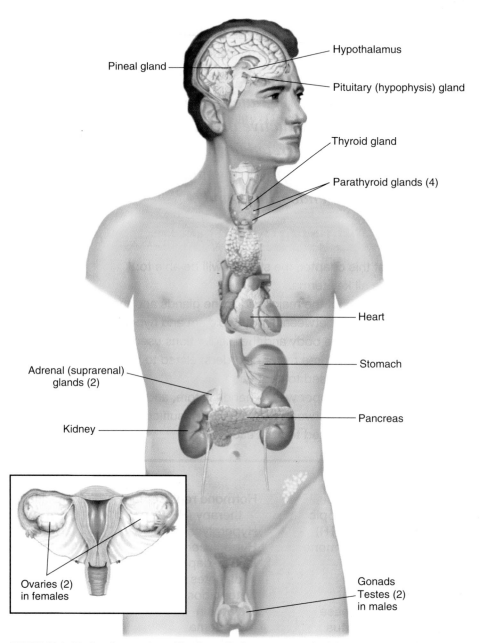

Pineal gland

Hypothalamus

Pituitary (hypophysis) gland

Thyroid gland

Parathyroid glands (4)

Heart

Stomach

Adrenal (suprarenal) glands (2)

Pancreas

Kidney

Ovaries (2) in females

Gonads Testes (2) in males

**FIGURE 15-1:** Endocrine system. The hypothalamus controls this system by telling the pituitary gland which hormones to secrete. Hormones have a wide range of effects on body organs, including the thyroid, pancreas, adrenals, and reproductive organs (testes and ovaries).

triggers thyroid gland function. Table 15.1 and Figure 15-2 provide a more in-depth look at all the hormones secreted by the pituitary gland. The hypothalamus is the body's switchboard—it tells the pituitary gland which hormones to send out to the body. When a hormone level becomes too high, the body tells the hypothalamus, which, in turn, tells the pituitary to stop producing the hormone. This is called a **negative feedback system.**

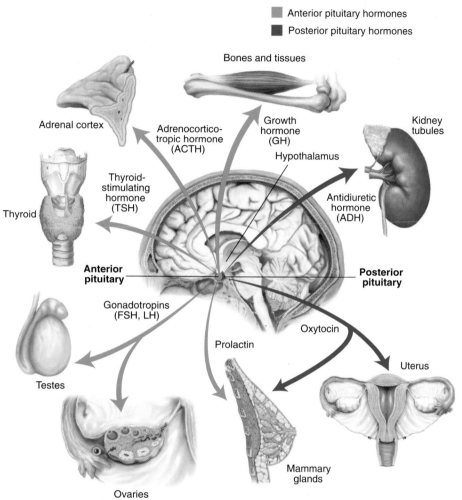

FIGURE 15-2:  Pituitary gland. Hormones and target glands.

## TABLE 15.1  Hormones Secreted by the Pituitary Gland

| Hormone | Target Organs and Effect | Overproduction Causes... | Underproduction Causes... |
| --- | --- | --- | --- |
| **Front or Anterior Pituitary** | | | |
| Adrenocorticotropic hormone (ACTH) | Regulates release of epinephrine and glucocorticoids from the adrenal glands, which determines fight or flight responses of the autonomic nervous system | Cushing's disease | Addison's disease |
| Thyroid-stimulating hormone (TSH) | Regulates release of hormones in the thyroid, which affects energy | Graves' disease | Myxedema in adults, cretinism in children |

*Continued*

**TABLE 15.1   Hormones Secreted by the Pituitary Gland—cont'd**

| Hormone | Target Organs and Effect | Overproduction Causes... | Underproduction Causes... |
|---|---|---|---|
| Somatotropin, or growth hormone (GH) | Regulates growth of bone, muscles, and other tissues by affecting the liver and adipose tissue | **Gigantism** (abnormally tall stature; patient becomes a "giant")<br>**Acromegaly** (growth of hands and feet after puberty when growth is supposed to stop)<br>Treatment of acromegaly: medications that suppress growth hormones | **Dwarfism** (abnormally short stature)<br>Treatment: growth hormone |
| Prolactin | Stimulates milk production in the mammary gland | Overproduction of breast milk in women<br>Milk production in a non-lactating patient can be a sign of a pituitary tumor<br>Parlodel is used to suppress lactation in women who choose not to breastfeed, but a side effect is increased fertility | Underproduction of milk in women; baby has difficulty nursing |
| Follicle-stimulating hormone (FSH) | Stimulates sperm production in men and egg production in women | Increased fertility | Men: sterility<br>Women: irregular or absent menses |
| Luteinizing hormone (LH) | Stimulates release of the ripened egg in women (ovulation); also helps in the production of female hormones (**estrogens** and **progestins**) | Multiple gestations (e.g., twins, triplets) | Infertility (woman cannot ovulate and therefore cannot conceive) |
| Interstitial cell–stimulating hormone (ICSH) | Stimulates production of androgens (the male hormone testosterone) | Aggressiveness, excess hair | Feminine attributes in men (e.g., high voice, small muscles) |
| **Back or Posterior Pituitary** | | | |
| Antidiuretic hormone (ADH) | Conserves fluids by changing the permeability of the kidneys | **Syndrome of inappropriate antidiuretic hormone (SIADH):** too much fluid is retained<br>Treatment: diuretics | **Diabetes insipidus**; too much fluid is excreted by the kidneys, with resulting dehydration<br>Treatment: desmopressin (DDAVP)* |
| Oxytocin | Contracts the uterus and milk ducts in the breasts; contracts the prostate gland in men | The uterus or prostate can contract so much that it ruptures (rarely) | Labor may be slowed or milk expulsion constricted<br>Treatment: Pitocin (oxytocin in synthetic form) may be given intramuscularly or intravenously to the laboring or postpartum patient to increase the force of contractions |

*DDAVP is also used to help chronic bedwetters stop urinating at night and to stop bleeding in patients with hemophilia.

The gonads (sex organs) consist of the ovaries in females and testes in males. These glands are responsible for secreting hormones in response to those released by the pituitary gland. The ovaries produce and release both estrogen and progesterone, and the testes produce and release androgens, which include testosterone. Chapter 20 covers the medications used to treat reproductive disorders.

The thyroid gland, which is located in the neck surrounding the esophagus, regulates metabolism, including temperature and body weight. The thyroid gland also regulates blood and bone calcium by secreting calcitonin. **Calcitonin** helps force calcium ions into bone. If the patient has insufficient calcitonin, the blood calcium level remains high and the bone calcium level remains low, thus leading to bone fractures. Replacement hormones help with both energy and calcium storage, but the prescriber may order only calcium supplements.

The four parathyroid glands are located on the surface of the thyroid gland and are responsible for the concentration of sodium and calcium in the blood and urine. The parathyroid glands, which are embedded in the thyroid gland, also help regulate calcium balance. They counter calcitonin with **parathormone,** which pulls calcium out of the bones into the bloodstream.

The pancreas, located in the abdominal cavity, has two major functions. First, it secretes digestive enzymes into the small intestine and thereby allows what we eat to be digested and used. The second function of the pancreas is achieved by secreting two hormones: insulin, which decreases blood glucose by moving it into the tissue, where it can be used; and glucagon, which increases blood glucose. The liver helps the pancreas determine blood glucose levels, so the liver and pancreas must be functioning properly to control blood glucose.

The adrenal glands are located above the kidneys. The secretion of **adrenocorticotropic hormone (ACTH)** by the pituitary gland stimulates the release of cortisol and glucocorticoids to control the fight or flight response. The **fight or flight response** is the automatic reaction that prepares the body to flee or stay and face an attack. The outer cortex of the adrenal gland secretes cortisol, which helps maintain blood pressure and cardiovascular function, slows the immune response of the body, and maintains steady glucose levels. Through the negative feedback system, when the cortisol level increases, the hypothalamus tells the pituitary to shut off the release of ACTH. The inner medulla secretes epinephrine, more commonly known as adrenaline, in response to stressful situations such as anger or fright.

The pineal gland, which is located in the brain, secretes **melatonin** in response to input from the eyes. The more light that enters, the less melatonin is released. Melatonin is what helps us to sleep; thus, in the darker hours of night and winter, we tend to feel sleepier. When the pineal gland fails, sleep is impaired, and melatonin or barbiturates (see Chapter 13) may be prescribed to correct this disorder (see the Master the Essentials table for descriptions of the most common endocrine system drug classifications).

## Master the Essentials: Endocrine Medications

This table shows the various classes of endocrine medications and key side effects, contraindications and precautions, interactions, and examples of each class.

| Class | Side Effects | Contraindications and Precautions | Interactions | Examples |
|---|---|---|---|---|
| Anabolic steroids | Acne, hirsutism, depression, altered libido, edema, glucose tolerance, aggression, liver cancer, atherosclerosis | Breast cancer, prostate cancer, pregnancy, hypercalcemia, liver failure | Oral anticoagulants, oral hypoglycemic agents | Nandrolone decanoate, oxandrolone |
| Antithyroid drugs | Paresthesia, headache, rash, agranulocytosis | Hypersensitivity, pregnancy, breastfeeding | Anticoagulants | Methimazole (Northyx, Tapazole), propylthiouracil I-131-RAI (Iodotope) |
| Cortisol-inhibiting medications | Dizziness, drowsiness, headache, nausea, vomiting | Pregnancy, breastfeeding | Insulin, oral hypoglycemic, corticosteroids, estrogen, hydantoins, acetaminophen | Metyrapone (Metopirone) |

*Continued*

## Master the Essentials: Endocrine Medications—cont'd

| Class | Side Effects | Contraindications and Precautions | Interactions | Examples |
|---|---|---|---|---|
| Corticosteroids | Adrenocortical insufficiency, anxiety, cessation of menses, constipation, decreased wound healing, decreased growth in children, diarrhea, dizziness, fluid and electrolyte imbalances, GI upset, headache, hyperglycemia, increased eye pressure, increased infection, muscle pain and weakness, osteoporosis, psychosis, petechiae | Pregnancy, lactation, children; history of clots, seizures, or immunosuppression; not used for long-term therapy; cautious use with infection, hypothyroidism, cirrhosis, increased blood pressure, congestive heart failure, emotional instability, diabetes, glaucoma, or GI upset; do not use in patients with a history of clots, seizures, or immunosuppression | Barbiturates, contraceptives, diuretics, NSAIDs, vaccines | Hydrocortisone USP, fludrocortisone acetate (Florinef) |
| Insulin | Headache, increased sweat, irritability, tingling, tremor, blurred or double vision, weakness, hypoglycemia, hypokalemia | Hypoglycemia, sensitivity, kidney impairment, liver impairment | Alcohol, MAO inhibitors, salicylates, anabolic steroids | Lispro (Humalog, NovoLog), regular insulin (Iletin I, Iletin II, Humulin R, Novolin R), isophane (NPH) insulin (Humulin N, Novolin N), lente insulin (Humulin L, Novolin L), ultralente insulin (Humulin U, Ultralente), glargine insulin (Lantus) |
| Oral antidiabetic agents | Hypoglycemia; abdominal pain (alpha-glucosidase inhibitors); nausea, vomiting, metallic taste (metformin); aplastic anemia, rash, nausea (sulfonylureas); swelling, weight gain (thiazolidinediones) | Hypersensitivity, diabetic ketoacidosis, cirrhosis; inflammatory bowel disease (alpha-glucosidase inhibitors); kidney or liver dysfunction (metformin) | Alcohol, MAO inhibitors, corticosteroids, salicylates, warfarin | **First Generation**<br><br>Acetohexamide (Dymelor), chlorpropamide (Diabinese), tolazamide (Tolinase), tolbutamide (Orinase)<br><br>**Second Generation**<br><br>Glimepiride (Amaryl), glipizide (Glucotrol), glyburide (Diabeta, Micronase Glynase) |
| Pancreatic enzymes | Nausea, vomiting, stomach pain, diarrhea, constipation, greasy stools, gas | Allergy to pork, pregnancy or lactation | None known | Pancrelipase (Pancrease, Ultrase or Creon) |

## Master the Essentials: Endocrine Medications—cont'd

| Class | Side Effects | Contraindications and Precautions | Interactions | Examples |
|---|---|---|---|---|
| Thyroid medications | Palpitations, fast heart rate, irregular heartbeat, increased blood pressure nervousness, tremor, headache, insomnia, weight loss, diarrhea, abdominal cramps, intolerance of heat, fever, menstrual irregularities | Adrenal insufficiency, diabetes, cardiovascular disease | Adrenergics, insulin, oral anticoagulants, oral hypoglycemics | Levothyroxine ($T_4$) (Levothroid), desiccated thyroid ($T_3$, $T_4$) (Armour) |

GI, gastrointestinal; MAO, monoamine oxidase; NSAIDs, nonsteroidal anti-inflammatory drugs.

## ENDOCRINE SYSTEM MEDICATIONS

Medications used to treat disorders of the endocrine system can be separated into three categories: medications for thyroid and parathyroid disorders, medications for pancreatic disorders, and medications for adrenal disorders.

### Medications for thyroid and parathyroid disorders

The thyroid gland cues individual cells to work. It is an "on" switch for the body. The thyroid has an integral role in the body's metabolism. It produces two hormones, **triiodothyronine ($T_3$)** and **thyroxine ($T_4$),** which stimulate every tissue in the body to produce proteins and increase the amount of oxygen used by cells. Therefore, when the thyroid fails to work properly, the patient has less energy, and every cell in the body is affected. Decreased levels of these two hormones indicate hypothyroidism. Prolonged hypothyroidism can lead to a skin and tissue disorder called **myxedema,** which may be difficult to treat. A decrease of thyroid hormone secretion in utero and early infancy causes **cretinism** (slowed brain growth) in children. Rapid treatment can prevent both mental retardation and growth retardation.

To treat hypothyroidism, patients take oral doses of these hormones. These medications are prepared from natural sources, such as dried porcine thyroid gland, which include thyroid (Armour Thyroid, Bio-Throid) and liothyronine (Cytomel), or they are synthetically manufactured tablets such as levothyroxine (Synthroid, Levoxyl). This is known as **hormone replacement therapy (HRT).** Because a naturally occurring substance is being replaced, this medication is safe for use during pregnancy, although breastfeeding should be discussed with the physician. Caution should be used in elderly patients and those with heart problems or diabetes.

Hyperthyroidism results from an excess of thyroid hormone, leading to **Graves' disease,** characterized by bulging eyes, hyperactive metabolism, **goiter** (enlarged thyroid), and weight loss. **Thyroid storm,** which is a life-threatening condition and includes such symptoms as tachycardia, hyperthermia, chest pain, sweating, weakness, heart failure, anxiety, shortness of breath, and disorientation, can occur if hyperthyroidism is untreated. The thyroid can be inhibited from secreting $T_3$ and $T_4$ by thyroidectomy. Radioactive sodium iodide I-131 (Iodotope) is taken by mouth; it is trapped within the thyroid gland and damages the thyroid's ability to function (Drug Spotlight 15.1). Other oral antithyroid drugs, such as propylthiouracil or methimazole (Northyx, Tapazole), can also be used. These medications should be avoided in pregnancy and in breastfeeding mothers.

### CRITICAL THINKING

How does removal of the thyroid gland affect calcium in the body?

**Drug Spotlight 15.1** *Iodotope (sodium iodide I-131)*

| | |
|---|---|
| Define | Radioactive agent available as a capsule given orally one time; category listed as antithyroid agent |
| Use | Treats overactive thyroid gland |
| Application | Damages thyroid gland to decrease activity to more normal levels; may be used after surgical removal of thyroid to destroy any remaining thyroid tissue that was not removed |
| Administered | Given only by a physician trained in nuclear medicine or radiation oncology |
| Side effects | Adverse reactions are rare and are from the iodine: nausea, vomiting, chest pain, tachycardia, and hypersensitivity |
| Contraindications | Preexisting vomiting and diarrhea; pregnancy is a contraindication; it is excreted in breast milk, so mothers taking this medication should not breastfeed |

## Medications to treat pancreatic disorders

The pancreas functions properly when it secretes the correct amount of both insulin and glucagon. When this does not happen, the patient may develop one of two serious conditions: hyperglycemia or hypoglycemia. **Hyperglycemia** results from an excess of glucose in the blood. This condition can lead to problems with wound healing, high blood pressure, and nerve damage, among others. **Hypoglycemia** is caused by too little glucose in the blood and can lead to death. If the patient has low blood glucose, energy to fuel the cells is insufficient. Signs and symptoms of hypoglycemia are restlessness, shaky hands, lethargy, seizures, and coma (Fast Tip 15.1). Hypoglycemia is normally treated with a small dose of glucose such as hard candy, but patients may also choose to carry glucose preparations such as Insta-Glucose (gel) or BD Glucose (chewable tablet) that they take by mouth at the first sign of hypoglycemia. If patients cannot tolerate anything by mouth or are unconscious, they may be given injections such as glucagon (GlucaGen).

**Diabetes mellitus** is a disease characterized by hyperglycemia, or excessive blood glucose. Diabetes is categorized as type 1 or type 2. In type 1 diabetes or **insulin-dependent diabetes mellitus (IDDM),** destruction of the beta cells of the pancreas causes a decrease or lack of insulin secretion. Insulin in a healthy body serves to move glucose into the body tissues where it is needed, to assist in all functions at the cellular level. When the insulin is missing, glucose is elevated in the blood and unavailable to the tissues. When insulin is unavailable to remove accumulating glucose from the bloodstream, cells excrete water to flush out the vessels and send the glucose to the kidneys. For that reason, signs and symptoms of hyperglycemia include increased urination (from diuresis), increased thirst (the cells are dehydrated), and increased hunger (glucose is in the bloodstream but does not make it into the cells that desperately need it). Worsening damage occurs in the eyes, kidneys, heart, and nerves as long as glucose levels are elevated. Eventually, body organs can become severely affected. Vision worsens, wounds do not heal

---

● *Fast Tip 15.1* Emergency Treatment of Hypoglycemia

If an insulin dose is too high and low blood glucose results, immediately give juice, oral glucose gel, or hard candy if the patient is awake. A physician may also order dextrose IV or glucagon IM or IV to correct low blood glucose levels, especially if the patient is not conscious.

normally, fingers and toes may become numb, and kidney functions may be impaired. When blood glucose is very high, the patient may become lethargic and exhibit fruity-smelling breath and ketoacidosis (inefficient burning of fat). This can lead to seizures, coma, and death. Although type 1 diabetes is typically diagnosed in childhood or adolescence, it can occur at any age. Genetics, virus exposure, and pancreatic injuries are the contributing factors to the development of this chronic disease.

In type 2 diabetes or **non–insulin-dependent diabetes mellitus (NIDDM),** patients are insulin resistant; that is, their bodies produce adequate amounts of insulin, but it does not lower the glucose levels as expected. The pancreas responds by increasing its production of insulin. Eventually, the pancreas cannot keep up with the body's need for insulin. Genetics, a sedentary life style, and obesity are the main contributing factors for type 2 diabetes. Type 1 and type 2 diabetes are summarized in Table 15.2.

Patients with type 1 diabetes require insulin for treatment, whereas patients with type 2 diabetes may be managed with diet alone or with oral diabetic (antihyperglycemic) agents. Some antihyperglycemic drugs encourage the pancreas to release insulin, and others encourage the liver to trigger the pancreas to release insulin. The choice of drug prescribed depends on the patient's individual problem. These medications are categorized as first or second generation, based on when they were released. First generation antihyperglycemic medications include acetohexamide (Dymelor), chlorpropamide (Diabinese), tolazamide (Tolinase), and tolbutamide (Orinase). The newer second generation antihyperglycemic medications are more potent and tend to be safer. They include glimepiride (Amaryl), glipizide (Glucotrol), and glyburide (Diabeta, Micronase Glynase). You must understand the types of insulin, its proper handling, and its proper injection to care safely for patients with diabetes mellitus.

 *CRITICAL THINKING*

Why may too much glucose in the blood affect wound healing and nerve health?

 *CRITICAL THINKING*

What would you do if a patient with diabetes mellitus came to your office and collapsed in the waiting room?

### Types of insulin

Insulin preparations are divided into three categories, based on how quickly they start working and the length of action: short-acting, intermediate-acting, and long-acting (Table 15.3). When a patient's blood glucose level is high, you may need to use short-acting insulin to lower it. Short-acting insulin is usually prescribed on a sliding scale, depending on the assessed blood glucose level. It may also be taken before meals so that it starts to work as food is being digested. If a patient is allowed nothing by mouth (NPO) for a test, insulin is not given because food is not given.

Intermediate-acting insulin is insulin mixed with a substance that makes the body absorb the insulin more slowly. This type of insulin looks cloudy in the bottle and must be mixed before injection.

---

**TABLE 15.2  Types of Diabetes**

| Diabetes Type | Contributing Factors | Insulin Production | Treatment |
|---|---|---|---|
| Type 1: insulin-dependent diabetes mellitus (IDDM) | Family history, pancreatic trauma | Pancreas makes little or no insulin | Insulin is destroyed in the stomach, so patients are dependent on subcutaneously injectable insulin; diet modification and exercise |
| Type 2: non–insulin-dependent diabetes mellitus (NIDDM) | Family history, obesity, poor diet | Pancreas does not secrete enough insulin, or body does not use insulin properly; if dietary fat intake is excessive, pancreas may not be able to keep up with demand | Diet modification and exercise may be enough; if not, oral antihyperglycemic agents; if these do not work, insulin |

**TABLE 15.3 Types of Insulin**

| Type | Action | Onset of Action (Hours) | Duration of Action (Hours) |
|------|--------|-------------------------|----------------------------|
| Insulin Lispro | Rapid | 0.25–.0.50 | 3–5 |
| Insulin Aspart | Rapid | 0.25 | 3–5 |
| Insulin Glulisine | Rapid | 0.25–0.50 | 1–1.5 |
| Regular | Short | 0.5.–1.0 | 5–8 |
| Velosulin (pump only) | Short | 1–1.0 | 2–3 |
| NPH | Intermediate | 1–2.0 | 18–24 |
| Lente | Intermediate | 1–2.5 | 18–24 |
| Levemir | Long | 6–8 | Up to 24 |
| Lantus | Long | 1–1.5 | 20–24 |
| Ultralente | Long | 0.5–3 | 20–36 |
| Humulin 70/30 | Premixed | 0.5 | 2–4 |
| Novolin 70/30 | Premixed | 0.5 | 2–12 |
| NovoLog 70/30 | Premixed | 0.25 | 1–4 |
| Humulin 50/50 | Premixed | 0.5 | 18–24 |
| Humalog 75/25 | Premixed | 0.25 | 16–20 |

Long-acting insulin can last up to a day and a half. It is usually taken in the morning or at bedtime. If a patient's diabetes is fairly stable, different categories of insulin can be mixed to cover the next meal and beyond in one dose. This is done by the patient or health-care worker, or a commercially prepared mixture can be used. The name of the insulin states the ratio of long-acting to short-acting insulin (e.g., 70/30).

Patients with a history of hypoglycemia or poor control of blood glucose levels may receive insulin through a pump. This small, rectangular device delivers insulin at a continuous rate 24 hours a day, 7 days a week. The pump also delivers a bolus at meal times to help with the size of each meal eaten. In addition, some pumps monitor the blood sugar level continuously and allow the patient to make needed adjustments. The only category of insulin used with a pump is rapid or short-acting insulin.

## Virtual Field Trip

Using your favorite search engine, find out the latest information about inhaled insulin. Is it currently on the market? If so, is it widely used?

### Handling insulin

Insulin should be refrigerated until the vial is opened because refrigeration extends the shelf life for 1 to 2 years (depending on manufacturer). Once the vial is opened, it may be kept at room temperature to avoid painful injections, but it must be discarded within 1 month. Insulin should never be kept at temperature extremes (freezing or very hot) because they will severely damage the insulin. Always label a container with the time and date that it was opened. After you have opened an insulin vial, gently roll it between your fingers (Fig. 15-3). Do not shake it.

### Injecting insulin

Rotate sites on the patient's body when injecting insulin. This is necessary for several reasons: (1) if a site is used too frequently, the body may develop scar tissue that thickens, thus preventing insulin absorption; (2) abscesses may form; and, most important, (3) rotating sites allows insulin to be evenly absorbed and thereby helps to maintain steady glucose levels and delay or minimize the complications of diabetes such as neuropathy, eye and kidney damage, and cardiovascular disease. You may need to help the patient develop a chart of site rotation, such as that shown in Figure 15-4. A good rule of thumb to teach patients is that each site should only be used once a month and each injection site should be one inch away from other sites.

**FIGURE 15-3:** Proper insulin handling. Be sure to roll the insulin vial in your fingers before drawing up the injection; do not shake the vial.

| Sunday | Monday | Tuesday | Wednesday | Thursday | Friday | Saturday |
|--------|--------|---------|-----------|----------|--------|----------|
| Above navel | Below navel | Left thigh | Right thigh | Left of navel | Right of navel | Back of either arm |

**FIGURE 15-4:** Site rotation for insulin injections. Use a chart to remind patients to rotate injection sites.

The patient is spared discomfort and cost if you draw up regular and longer-acting insulin into one syringe before injection. Follow your agency protocol, but typically, the ordered amount of the clear, regular insulin is drawn up first, followed by the cloudy, longer-acting insulin. Following these directions ensures that you do not inadvertently put some of the cloudy, longer-acting insulin into the clear, regular insulin vial.

Another method of delivering insulin to patients with type 1 diabetes is the insulin pump (Fig. 15-5). This method uses a small needle, small-bore tubing, and a small, pager-sized pump that delivers a steady dose of insulin to the patient. Only short-acting insulin may be used with this method, and it is delivered at a base rate with programming available to provide extra insulin as needed. The newest pumps provide continuous glucose monitoring and allow insulin to be adjusted as needed. This method allows for injections to be reduced to once every few days instead of multiple times per day.

One other major function of the pancreas is the secretion of digestive enzymes. In patients with cystic fibrosis, the ducts in the pancreas become blocked with thick mucus and are unable to secrete these enzymes. For this reason, these patients must take replacement enzymes such as pancrelipase (Pancrease, Ultrase, or Creon) for the rest of their lives with every bite of food they ingest.

Insulin injected through catheter

Tubing delivers insulin

Insulin pump

0.5 U/h

**FIGURE 15-5:** Insulin pump. This provides continuous and steady administration of insulin to the patient with type 1 diabetes.

## Virtual Field Trip

Go to the American Diabetes Association Web site (www.diabetes.org) to find information to help you to create a teaching aid for diabetic patients.

## Medications that treat adrenal disorders

As with the thyroid gland, treatments for adrenal disorders are a response to the secretion of either too much or too little hormone. If too little hormone is secreted, then it must be replaced, and if too much is secreted, it must be controlled before damage is done to the body.

### Corticosteroid medications

Glucocorticoid hormones available as medications are known as corticosteroids because their actions are exactly the same as those of the naturally occurring hormones hydrocortisone and cortisol. Chemically, these medications are steroids and are used as replacement therapy when these hormones are absent or diminished. Corticosteroid medications are used to treat Addison's disease, autoimmune diseases, inflammatory reactions, cerebral edema, dermatologic disorders, allergies, asthma, cancer, Crohn's disease, dermatitis, edema, rashes, rheumatoid arthritis, rhinitis, shock, transplant rejection, and ulcerative colitis.

Addison's disease occurs when the adrenal cortex undersecretes glucocorticoid hormones. Patients with Addison's disease suffer from chronic fatigue that eventually worsens, muscle weakness, anorexia, nausea, vomiting, diarrhea, hypotension, hypoglycemia, sweating, irritability, and weight loss. The disease is treated with hydrocortisone USP tablets, a synthetic corticosteroid. If the level of aldosterone is also insufficient, it is replaced with oral doses of fludrocortisone acetate (Florinef).

In Cushing's disease, the adrenal cortex oversecretes the glucocorticoids mentioned earlier. Patients with Cushing's disease have symptoms similar to those of Addison's disease, except these patients suffer hypertension and hyperglycemia instead of hypotension and hypoglycemia. They also develop a fatty hump between their shoulders. Most patients have upper body obesity and a rounded face, and women have excessive hair growth on their face, chest, abdomen, and thighs. Treatment is based on the cause of the excess production and may include surgery, irradiation, chemotherapy, and cortisol-inhibiting drugs such as metyrapone (Metopirone).

### Anabolic steroids

Anabolic steroids are mainly composed of male hormones called androgens, which change the natural balance between tissue breakdown and building. They can be used to prevent muscle wasting in patients with AIDS or to help patients with severe trauma to rebuild tissue. Examples of anabolic steroids are oxandrolone and nandrolone decanoate. Side effects of these medications include aggressive behavior, rage, atherosclerosis, sterility, and liver cancer. Because of these side effects and because anabolic steroids are frequently abused by athletes trying to build muscle mass, they are Schedule III controlled substances.

●●● SUMMARY

The endocrine system controls many of the body's functions; therefore, disorders affecting this system can have profound implications for the health of the patient. Extremely high or extremely low hormone levels can cause various illnesses, so it is important to be aware of the various types of hormones and their functions. Patients may need to take medications to suppress hormone secretion or hormone supplements to compensate for missing hormones.

Medications for thyroid gland disorders are required to prevent mental and growth retardation when hormones are lacking and to treat life-threatening situations resulting from too much thyroid hormone in the body. Both the thyroid and parathyroid glands regulate blood and bone calcium; thus, medication is required to maintain proper levels of calcium when thyroid or parathyroid hormones are present in either excess or reduced amounts. Pancreatic dysfunction causes two major problems that require medication. The first is the inability to digest food, and the second is the inability to regulate blood sugar. In the first instance, pancreatic enzymes must be taken with every bite of food for the remainder of the patient's life. With blood sugar regulation difficulties resulting from diabetes mellitus, insulin or oral antidiabetic medications are required to lower blood glucose levels. For those patients diagnosed with hypoglycemia, antihypoglycemic agents must be kept on hand to take at the first sign of the condition.

The adrenal gland helps to stimulate the fight or flight response and slows the immune response. If the levels hormones naturally secreted are missing, they must be replaced to help with symptoms such as weakness, hypoglycemia, and hypotension. If the adrenal gland is oversecreting hormones, the patient needs medication to inhibit cortisol to treat hypertension and hypertension symptoms.

Overall, patients need normally functioning endocrine glands. If this is not the case, the physician will use medication along with surgery and/or radiation to return hormones to levels as close to normal as possible, to maintain optimum health.

# Activities

To make sure that you have learned the key points covered in this chapter, complete the following activities.

## True or False
Write true if the statement is true. Beside the false statements, write false, and correct the statement to make it true.

Hypoglycemia is low blood sugar. _____

Cushing's disease is caused by too much thyroid hormone. _____

Lack of insulin causes hypoglycemia. _____

A goiter may be a symptom of Graves' disease. _____

Ketoacidosis is the inefficient burning of fat. _____

Different categories of insulin cannot be mixed in one injection. _____

Insulin pumps are used for 8 hours of every day. _____

Regular short-acting insulin can be used on a sliding scale. _____

Anabolic steroids are never legal to use. _____

Addison's disease is caused by too little adrenal cortex hormone. _____

## Multiple Choice
Choose the best answer for each question.

**1. Which of the following is a symptom or sign of Addison's disease?**
   A. Tremor
   B. Dehydration
   C. Restlessness
   D. Weight loss

**2. Which organ secretes insulin?**
   A. Pancreas
   B. Renal
   C. Adrenal
   D. Thyroid

**3. What hormone triggers the release of hormones from the thyroid gland?**
   A. FSH
   B. TSH
   C. GH
   D. ICSH

**4. When should insulin be refrigerated?**

A. Before opening (while storing)

B. After opening

C. Never

D. Always

**5. Which is a common reason for an insulin pump to be prescribed?**

A. Patient's aversion to shots

B. Good insurance

C. History of hyperglycemia

D. Poor control of blood sugar

## Application Exercises

Respond to the following situations on a separate sheet of paper.

1. Barbara is a 10-year-old patient with newly diagnosed diabetes. Her mom wants to know why Barbara needs to have injections three to five times a day while her father just has to take pills. Explain the reason for this.

2. Steve was in a devasting car accident. He is taking anabolic steroids to help repair the body tissues injured in the accident. His wife is concerned about the serious side effects of these drugs. What are the side effects, and is she justified in being concerned? What would you say to her?

3. David has been recently diagnosed with IDDM. He is a traveling salesman and states that he leaves his insulin and injection supplies in the car for convenience. Explain to him the reason this is a bad idea and give him some suggestions on better ways to handle his insulin needs.

4. Cindy is told that she has hyperparathyroidism. She has had two episodes of kidney stones. She is confused about how these two things are connected; what would you say to her?

# Essentials Review

For further study and practice with drug classifications learned in this chapter, complete the following table to the best of your ability. Use resources such as the *PDR,* the Internet, or printed drug guides for help.

| Example | Generic Name | Classification | Purpose | Side Effects | Contraindications and Precautions | Examples | Patient Education |
|---|---|---|---|---|---|---|---|
| Oxandrin |  |  |  |  |  |  |  |
| Solu-Medrol |  |  |  |  |  |  |  |
| Iletin I |  |  |  |  |  |  |  |
| Glucotrol XL |  |  |  |  |  |  |  |
| Levothroid |  |  |  |  |  |  |  |

C H A P T E R

16

# Cardiovascular System Medications

*This chapter discusses medications that affect the cardiovascular system. The heart is a vital organ, and cardiovascular disorders can cause serious conditions, such as chest pain or even death. Fortunately, cardiovascular disease has been well researched, and many medications exist to help patients. Medications that affect this system are prescribed for a variety of illnesses. This section covers medications used for the following: to prevent myocardial infarction, stroke, and clotting; to promote blood cell development; to lower blood pressure; to treat heart failure; to regulate heart rhythm; to treat shock; and to treat lipid disorders.*

*In addition, many other medications that patients take have implications for the cardiovascular system. Medications taken for migraine, for example, may cause severe hypotension, which puts the patient at risk for falls. Patients taking aspirin for chronic back pain are at increased risk for bleeding. Therefore, finding out what medications (both over-the-counter and prescription) your patients are taking is extremely important to providing the best care and education possible.*

## LEARNING OUTCOMES

At the end of this chapter, the student will be able to:

16.1   Define all key terms.
16.2   Discuss how the cardiovascular system functions.
16.3   Describe 10 categories of cardiovascular medications and their uses and actions.

**KEY TERMS**

ACE inhibitors
Angina pectoris
Angiotensin receptor
  blockers (ARBs)
Anoxia
Atherosclerosis
Cerebrovascular
  accident (CVA)
Congestive heart
  failure (CHF)

Contractility
Cyanosis
Deep vein thrombosis
  (DVT)
Dysrhythmias
Embolus
Hemostasis
High-density lipoprotein
  (HDL)
Hypertension (HTN)

Hyperlipemia
Hypoxia
Ischemia
Low-density lipoprotein (LDL)
Myocardial infarction (MI)
Pulmonary circulation
Shock
Thrombus
Very low-density lipoprotein
  (VLDL)

# ■ THE CARDIOVASCULAR SYSTEM

The cardiovascular system consists of the heart and blood vessels. The heart (Fig.16-1) consists of four chambers, called the left and right atrium and the left and right ventricles, which are continuously contracting and relaxing in a coordinated rhythm. This rhythmic pumping of the heart sends the blood out to the lungs via the pulmonary artery to obtain oxygen, which the heart and body tissues need to

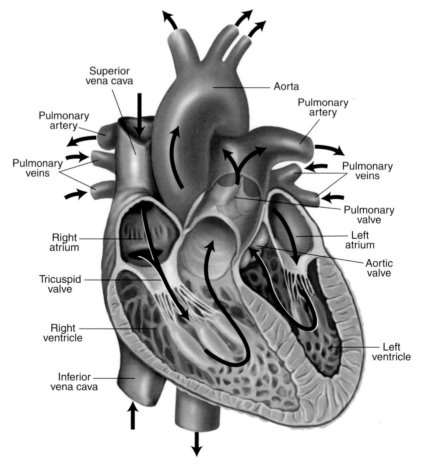

**FIGURE 16-1:** The heart. The heart is made up of four basic chambers: the left and right atrium and the left and right ventricle. In addition, the major blood vessels are attached to the heart to circulate blood from heart to the body and back again.

survive (Fig. 16-2). This oxygen-rich blood is then returned to the heart via the pulmonary veins. This is known as the **pulmonary circulation.** The oxygenated blood is then sent out to the upper and lower parts of the body via the aorta, which subdivides into a system of arteries. Finally, the blood, which is now depleted of oxygen and rich in carbon dioxide, returns from the body to the heart via a network of veins, where it again is pumped to the lungs to exchange the carbon dioxide for more oxygen in a never-ending cycle.

The cardiovascular system plays two major roles in the human body. One is to deliver much needed nutrients such as oxygen, hormones, and immune and clotting factors to every part of the body including the heart (see Fig. 16-1). The other role is to carry waste products such as carbon dioxide out of the cells. If any area of this system is damaged through accident or disease, the effects on health can be devastating.

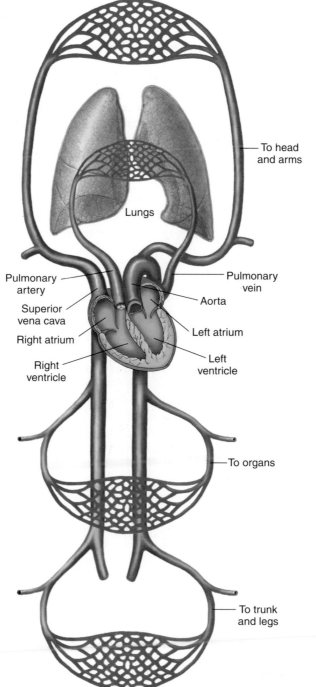

To head and arms

Lungs

Pulmonary artery

Superior vena cava

Right atrium

Right ventricle

Pulmonary vein

Aorta

Left atrium

Left ventricle

To organs

To trunk and legs

**FIGURE 16-2:** Cardiopulmonary circulation. The *red blood vessels* represent oxygen-rich blood, and the *blue blood vessels* represent oxygen-poor blood.

# MYOCARDIAL INFARCTION, STROKE, AND CLOTTING

**Myocardial infarction (MI)** or heart attack, stroke, and clots all cause damage when blood flow is impeded to the chest, brain, or lungs. Chest pain can be a symptom of a total lack of oxygen, called **anoxia,** or significantly reduced oxygen, called **hypoxia,** in the heart muscle (myocardium). The lack or reduction of oxygen prevents the tissues of the heart from receiving enough nourishment, and this can lead to tissue injury or **ischemia** or even death, referred to as an **infarction.** The classic signs of MI are chest pain, sweating, pale skin, and **cyanosis** (a bluish tint to the skin), particularily around the mouth. Chest pain can also be caused by noncardiovascular conditions, including broken ribs, gastrointestinal (GI) disorders, anxiety, or injured skeletal muscles (A Closer Look 16.1).

---

### A CLOSER LOOK 16.1: Heart Attacks and Women

Women tend to have atypical symptoms, such as upper back or shoulder pain, light-headedness, and unusual fatigue that lasts for several days. These atypical symptoms make rapid diagnosis more difficult. Health-care professionals and the public are becoming more educated about these atypical symptoms to help with quick diagnosis and treatment in women.

---

A stroke or **cerebrovascular accident (CVA)** occurs when the brain is deprived of oxygen and blood flow for several minutes. CVAs are a major cause of death and disability. MIs are caused by ischemia of heart muscle; CVAs are caused by ischemia of the brain. For this reason, medications that prevent ischemia can be prescribed to prevent stroke as well as MI.

# CARDIOVASCULAR MEDICATIONS

Cardiovasular medications function in a few basic ways. Certain medications, such as atropine, increase the heart rate. Others, such as diltiazem (Cardizem) or verapamil (Calan), slow the heart rate. Drugs such as Lanoxin (digoxin) make the heart function more efficiently. Other medications, such as propafenone (Rhythmol) and sotalol (Betapace), make it less irritable. In addition, drugs may be given to make the environment in which the heart functions less hostile. For example, if the heart is having a difficult time pumping, a backup of fluid may occur, leading to breathing problems. In this instance, administration of a diuretic such as furosemide (Lasix) decreases the amount of fluid that the heart must circulate through the body. This reduces the workload of the heart (see the Master the Essentials table for descriptions of the most common cardiovascular system drugs).

### Antianginal medications

**Angina pectoris** is chest pain caused by a lack of oxygen and nutrients in the heart tissue. As discussed earlier, ischemia (damage) occurs, and if continued, infarction, or the death of heart tissue, will ensue. Antianginal drugs decrease angina pectoris by dilating arteries and veins. An example is nitroglycerin (Nitrolingual, Nitroquick, Nitrostat, Nitro-Bid, Nitro-Dur), which can be administered via different routes such as sublingual, buccal, spray, or IV, depending on the patient's circumstances. The most common route is sublingual. The patient places a tablet or sprays the medication under the tongue at home when chest pain begins, with instructions to repeat the procedure every 5 minutes, for a maximum of three times. If pain continues, the patient should call emergency medical services (EMS) so that he or she can be evaluated for a possible MI.

A transdermal patch such as nitroglycerin topical (Nitro-Bid or Nitrol Appli-Kit) may also be used for prevention of angina pectoris. This patch is used daily as maintenance to prevent tissue ischemia and infarction. Angina can be treated with more than just medicine (Fast Tip 16.1). Nitroglycerin is also given in an IV form by EMS or in the hospital setting for acute chest pain.

*(Text continues on page 288)*

# Master the Essentials: Cardiovascular Medications

This table shows the various classes of cardiovascular medications and key side effects, contraindications and precautions, interactions, and examples of each class.

| Class | Indications for Use | Side Effects | Contraindications and Precautions | Interactions | Examples |
|-------|--------------------|--------------|----------------------------------|--------------|----------|
| Nitrates | Angina | Blurred vision, dry mouth, flushing, headache, hypersensitivity reaction, postural hypotension | Severe anemia, GI disease, glaucoma, intracranial pressure, hypotension | Alcohol, Viagra | Nitroglycerin (Nitrolingual, Nitroquick, Nitrostat, Nitro-Bid, Nitro-Dur), nitro-glycerin topical (Nitro-Bid or Nitrol Appli-Kit) |
| Anticoagulants | Prevention of heart attack and strokes by preventing blood clots in veins and arteries | Increased bleeding; blood irregularities; GI, liver, and kidney disease | Uncontrolled bleeding, heparin (an anti-coagulant does not cross the placenta but is used during pregnancy with caution) | Acetaminophen, alcohol, anabolic steroids, anti-infectives, barbiturates, chloral hydrate, corti-costeroids, estrogen, NSAIDs, tricyclic antide-pressants, thyroid drugs | Warfarin (Coumadin), heparin, enoxaparin (Lovenox) |
| Antiplatelet agents | History of heart attack and/or stroke, to prevent further clots | Diarrhea, dizziness, flushing, headache, nausea, rash, vomiting, weakness | Other medications that increase bleeding | ACE inhibitors, antico-agulants, anticonvul-sants, NSAIDs, beta blockers, diuretics, methotrexate, oral hypoglycemics | Aspirin, ticlopidine (Ticlid), clopido-grel (Plavix), abciximab (ReoPro), eptifibatide (Integrilin), tirofiban (Aggrastat) |
| Thrombolytics | Stroke symptoms, clotted central venous devices | Allergic reactions, bleeding, respiratory depression | Active bleeding, CVA within 2 months, recent intracranial or intraspinal sur-gery, intracranial neoplasm, uncon-trolled hypertension | Antiplatelet agents, anticoagulants | **Tissue plasminogen activators (tPA):** tenecteplase (TNKase), alteplase (Cathflo Activase), reteplase (Retavase) |
| Antifibrinolytics | Bleeding caused by aplastic anemia, cirrhosis of the liver, placenta abruption, cancer | Allergic reaction, anaphylaxis, dyspnea, confusion, bradycar-dia, rash | Known hypersensi-tivity, active intravas-cular clotting | Oral contraceptives | Aminocaproic acid (Amicar), tranexamic acid (Cyklokapron) |

Continued

## Master the Essentials: Cardiovascular Medications—cont'd

| Class | Indications for Use | Side Effects | Contraindications and Precautions | Interactions | Examples |
|---|---|---|---|---|---|
| Hematopoietics | Anemia | Gastric irritation, liquid iron preparations can stain teeth, allergic reactions | Known hypersensitivity, primary hemochromatosis, hemosiderosis, and hemolytic anemia (iron) | Antacids, tetracycline, H$_2$ blocker (iron); alcohol, neomycin, colchicines (vitamin B$_{12}$) | Ferrous sulfate (Feosol, Fer-in-Sol, Ferra-TD), cyanocobalamin (vitamin B$_{12}$) |
| ACE inhibitors | Hypertension | Blood irregularities, decreased blood pressure, light sensitivity, increased potassium, rash, decreased taste | Children (increased risk of side effects), collagen disease, kidney impairment, lactation, pregnancy, vessel swelling | Antacids, digoxin, diuretics, lithium, NSAIDs, vasodilators | Benazepril (Lotensin), captopril (Capoten), enalapril (Vasotec), fosinopril (Monopril), lisinopril (Prinivil, Zestril), moexipril (Univasc), perindopril (Aceon), quinapril (Accupril), ramipril (Altace), trandolapril (Mavik) |
| Beta-adrenergic blockers | Angina, hypertension, cardiac arrhythmias, acute MI | Bronchodilation, uterine relaxation, vasodilation | Bronchospasm, heart failure, heart block, bradycardia, some valvular diseases; use with caution in diabetes mellitus, lactation, liver disease, pregnancy | Bronchodilators, cimetidine, diabetic medications, digoxin | Acebutolol (Sectral), atenolol (Tenormin), betaxolol (Kerlone), bisoprolol (Zebeta), carvedilol (Coreg), esmolol, metoprolol (Toprol, Lopressor), nadolol (Corgard), nebivolol (Bystolic), propranolol (Inderal LA), timolol (Blocadren) |
| Diuretics | Hypertension, congestive heart failure, renal disease | Hypotension, hyponatremia, hypokalemia, anorexia, nausea | Known hypersensitivity, anuria, breast-feeding, pregnancy | Oral hypoglycemics, lithium, corticosteroids, cardiac glycosides, NSAIDs | **Thiazide diuretics:** bendroflumethiazide (Naturetin), chlorthalidone (Thalitone), chlorothiazide (Diuril, Diuril Sodium), hydrochlorothiazide (HydroDIURIL, Aquazide H, Esidrix, Microzide), indapamide (Lozol, methyclothiazide (Aquatensen, Enduron), metolazone (Mykrox, Zaroxolyn), polythiazide (Renese) **Postassium-sparing diuretics:** amiloride (Midamor), spironolactone (Aldactone), triamterene (Dyrenium) **Loop diuretics:** bumetanide (Bumex), ethacrynic acid (Edecrin, Sodium Edecrin), furosemide (Lasix), torsemide (Demadex) |

| Class | Uses | Side Effects | Contraindications/Cautions | Interactions | Examples |
|---|---|---|---|---|---|
| Calcium channel blockers | Angina, hypertension | Hypotension, constipation, bradycardia, edema | Children, lactation, liver or kidney disease, and pregnancy | ACE inhibitors, barbiturates, diuretics, lithium, rifampin, salicylates, sulfonamides | Amlodipine (Norvasc), diltiazem (Cardizem, Dilacor, Tiazac, Diltia XL), felodipine (Plendil), isradipine (Dynacirc), nicardipine (Cardene), nifedipine (Procardia XL, Adalat), nisoldipine (Sular), verapamil (Isoptin, Calan, Verelan, Covera-HS) |
| Phosphodiesterase inhibitors | Congestive heart failure | Arrhythmias, nausea, vomiting, headache, fever, chest pain, hypotension | Known hypersensitivity, severe aortic or pulmonic valvular disease | Disopyramide, potassium-wasting diuretics | Inamrinone (Inocor) |
| Cardiac glycosides | Congestive heart failure, arrhythmias | Arrhythmias, dizziness, electrolyte imbalances, GI upset, headache, irritability, lethargy, muscle weakness, tremors, seizures | Hypothyroidism, lactation, MI, pregnancy, impaired renal function; monitor for high or low potassium, irregular rhythm, severe bradycardia; if noted, discontinue drug | Adrenergics, antacids, antiarrhythmics, diuretics, neomycin, phenobarbital, rifampin, sulfa drugs | Digoxin (Cardoxin, Digetek, Lanoxicaps, Lanoxin), digitoxin |
| Angiotensin receptor blockers | Hypertension, vasodilation | Dizziness, upper respiratory tract infection, palpitations | Known hypersensitivity, volume depletion, children | Cimetidine, fluconazole, digoxin, phenobarbital | Candesartan (Atacand), eprosartan (Teveten), irbesartan (Avapro), losartan (Cozaar), olmesartan (Benicar), telmisartan (Micardis), valsartan (Diovan) |
| Sodium channel blockers | Ventricular and atrial arrhythmias | New or worsened arrhythmia, dizziness, nausea, headache, fatigue, palpitations, dyspnea | Breastfeeding, heart block, pregnancy, known hypersensitivity, severe renal or liver disease | Other antiarrhythmics, anticholinergics, digoxin, warfarin, cimetidine | Disopyramide (Norpace), flecainide (Tambocor), lidocaine (Xylocaine) **(emergency IV use only)**, mexiletene (Mexitel), phenytoin (Dilantin), procainimide (Procainimide HCl, Procan, Procanabid, Pronestyl), propafenone (Rhythmol), quinidine (Cardioquin, Quinaglute Dura-Tabs, Quinidex), tocainide (Tonocard) |

*Continued*

## Master the Essentials: Cardiovascular Medications—cont'd

| Class | Indications for Use | Side Effects | Contraindications and Precautions | Interactions | Examples |
|---|---|---|---|---|---|
| Potassium channel blockers | Life-threatening ventricular arrhythmia | Hypotension, nausea, anorexia, malaise, fatigue, tremor, pulmonary toxicity | Known hypersensitivity, severe sinus node dysfunction, second- or third-degree heart block, severe aortic stenosis, severe pulmonary hypertension | Sympathomimetics, antihypertensives, warfarin, digoxin, procainamide | Amiodarone (Cordarone), azimilide (Stedicor), bepridil, bretylium tosylate, dofetilide (Tikosyn), ibutilide (Corvert), sotalol (Betapace), tedisamil |
| Vasopressors | Hypotension | Angina, apnea, dyspnea, dizziness, headache, necrosis, pallor, palpitations, tremor, weakness, arrhythmias | Ventricular arrhythmias, hypoxia, acidosis | MAO inhibitors, phenytoin, tricyclic antidepressants, oxytocic drugs | Epinephrine, norepinphrine (Levophed), dopamine (Intropin) |
| Inotropic agents | Cardiac decompensation | Increased blood pressure, increased heart rate, premature ventricular beats, allergic reactions | Hypersensitivity, caution with pregnancy and breastfeeding, children | Beta blockers, nitroprusside | Dobutamine (Dobutrex) |
| Vasodilators | Hypertension, angina pectoris | Nausea, vomiting, loss of appetite, diarrhea, constipations, headache, dizziness, anxiety, muscle or joint pain, runny or stuffy nose, mild itching or skin rash | Hypersensitivity, coronary artery disease, rheumatic heart disease | Dizoxide, MAO inhibitors, erectile dysfunction medications | Isorbide dinitrate (Dilatrate-SR, Iso-Bid, Isonate, Isorbid, Isordil, Isotrate, Sorbitrate), isosorbide mononitrate (IMDUR), hydralazine (Apresoline) |

| Drug Class | Use | Adverse Effects | Contraindications | Interactions | Examples |
|---|---|---|---|---|---|
| **HMG-CoA reductase inhibitors** | Hyperlipidemia | Weakness, headache, abdominal pain, nausea, vomiting, constipation, diarrhea, myalgia, rash | Known hypersensitivity, liver disease, elevated liver enzymes, pregnancy, lactation | Itraconazole, erythromycin, protease inhibitors, nefazodone, cyclosporine, antacids, cimetidine | Atorvastatin (Lipitor), cerivastatin (Baycol), fluvastatin (Lescol, Lescol XL), lovastatin (Altocor, Altoprev, Mevacor), pitavastatin (Livalo), pravastatin (Pravachol), rosuvastatin (Crestor), simvastatin (Zocor) |
| **Bile acid sequestrants** | Hyperlipidemia | Constipation, abdominal pain, nausea, vomiting, headache, dizziness | Complete biliary obstruction, known hypersensitivity, pregnancy, lactation | Anticoagulants, corticosteroids, cardiac glycosides, iron | Such as cholestyramine (Questran, Questran Light, Prevalite, Cholestyramine Light, Locholest, Locholest Light), colesevelam (Wechol), colestipol (Colestid, Colestid Flavored) |
| **Fibric acid derivatives** | Hyperlipidemia | Hypersensitivity, adverse GI effects similar to bile acid sequestrants, arrhythmias, gallstones with prolonged use | Gallbladder disease, hepatic or renal dysfunction, pregnancy, peptic ulcer disease, breastfeeding | Anticoagulants, sulfonylureas | Clofibrate (Atromid-S), fenofibrate (Antara, Fenoglide, Lipofen, Lofibra, TriCor, Triglide), fenofibric acid (Tilipix, Fibricor), gemfibrozil (Lopid) |

ACE, angiotensin-converting enzyme; CVA, cerebrovascular accident; GI, gastrointestinal; HMG-CoA, 3-hydroxy-3-methyl-glutaryl-coenzyme A; MAO, monoamine oxidase; MI, myocardial infarction; NSAIDs, nonsteroidal anti-inflammatory drugs

> **● *Fast Tip 16.1*** Nonpharmacological Treatment for Angina Pectoris
>
> All the following strategies can help treat angina: decrease dietary fats, lower blood pressure, develop coping mechanisms for stress, exercise, decrease alcohol consumption, stop smoking, and decrease dietary sodium. If these changes do not improve heart function, nitrates may be prescribed.

If chest pain is caused by a skeletal muscle condition rather than by heart muscle problems, pain relievers such as nonsteroidal anti-inflammatory drugs (NSAIDs) may be effective. Be sure to teach patients to rule out heart problems (excluded as a diagnosis) before medicating chest pain with NSAIDS.

**Virtual Field Trip**

Visit the Web site of the American Heart Association (www.heart.org) and find:
A support group for heart patients in your area
Information to allow you to create an educational tool to decrease behaviors that could lead to heart attacks

## Anticoagulants, antiplatelet, thrombolytic, and antifibrinolytic medications

Anticoagulants and antiplatelet medications prevent the formation of clots. Thrombolytics dissolve clots that have already formed. Aggressive treatment of thrombolytic stroke with anticoagulants and thrombolytics (as well as antihypertensives, discussed later) can increase survival by increasing blood flow to the brain. Thrombolytics can also be used to prevent CVAs and MIs. Antifibrinolytics prevent the destruction of fibrin and thus promote clot formation, which has the opposite effect. This effect is useful, for example, in women with unusually heavy menstrual bleeding because it decreases the amount of blood lost each month.

### Anticoagulants and antiplatelet medications

Anticoagulants such as warfarin (Coumadin), heparin, and enoxaparin (Lovenox) prevent blood from clotting by interrupting the production of proteins called cofactors that work together in the clotting process. Vitamin K controls creation of these cofactors. Coumadin, which is taken orally, decreases the body's vitamin K levels and thus reduces clot formation. Heparin blocks the cofactors thrombin and fibrin from functioning to form clots. Exactly how Lovenox works is not clearly understood. It is believed that the drug attaches to one of the cofactors and neutralizes its effectiveness. Heparin and Lovenox are given by subcutaneous injection several times a day in patients at risk of developing **deep vein thrombosis (DVT).** DVT is the formation of a blood clot in a vein that is located deep inside the body. Most commonly, this occurs in the lower extremities. However, portions of a clot can break off and travel to the brain, heart, or lungs and can cause serious injury or death. Patients at risk are those that are on bedrest and those with fractures to the pelvis, obesity, recent surgery, and a family history of blood clots.

After surgery, a patient may develop DVT because of inactivity. Physicians may prescribe not only anticoagulants to prevent clots but also tight stockings that cover most of the leg. These stockings compress the veins and aid the smooth return of blood to the heart, even if the veins in the leg are weakened. These antiembolic stockings are usually prescribed in addition to, not instead of, medications. Patients taking anticoagulants must have their blood monitored for safety.

The clotting process is complex and has several stages. Anticoagulants interrupt the clotting process and ensure that blood flows smoothly through the vessels. However, if a patient taking anticoagulants has a break in the skin or mucosal integrity, profuse bleeding can occur because the clotting mechanism is disturbed (Fast Tip 16.2).

---

**● Fast Tip 16.2** Patient Teaching About Anticoagulants

Patients taking an anticoagulant should be educated about the risks of this medication. If these patients are injured, clotting will likely be delayed. The following precautions should be taken to avoid injury and thus clotting delays.

- Use an electric razor to avoid injury.
- Reduce intake of green leafy vegetables, green tea, hummus, and other foods that are high in vitamin K, a vitamin necessary for coagulation.
- Watch for signs of abnormal bleeding, such as frequent bruising, bleeding gums, and black, tarry stool.
- Keep appointments to have blood drawn to monitor the effect of anticoagulants.

---

Antiplatelet medications such as aspirin, ticlopidine (Ticlid), clopidogrel (Plavix), abciximab (ReoPro), eptifibatide (Integrilin), and Tirofiban (Aggrastat) prevent platelets from clumping together to form clots. Because aspirin is an over-the-counter (OTC) medication, patients may not understand its potency relative to interfering with clotting. Always ask a patient whether OTC medications, including aspirin, are being taken. Aspirin is showing promise in the survival rates of heart attack victims when the drug is taken when initial symptoms occur and in prevention of subsequent heart attacks when it is taken routinely following an initial heart attack (Drug Spotlight 16.1).

Two other types of antiplatelet medications are adenosine diphosphate (ADP) receptor blockers and glycoprotein IIb/IIIa inhibitors. ADP receptor blockers interfere with the plasma membrane of platelets that prevents clots from forming. An example of this thrombus prevention drug is clopidogrel (Plavix). These medications provide long-term prevention against clot formation.

Glycoprotein IIb/IIIa inhibitors prevent the enzyme that aggregates platelets from working. They are sometimes given before cardiac procedures to prevent clots from forming during surgery or a procedure.

Patients taking antiplatelet medications should also learn the signs of bleeding and precautions. In addition, patients should be educated to avoid foods high in vitamin K because they interfere with anticoagulant therapy. These foods include cabbage, cauliflower, spinach, and other leafy green vegetables, cereals, and soybeans.

### Thrombolytic medications

If other medications fail to prevent clots from blocking blood vessels, thrombolytics can dissolve them. A clot in a vessel such as in DVT is known as a **thrombus**. A clot that breaks loose and travels is an **embolus**. A clot can form in the heart, lung, or brain or in the peripheral circulation. If a thrombus forms in a peripheral vein, as in DVT, the patient will complain of pain and swelling of the extremity.

---

**Drug Spotlight 16.1** *Aspirin (acetylsalicylic acid)*

| | |
|---|---|
| Definition and history | A substance used for pain relief and fever reduction in the form of a powder made from willow bark as far back as 400 to 500 B.C.; patented February 27, 1900 by a German company named Bayer; Bayer forced to give up patent as a result of the treaty of Versailles in 1919 |
| Uses | Used today for pain, inflammation, and fever reduction; taken in high doses for arthritis therapy; side effects must be monitored closely; also taken in low doses to decrease the risk of heart attack and strokes in older adults |
| Side effects | Stomach upset, stomach ulcerations, increased bleeding time |
| Contraindications | Cited as a link in Reye's syndrome in children when taken after a viral infection; therefore, aspirin is not routinely given to children |

When this clot breaks loose, the embolus can travel and cause a heart attack (MI), a pulmonary embolus (blood clot in the lung), or a stroke (blood clot in the brain). In addition, a clot that lodges in the kidney, liver, or other organ may cause damage resulting from lack of blood flow to that organ.

A patient who can be diagnosed and treated within 60 minutes of the onset of symptoms of a CVA can be given a treatment called tissue plasminogen activator (tPA). This thrombolytic medication is given by the IV route and is approved for use in acute stroke. If it is given within 60 minutes of the onset of symptoms, the effects of the stroke are minimized.

Thrombolytics can also be used to clear IV catheters and cannulas blocked with blood, but these medications must be used with extreme caution. If the blood has been in the cannula too long, injecting the drug can break off the clot rather than dissolve it.

Uncontrolled bleeding is just as dangerous as clotting. Clots must be dissolved quickly to prevent ischemia and infarction; however, a patient can die of uncontrolled bleeding as well. Therefore, frequent testing is necessary to ensure that the dose of anticoagulants, antiplatelets, or thrombolytics is therapeutic. The most common tests are prothrombin time (PT), activated partial thromboplastin time (aPTT), and international normalized ratio (INR). These tests are also used with anticoagulant, antiplatelet, and antithrombolytic therapy. PT is a blood test done to evaluate the ability of blood to clot and is often performed before surgical procedures. The aPTT blood test is usually done to evaluate the effectiveness of heparin therapy. An INR is a blood test performed to determine how long it takes blood to clot and is used primarily in patients taking Coumadin.

### Antifibrinolytic medications

Antifibrinolytic medications have an effect opposite to that of thrombolytics in that they help form clots when the patient is losing too much blood (hemorrhaging) and thereby provide **hemostasis** (stops the bleeding). "Anti" means against, and "lytic" means to break down. These drugs work against the breakdown of fibrin and thus allow fibrin to form a clot. Examples include aminocaproic acid (Amicar) and tranexamic acid (Cyklokapron).

Blood loss can also be treated with other hemostatic drugs, such as vitamin K, protamine sulfate, and desmopressin acetate (DDAVP). They help regulate the clotting process. As described earlier, vitamin K is responsible for the formation of the cofactors responsible for clotting. Vitamin K is an antidote for anticoagulant overdose because it increases the production of those cofactors. Protamine sulfate is specifically administered by the IV route as an antidote to heparin overdose. DDAVP is an artificially made hormone that naturally occurs in the pituitary gland. This medication is used specifically in the treatment of hemophilia (bleeding disorders) in which the patient is lacking factor VIII and von Willebrand factor. DDAVP can raise the levels of these necessary clotting factors without the administration of blood products.

## Medications that promote blood cell development (hematopoietic stimulants)

Some medications stimulate the growth of blood cells. Hematopoietic stimulant medications are used to treat anemias such as sickle cell and pernicious anemia (vitamin $B_{12}$ deficiency). They are also used to treat patients with low blood iron levels, which decrease the ability of the red blood cells to carry oxygen. In addition, patients who are receiving chemotherapy often have lowered blood levels resulting from the bone marrow suppressing effects of that treatment.

One example of a hematopoietic stimulant is ferrous sulfate (Feosol, Fer-in-Sol, Ferra-TD). This medication is taken by mouth and specifically treats iron deficiency anemia. Another medication is cyanocobalamin (vitamin $B_{12}$) and is used in patients who cannot absorb vitamin $B_{12}$ in the GI tract, such as those with pernicious anemia. Therefore, injectable vitamin $B_{12}$ is usually administered to facilitate blood cell development for the remainder of their lifetime. This, in turn, promotes oxygen delivery to the cells and boosts the patient's energy. Medications such as filgrastim (Neupogen), pegfilgrastim (Neulasta), and sargramostim (Leukine) are given to stimulate blood cell development (see the Master the Essentials table for contraindications to and precautions for these medications).

### Virtual Field Trip

Search the Internet for a list of side effects of cancer medications on blood cells. Print the list, and bring it to class for discussion.

## Medications that decrease blood pressure

Cardiac output, peripheral resistance, and blood volume interact to create blood pressure. Cardiac output is the product of the heart rate and the stroke volume (amount of blood that is pumped with each heartbeat). Peripheral resistance is determined by the size and flexibility of the arteries. Therefore, the force of the heart's contraction, the amount of blood that is pumped, and the resistance, or "give," of the blood vessels all influence blood pressure. The kidneys also play a key role by regulating circulating fluid volume (A Closer Look 16.2).

---

### A CLOSER LOOK 16.2: Cardiac Output, Peripheral Vascular Resistance, Blood Volume, and Blood Pressure

Cardiac output (CO), peripheral resistance, and blood volume all interact to create blood pressure (BP). CO relates to the volume of blood that fills the heart, the force of the heart contraction, and the ability of the heart to relax. It is calculated by multiplying heart rate (HR) and stroke volume (SV), the amount of blood in the left ventricle.

$$CO = HR \times SV$$

The sympathetic and parasympathetic nervous systems control the HR, so medications that affect the HR may also affect CO. BP is the product of CO and peripheral vascular resistance (PVR).

$$BP = CO \times PVR$$

PVR is the amount of force in the peripheral blood vessels. If the PVR is higher than normal, the heart has to work harder to maintain appropriate CO, which is the volume of blood the heart pumps each minute.

SV may be referred to as preload, and PVR is referred to as afterload. If a medication decreases the preload of the heart, the **contractility** (ability of the heart to contract) improves. If a medication decreases the afterload, the heart works more efficiently.

---

Poor heart action, **atherosclerosis** (fatty plaques in the arteries), kidney failure, narrowed peripheral blood vessels caused by diabetes mellitus, and chronic stress can cause hypertension.

**Hypertension (HTN),** or high blood pressure, is a major cause of death and disability. Chronic high blood pressure can reduce the kidney's ability to remove excess fluid and consequently puts a strain on circulatory organs.

Antihypertensives, which reduce blood pressure, include angiotensin-converting enzyme (ACE) inhibitors, autonomic nervous system agents, diuretics, and calcium channel blockers. Many of these drugs are also used to treat heart failure and are discussed later. To help you understand where in the process each class of medications works, please review A Closer Look 16.3 to refresh your understanding of blood pressure regulation.

---

### A CLOSER LOOK 16.3: Blood Pressure Regulation

Blood pressure regulation is a complex process. The primary regulation is carried out by the medulla oblongata (the vasomotor center in the brain), chemoreceptors, and baroreceptors. Chemoreceptors recognize oxygen and carbon dioxide levels and pH in the blood. Baroreceptors sense pressure in the large blood vessels. Both types of receptors pass on their information to the medulla, which then tells the body how to respond.

The endocrine system also plays a role through the renin-angiotensin system, illustrated here. This system increases blood pressure through its effects on the blood vessels and the kidneys.

---

*Continued*

## A CLOSER LOOK 16.3: **Blood Pressure Regulation—cont'd**

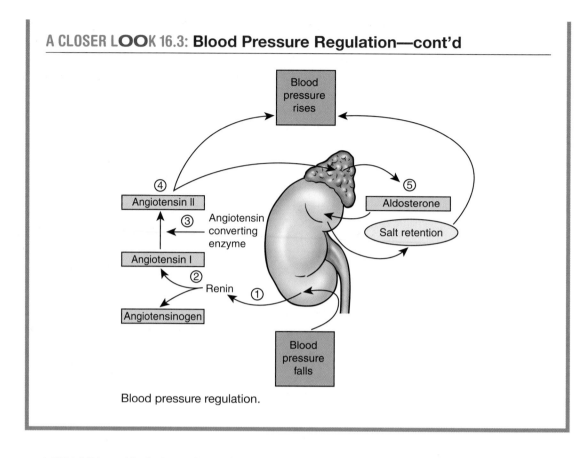

Blood pressure regulation.

ACE inhibitors block the renin-angiotensin pathway from the kidneys to decrease blood pressure. They also help reduce the possibility of heart failure by blocking the action of the renin-angiotensin system. These drugs stop the enzyme that converts angiotensin I to angiotensin II. Angiotensin II is a polypeptide in the blood that causes constriction of the blood vessels that, in turn, increases blood pressure. If there is less angiotensin II, the blood vessels will not constrict, and the blood pressure will not increase. ACE inhibitors include benazepril (Lotensin), captopril (Capoten), enalapril (Vasotec), and fosinopril (Monopril) (for further examples, see the Master the Essentials table).

Angiotensin receptor blockers (ARBs) block the action of angiotensin. These medications work similarly to ACE inhibitors. ARBs prevent angiotensin from attaching to receptors and thus prevent blood vessels from contracting and increasing blood pressure. These medications are sometimes are used when patients are unable to tolerate the side effects of ACE inhibitors. Examples of ARBs include candesartan (Atacand), eprosartan (Teveten), irbesartan (Avapro), losartan (Cozaar), olmesartan (Benicar), telmisartan (Micardis), and valsartan (Diovan).

Autonomic nervous system agents, such as adrenergic blockers (see Chapter 13), relax the fight or flight stress response. They can act on alpha- and beta-adrenergic receptors. Beta-adrenergic blockers such as acebutolol (Sectral), atenolol (Tenormin), bisoprolol (Zebeta), metoprolol, nadolol (Corgard), nebivolol (Bystolic), and propranolol (Inderal LA) are autonomic nervous system agents that decrease the fight or flight response, which causes blood vessels to constrict and the heart to beat faster (see the Master the Essentials table for a full list of beta-blocker medications). These drugs are used to manage hypertension and angina pectoris, slow the heart rate, prevent MIs, reduce congestion associated with heart failure, and treat glaucoma. Reducing the body's perception that it is in a threatening situation can improve cardiovascular function.

Diuretics clear excess fluid from the body and regulate blood pressure by encouraging the kidneys to excrete fluid. Less fluid in the body creates less blood volume and thus less pressure in the blood vessels (decreased peripheral vascular resistance). Diuretics are also used in the treatment of heart failure. The three major classifications of diuretics are thiazides, potassium-sparing diuretics, and loop diuretics. They are classified based on their site of action in the kidney.

■ Thiazide diuretics such as hydrochlorothiazide (HydroDIURIL, Aquazide H, Esidrix, Microzide) and chlorothiazide (Diuril, Diuril Sodium) are the most common classification of diuretic prescribed. Thiazide diuretics work by diminishing the amounts of sodium and chloride reabsorbed by the distal tubule of the kidneys. This effect increases fluid loss and thus decreases blood volume.

- Potassium-sparing diuretics such as amiloride (Midamor), spironolactone (Aldactone), and triamterene (Dyrenium) produce diuresis by interrupting the sodium-potassium exchange in the distal tubule as do the thiazide diuretics, but they spare potassium from being lost, as occurs with thiazide medications.

- Loop diuretics are the most potent of the three classifications. These medications act on the loop of Henle to inhibit the reabsorption of sodium and chloride. This effect, in turn, causes less water to be reabsorbed into the blood and is thus excreted into the urine, to reduce blood volume. Examples of loop diuretics include bumetanide (Bumex), ethacrynic acid (Edecrin, Sodium Edecrin), furosemide (Lasix), and torsemide (Demadex).

When thiazide and loop diuretics work effectively, the patient may lose valuable potassium, so potassium is usually prescribed as a supplement to prevent imbalances that could lead to severe arrhythmias, seizures, and death. Although diuretics relieve heart failure symptoms and decrease blood pressure, they can also significantly disrupt the lives of patients by necessitating frequent trips to the bathroom. A patient may need assistance in planning activities around dosing.

Calcium channel blockers block calcium from passing into the heart muscle and the blood vessel walls. Calcium allows muscles and blood vessels to contract and narrow, thus increasing blood pressure. These medications decrease the level of contraction in the muscles in the arteries and trigger a series of responses: dilation of the arteries, decreased peripheral vascular resistance, reduced workload for the heart, and, ultimately, reduced blood pressure. Calcium channel blockers are used to treat angina and certain tachyarrhythmias, as well as hypertension. Drugs in this class that are indicated for the treatment of hypertension include amlodipine (Norvasc), diltiazem (Cardizem, Dilacor, Tiazac, Diltia XL), nifedipine (Procardia XL, Adalat), and verapamil hydrochloride (Isoptin, Calan, Verelan, Covera-HS) (additional calcium channel blocker medications are included in the Master the Essentials table).

Ways to decrease or regulate blood pressure without medications include losing weight, ceasing tobacco use, decreasing salt (sodium) intake, limiting alcohol, reducing stress, and exercising.

### *CRITICAL THINKING*

What do you think is the role of stress in hypertension?

## Medications for heart failure

Chronic high blood pressure can place great stress on the heart muscle. The muscle can weaken and fail to push a normal amount of blood around the body, thus leading to a condition called **congestive heart failure (CHF).** When that happens, the kidneys do not receive enough blood, and fluid that would normally be flushed out of the body builds back up in the blood. This additional fluid puts even greater strain on the heart and leads to worsening heart failure.

Although CHF has no cure, some drugs can decrease the symptoms caused by the weakened heart muscle. Drugs used to treat heart failure include vasodilators, which decrease the amount of pressure the heart has to exert to pump blood through the vascular system, and cardiac glycosides, which help the heart to beat more strongly and more efficiently. ACE inhibitors, angiotensin receptor blockers, beta blockers, and diuretics, discussed earlier in the chapter, are also used for the treatment of CHF. They work to slow the heart rate, relax the blood vessels, and decrease the amount of blood that the heart has to push through the vascular system.

Signs and symptoms of CHF are anxiety, restlessness, cyanotic and clammy skin, tachycardia, lower leg edema, tachypnea, persistent cough, and a forward-leaning posture.

### Virtual Field Trip

Locate a drug information Web site, and record the classifications of the following drugs:
Lasix, Apresoline, Lanoxin, Nitrobid, Zocar, Streptase, Plavix, Inderal, quinidine, and heparin sodium.

In addition to taking medications, patients can decrease their symptoms and risk of complications by quitting smoking, exercising, reducing weight, decreasing salt consumption, and minimizing stress. The nicotine in tobacco contracts the blood vessels and increases blood pressure. Exercise decreases stress and causes increased blood flow to the tissue. Reducing body fat reduces the workload required to move an overweight body. With salt goes water; therefore, if the patient retains salt, water is also retained. Increased fluid retention raises blood pressure. Decreasing stress reduces the fight or flight mechanism and thus lowers blood pressure.

## Vasodilators

Vasodilators taken by mouth, such as isosorbide dinitrate (Dilatrate-SR, Iso-Bid, Isonate, Isorbid, Isordil, Isotrate, Sorbitrate), isosorbide mononitrate (IMDUR), and hydralazine (Apresoline), decrease oxygen demand on the heart by decreasing resistance in the vessels (vascular resistance), thereby making it easier for the heart to pump more effectively. In essence, blood vessels open, blood pressure drops, and there is less pressure on the heart. Phosphodiesterase inhibitors, a type of vasodilator, cause vasodilation and increase the force of contraction by blocking the enzyme phosphodiesterase.

## Cardiac glycosides

Cardiac glycosides, which are made up of three sugars, called glycosides, strengthen the heart's **contractility.** In a fight or flight situation, constricting peripheral blood vessels would reduce blood loss if injury occurred. However, this is not a desired effect in the presence of cardiovascular disease. Cardiac glycosides increase the strength of heart contractions, whereas other drugs relax the resistance in the peripheral vessels (reduce afterload). Therefore, combining these drugs makes the cardiovascular system more efficient. Cardiac glycosides such as digoxin (Cardoxin, Digetek, Lanoxicaps, Lanoxin) and digitoxin come from plants, such as purple and white foxglove (Drug Spotlight 16.2).

## Drugs for abnormal heart rhythms

**Dysrhythmias** (heart rhythm irregularities) can be caused by increased blood pressure, cardiac valve disease, coronary artery disease, decreased or increased potassium consumption, heart failure, diabetes mellitus, stroke, MI, and certain medications (Fast Tip 16.3).

Drugs used to treat dysrhythmias are classified by how they act to improve the heart rhythm.

- Sodium channel blockers (class I antiarrhythmics)
- Beta-adrenergic blockers (class II antiarrhythmics)

### Drug Spotlight 16.2 *Lanoxin (digoxin)*

| | |
|---|---|
| Definition and history | Used since the 1700s; obtained from the foxglove plant; chemists have been able to obtain purified drug from the plant so that the dosage and additives can be controlled for better safety |
| Uses | Used today mainly for congestive heart failure by helping the heart to beat more slowly and more strongly |
| Signs of toxicity | Nausea, vomiting, diarrhea, stomach pain, slow heart rate, greenish halo around lights |
| Special considerations? | Digoxin has a narrow therapeutic window; therefore, checking blood levels routinely is necessary |
| Patient education | Must include checking the pulse before taking medication, and if less than 60 beats per minute, do not take medication and call prescriber; call physician if any symptoms of toxicity occur; have blood levels drawn as advised; bulk laxatives and antacids containing aluminum will decrease digoxin levels in body, so avoid these |

> ● *Fast Tip 16.3*  Do Not Miss Dysrhythmias
>
> Be sure you accurately check a patient's pulse for a full minute so you do not miss a dysrhythmia that would prevent the patient from benefiting from medication therapy.

- Potassium channel blockers (class III antiarrhythmics)
- Calcium channel blockers (class IV antiarrhythmics)

Each class of medications is described here.

### Sodium channel blockers (class I)

Sodium channel blockers slow the rate of electrical conduction by inhibiting sodium. Sodium is necessary to facilitate nerve impulses and muscular contraction. Blocking sodium transfer therefore inhibits irregular rhythms. Sodium also is the main contributor to osmotic pressure and hydration. Class I antiarrhythmic medications are used to treat those irregular heart beats that originate above the ventricles; these are also called supraventricular rhythms. Some medications in class I include flecainide (Tambocor TM), propafenone (Rhythmol), and quinidine (Cardioquin, Quinaglute Dura-Tabs, Quinidex). All these medications are taken orally. In the case of emergencies with a life-threatening ventricular arrhythmia, lidocaine (Xylocaine) may be administered via the IV route to decrease the sensitivity of the heart muscle.

### Beta-adrenergic blockers (class II)

Beta-adrenergic blockers slow electrical conduction in the heart and return the heart rhythm to normal. They can also be used to decrease oxygen demands for the heart by decreasing the fight or flight response. This is the same class of medications discussed earlier under medications that lower blood pressure. Some class II medications include atenolol (Tenormin), esmolol, and propranolol (Inderal).

### Potassium channel blockers (class III)

Potassium channel blockers are very successful in treating both ventricular and supraventricular arrhythmias. Patients with internal defibrillators are prescribed this class of medications if they are at high risk for sudden cardiac arrest because these medications will reduce the occurrence and severity of arrhythmias. Potassium channel blockers change the heart rhythm by affecting potassium, a necessary element for contraction of cardiac muscle. If too much potassium is lost through the use of diuretics or a poor diet, the patient may need to take potassium supplements or eat foods high in potassium, such as oranges, sweet potatoes, and bananas. Examples of class III antiarrhythmics include amiodarone (Cordarone), azimilide (Stedicor), bepridil, bretylium tosylate, dofetilide (Tikosyn), ibutilide (Corvert), sotalol (Betapace), and tedisamil.

### Calcium channel blockers (class IV)

As discussed earlier, calcium channel blockers block calcium ions, dilate heart vessels, and thus decrease the workload of the heart. This class of antiarrhythmics is generally used for those patients with very rapid arrhythmias. The specific calcium channel blocker medications used for arrhythmias include diltiazem (Cardizem, Tiazac) and verapamil (Dovera, Isoptin, Calan).

## Medications for shock

**Shock** is the collapse of the cardiovascular system, and it can be of cardiogenic origin (heart stops pumping), hypovolemic origin (loss of blood volume), neurogenic origin (central nervous system fails leading to vasodilation), or septic origin (invasion of a microorganism). Treatment of shock primarily targets the underlying causes, as well as supports the cardiovascular system while that cause is treated. Signs and symptoms of shock affect every portion of the body. In the early stages, the metabolism slows, causing the temperature to drop and the patient to complain of thirst. The skin becomes cold, clammy, and pale. Urine output diminishes because of the lack of circulating blood volume. As blood

# Essentials Review

For further study and practice with drug classifications learned in this chapter, complete the following table to the best of your ability. Use resources such as the *PDR,* the Internet, or printed drug guides for help.

| Classification | Purpose | Side Effects | Contraindications and Precautions | Examples | Patient Education |
|---|---|---|---|---|---|
| Anticoagulants | | | | | |
| Antiplatelet agents | | | | | |
| ACE inhibitors | | | | | |
| Diuretics | | | | | |
| Calcium channel blockers | | | | | |
| Vasopressors | | | | | |

ACE, angiotensin-converting enzyme.

# Immunological System Medications

*The immunological system protects the body from disease. Specialized cells attack invading microbes and then eliminate the damaged cells. Most often, medications are used to enhance or strengthen the body's immune system; however, at other times, drugs are used to suppress an immune response, such as in allergic reactions and rejection of transplanted organs. A healthy immune system means a healthy body.*

## LEARNING OUTCOMES

At the end of this chapter, the student will be able to:

17.1  Define key terms.

17.2  Discuss five categories of anti-inflammatory medications, when they are used, and their actions in the body.

17.3  Differentiate among the five classifications of anti-infectives, and describe when each is used and their actions in the body.

17.4  Compare the four types of acquired immunity a body develops and how they occur.

17.5  Identify at least three types of antineoplastic medications, and describe when each is used and their actions in the body.

17.6  Discuss the toxic effects of antineoplastic medications on patients and health-care workers, including the proper handling of both medications and patients' secretions.

---

### KEY TERMS

| | | |
|---|---|---|
| Active artificial immunity | Bactericidal | Metastasis |
| Active natural immunity | Bacteriostatic | Nosocomial |
| Aerobe | Chemotherapy | Passive artificial immunity |
| Antibodies | Culture and sensitivy | Passive natural immunity |
| Antigen | (C & S) | Pathogenic |
| Autoimmune | Host | Superinfection |

---

# ■ THE IMMUNE RESPONSE

When microbes or other **antigens** (foreign substance) invade the body, the body responds by attacking the antigen. The natural response against any microbe invasion is inflammation (Fig. 17-1), which helps limit the spread of microbes or injury. Several phases occur during this attack.

The first response occurs at the site of the invasion (e.g., a cut), where chemicals are released such as bradykinin (a vasodilator that causes pain), complement, (a protein that destroy antigens), and three chemicals released by mast cells: histamine; leukotrienes, both of which cause smooth muscle contraction, blood vessel dilation, and itching; and prostaglandins, which increase capillary permeability, attract leukocytes to the inflammation site, and increase pain.

The second phase occurs as the immune system launches an attack throughout the body by secreting **antibodies** (immunoglobins that fight antigens) that are specific to the invading antigen.

Additionally, some B cells (memory cells) record the attack and help guard against those particular microbes if they enter the body again. Vaccines are administered to encourage the production of these memory cells.

T cells (CD cells) are lymphocytes and do not produce antibodies but instead create cytokines. Some cytokines create inflammation, and others attack the invader directly.

# ■ MEDICATIONS THAT AFFECT THE IMMUNE SYSTEM

Medications are used to support or inhibit the immune response, depending on the patient's condition. Various anti-inflammatory medications may be given to suppress the immune response when a patient is faced with allergies, asthma attacks, or autoimmune disorders. Anti-infective medications may be given to combat bacterial infections. Antitoxin, antifungal, antiviral, and antiparasitic medications fight off other invading microorganisms. Vaccines are given from birth to very old age in an effort to prevent microorganisms from causing disease. The last category of medication discussed in this chapter comprises antineoplastic medications, more commonly known as chemotherapy. Chemotherapy is used to combat cancer (see the Master the Essentials table for descriptions of the most common immunological system drugs).

### Anti-inflammatory medications

Anti-inflammatory medications shut off or reduce the body's inflammatory response. They may be used in patients with such conditions as anaphylaxis, ankylosing spondylitis, rheumatoid arthritis, ulcerative colitis, Crohn's disease, dermatitis, type 1 diabetes mellitus, glomerulonephritis, Hashimoto's thyroiditis, multiple sclerosis, peptic ulcers, allergic rhinitis, and systemic lupus erythematosus. These diseases are called **autoimmune** disorders, in which the body's immune system attacks itself and must be stopped to halt the damage caused by this attack.

Allergies are an overresponse of the body's defense to substances that may not be an actual threat to the body. Examples of sensitizing substances are pollen, animal dander, mold, mildew, dust, and cigarette smoke. Patients may also have allergic reactions to food or medications.

*(Text continues on page 312)*

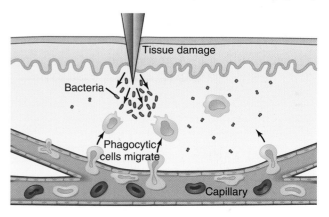

**FIGURE 17-1:** The inflammatory response. When bacteria or other antigens invade the body, the first response is inflammation, which helps limit the spread of the invading microorganisms.

## Master the Essentials: Immunological System Medications

This table shows the various classes of immunological medications and key side effects, contraindications and precautions, interactions, and examples of each class.

| Class | Indications for Use | Side Effects | Contraindications and Precautions | Interactions | Examples |
|-------|---------------------|--------------|-----------------------------------|--------------|----------|
| Antihistamines | Allergies, prophylactic use before medications likely to cause allergic reaction | CNS depression (sedation, dizziness, muscle weakness), epigastric distress, dry mouth | Known hypersensitivity, breastfeeding, MAO inhibitors, glaucoma, hypertension | CNS depressants, anticholinergics, aminoglycosides, salicylates, epinephrine | Diphenhydramine (Benadryl), loratadine (Claritin, Tavist), cetirizine (Zyrtec) |
| Glucocorticoids | Suppression of immune response; severe inflammation | Behavioral changes, hyperglycemia, increased susceptibility to infection, osteoporosis, hypertension | Known hypersensitivity, systemic fungal infection | Phenytoin, salicylates, NSAIDs, vaccines, estrogen, antihypertensives | Beclomethasone (Beclovent, Qvar, Vanceril, Vanceril DS), budesonide (Entocort EC), ciclesonide (Omnaris), flunisolide (AeroBid, AeroBid-M), fluticasone (Flovent), triamcinolone (Aristocort), dexamethasone (Decadron), hydrocortisone (Cortef, Solu-Cortef), methylprednisolone (Medrol, Solu-Medrol), prednisolone (Pediapred, Prelone), prednisone |
| Nasal decongestants | Nasal congestion | Arrhythmias, hypertension, headaches, nausea, sneezing, dryness (topical) | Known hypersensitivity, MAO inhibitors, hypertension | Beta blockers, MAO inhibitors, tricyclic antidepressants | Naphazoline (Privine), phenylephrine (Dimetapp Cold Drops, PediaCare Children's Decongestant, Sudafed PE Quick Dissolve, Triaminic Thin Strips Cold, Lusonal, Nasop), phenylpropanolamine (Rhindecon), propylhexedrine (Benzedrex), pseudoephedrine (Sudafed, Suphedrin), tetrahydrozoline (Tyzine Nasal) |
| NSAIDs | Inflammation, pain, fever | Nausea, vomiting, hypersensitivity reactions, vertigo, insomnia, rash | Known hypersensitivity, renal disease, GI bleeding, allergic reaction to sulfonamides | ACE inhibitors, fluconazole, phenobarbital, phenobarbital, cyclosporine, corticosteroids, anticoagulants | Aspirin, celecoxib (Celebrex), diclofenac (Voltaren), diflunisal (Dolobid), etodolac (Lodine), ibuprofen (Advil, Motrin, Nuprin, Haltran), indomethacin (Indocin), ketoprofen (Actron, Orudis, Oruvail), ketorolac (Toradol), nabumetone (Relafen), naproxen (Aleve, Anaprox, Naprosyn), oxaprozin (Daypro), piroxicam (Feldene), salsalate (Amigesic, Disalcid Salsitab, Marthritic), sulindac (Clinoril), tolmetin (Tolectin) |

Continued

## Master the Essentials: Immunological System Medications—cont'd

| Class | Indications for Use | Side Effects | Contraindications and Precautions | Interactions | Examples |
|---|---|---|---|---|---|
| Immunosuppressants | Autoimmune diseases such as lupus or rheumatoid arthritis; organ transplant | Leukopenia, thrombocytopenia, nephrotoxicity, hyperkalemia, hypertension, diarrhea, nausea | Known hypersensitivity, pregnancy, breastfeeding | Allopurinol, aminoglycosides, other immunosuppressants, calcium channel blockers, cardiac glycosides | Azathioprine (Imuran, Azasan), corticosteroids, cyclosporine (Neoral, Sandimmune, Gengraf), sirolimus (Rapamune) |
| Penicillins | Common infections with gram-positive and gram-negative bacteria | Blood changes, CNS effects, diarrhea, hypersensitivity, kidney and liver disorders, nausea, vomiting | Known hypersensitivity, decreased renal function, electrolyte imbalances | Antagonizes antacids and foods; probenecid potentiates penicillin; may decrease the action of oral contraceptives | Ampicillin (Omnipen, Principen), amoxicillin (Amoxil), carbenicillin (Geocillin), dicloxacillin (Dycill, Dynapen), nafcillin (Nallpen, Unipen) oxacillin (Bactocill), penicillin (Pen VK) penicillin g benzathine/potassium/sodium (Bicillin), piperacillin, ticarcillin (Ticar) |
| Cephalosporins | **First generation:** gram-positive bacterial infections in patients' allergic to penicillins **Second generation:** nosocomial pneumonia **Third generation:** gram-negative bacterial infections **Fourth generation:** severe nosocomial surgical infections | Bleeding, diarrhea, hypersensitivity, liver dysfunction, kidney disease, nausea, phlebitis, respiratory distress, seizures, vomiting, vaginal itching or discharge, headache | Known hypersensitivity, children, kidney impairment, lactation, pregnancy; not for long-term use | Alcohol and diuretics | **First generation:** cefazolin (Ancef, Kefzol), cefadroxil (Duricef), cephalexin (Biocef, Keflex), cephalothin (Keflin), cephapirin (Cefadyl), cephradine (Velosef) **Second generation:** cefaclor (Ceclor, Raniclor), cefprozil (Cefzil), cefotetan (Cefotan), cefuroxime (Ceftin, Zinacef), cefoxitin (Mefoxin), loracarbef (Lorabid) **Third generation:** cefdinir (Omnicef), cefditoren (Spectracef), cefixime (Suprax), cefoperazone (Cefobid), cefotaxime (Claforan), cefpodoxime (Vantin), ceftazidime (Ceptaz, Fortaz, Tazicef), ceftibuten (Cedax), ceftriaxone (Rocephin), ceftizoxime (Cefizox) **Fourth generation:** cefepime (Maxipime) |

| Class | Uses | Side Effects | Contraindications | Interactions | Examples |
|---|---|---|---|---|---|
| **Tetracyclines** | Gram-negative and/ or gram-positive bacterial infections | Allergic hypersensitivity, CNS malfunction, diarrhea, decreased bone growth in a fetus or child, discolored teeth in fetus or child, light sensitivity, thrombophlebitis, nausea, superinfection, vomiting | Children, direct sunlight, esophageal illness, kidney and liver disease, lactation, pregnancy | Antacids, antidiarrheal agents, calcium, dairy products, iron, magnesium, oral contraceptives, zinc | Doxycycline (Adoxa, Alodox, Avidoxy, Doryx, Monodox, Oracea, Oraxyl, Periostat, Vibramycin, Morgidox), minocycline (Dynacin, Minocin, Myrac, Solodyn, Vectrin), tetracycline (Ala-Tet, Panmycin, Sumycin) |
| **Macrolides** | Bacterial infections resistant to penicillin | Anorexia, cramps, diarrhea, nausea, superinfection, urticaria, vomiting | Alcoholism and liver damage | Cyclosporine, digoxin Halcion, Tegretol, theophylline, warfarin | Erythromycin (E.E.S. Granules, Ery-Tab, Erythrocin Stearate Filmtab), clarithromycin (Biaxin), azithromycin (Zithromax, Zithromax, Z-Pak) |
| **Aminoglycosides** | Aerobic gram-negative bacteria, mycobacteria, or some protozoal infections | Blurred vision, CNS symptoms, ear damage, kidney disease, paralysis (including respiratory paralysis), rash urticaria | Decreased kidney function, dehydration, infancy, high-frequency hearing loss, lactation, pregnancy, tinnitus, vertigo | Antiemetics, general anesthesia, ototoxic drugs | Amikacin (Amikin), gentamicin (Cidomycin, Garamycin, Septopal), kanamycin (Kantrex), neomycin (Mycifradin, Neo-Fradin, Neo-Tab), paromomycin (Humatin, Paromycin), tobramycin (Nebcin, Tobi) |
| **Quinolones** | Chronic urinary tract infections | CNS effects, diarrhea, toxicity in sunlight, nausea, superinfections, vomiting | Cardiovascular disorders, children, kidney disease, lactation, pregnancy | Antacids, calcium, Coumadin, iron, magnesium, probenecid, theophylline, zinc | Ciprofloxacin (Ciloxan Ophthalmic, Cipro), enoxacin (Penetrex), gatifloxacin (Tequin), levofloxacin (Levaquin, QUIXIN Ophthalmic), lomefloxacin (Maxaquin), moxifloxacin (Avelox), norfloxacin (Chibroxin Ophthalmic, Noroxin Oral), ofloxacin (Floxin, Ocuflox Ophthalmic), sparfloxacin (Zagam), trovafloxacin (Trovan) |
| **Sulfonamides** | Acute urinary tract infections | Fever, crystalluria, nausea, vomiting, diarrhea, rash, photosensitivity | Known hypersensitivity, impaired kidney or liver function, lactation, pregnancy | Anticoagulants, antidiabetics, local anesthesia, cyclosporine | Erythromycin-sulfisoxazole (Pediazole), sulfadiazine, sulfamethizole (Thiosulfil Forte), sulfamethoxazole (Gantanol), sulfasalazine (Azulfidine), sulfisoxazole (Gantrisin), trimethoprim-sulfamethoxazole (Septra, Bactrim) |

*Continued*

## Master the Essentials: Immunological System Medications—cont'd

| Class | Indications for Use | Side Effects | Contraindications and Precautions | Interactions | Examples |
|---|---|---|---|---|---|
| Antitoxins | Exposure to toxin in at-risk patient | **Diphtheria:** Fever, inflammation of joints, muscle aches, reddening of skin around ears, swollen lymph glands, weakness **Tetanus:** Pain at injection site, hypersensitivity | Known hypersensitivity, caution in pregnancy and breastfeeding | None reported | Botulism antitoxin (Heptavalent (HBAT), diphtheria antitoxin tetanus immune globulin (Baytet, HyperTET S/D) |
| Antituberculosis Agents | Tuberculosis infection and/or exposure | Allergic reaction, dizziness, seizures, numbness or tingling in extremities, rash, confusion, tremors, headache, drowsiness, irritability, fatigue, red/orange urine, stool, tears, sweat, saliva (rifampin, rifabutin), liver damage (INH), nausea, vomiting, anorexia | Epilepsy, psychiatric disorders, kidney disorder, alcoholism, children, lactation, liver or kidney disease, pregnancy | Ethionamide, rifampin may make birth control pill less effective; alcohol, anticoagulants, corticosteroids, digoxin, estrogen, phenytoin | Cycloserine (Seromycin), ethambutol (Myambutol), ethionamide (Trecator SC), isoniazid (Nydrazid), pyrazinamide, rifabutin (Mycobutin), rifampin (Rifadin, Rimactane) |
| Antifungals | Fungal infections | Anemia, chills, hypotension, dizziness, fever, headache, hypokalemia, kidney damage, malaise, muscle and joint pain and weakness, tachycardia, photosensitivity | Children, liver damage, penicillin hypersensitivity, pregnancy, porphyria | Alcohol, anticoagulants, oral contraceptives, phenobarbital | **Topical:** amphotericin B (Fungizone), benzoic acid/salicylic acid (Bensal HP), ciclopirox (CNL8 Nail, Loprox, Penlac), clotrimazole (Canesten, Lotrimin, Mycelex), econazole (Spectazole), haloprogin (Halotex), ketoconazole (Extina, Nizoral, Xolegel), miconazole (Aloe Vesta, Baza, Dermagran AF, Desenex, Lotrimin, Micatin, Monistat, Zeasorb-AF), miconazole/zinc oxide (Vusion), naftifine (Naftin), nystatin (Mycostatin, Pedi-Dri), oxiconazole (Oxistat), sertaconazole (Ertaczo), sulconazole (Exelderm), terbinafine (Lamisil), tolnaftate (Absorbine, Aftate, Blis-To-Sol, Tinactin), undecylenic acid (Blis-To-Sol Powder, Cruex, Trifungol) |

| Category | Uses | Side Effects | Contraindications | Interactions | Examples |
|---|---|---|---|---|---|
| | | | | | **Systemic:** amphotericin B (Fungizone), caspofungin (Cancidas), flucytosine, fluconazole (Diflucan), itraconazole (Sporanox), ketoconazole (Nizoral), miconazole (Monistat I.V.) |
| Antivirals | Viral infections | Confusion, diarrhea, headache, kidney disease, nausea, rash, urticaria, vomiting | Children, dehydration, lactation, kidney disease, neurological disease, pregnancy | Probenecid, nephrotoxic agents, cytotoxic agents, anticholinergics | Acyclovir (Acivir, Acivirax, Cyclovir, Herplex, Zovirax, Zovir), amantadine (Symmetrel), cidofovir (Vistide), oseltamivir (Tamiflu), ribavirin (Copegus, Rebetol, RibaPak, Ribasphere, Ribatab, Virazole), zanamivir (Relenza) |
| Antiretrovirals | HIV infection | Fat redistribution, hypoglycemia, GI upset, kidney stones | Known hypersensitivity, breastfeeding, pregnancy, kidney or liver impairment | Alcohol, oral contraceptives | **Multiclass combination medications:** efavirenz/emtricitabine/tenofovir (Atripla), emtricitabine/rilpivirine/tenofovir (Complera) **Nucleoside reverse transcriptase inhibitors (NRTIs):** abacavir/lamivudine (Epzicom), abacavir sulfate/ABC (Ziagen), abacavir/zidovudine/lamivudine (Trizivir), emtricitabine/FTC (Emtriva), didanosine/dideoxyinosine (Videx), lamivudine/zidovudine (Combivir), lamivudine/3TC (Epivir), stavudine/d4T (Zerit), tenofovir disoproxil fumarate/emtricitabine (Truvada), tenofovir disoproxil fumarate (Viread), zidovudine/azidothymidine (Retrovir) **Nonnucleoside reverse transcriptase inhibitors (NNRTIs):** delavirdine (Rescriptor), efavirenz (Sustiva), etravirine (Intelence), nevirapine (Viramune), rilpivirine (Edurant) **Protease inhibitors:** amprenavir (Agenerase), atazanavir sulfate (Reyataz), darunavir (Prezista), indinavir (Crixivan), fosamprenavir calcium (Lexiva), lopinavir/ritonavir (Kaletra), nelfinavir mesylate (Viracept), ritonavir (Norvir), saquinavir mesylate (Invirase), tipranavir (Aptivus) **Fusion inhibitors:** enfuvirtide (Fuzeon) **Entry inhibitors-CCR5 coreceptor antagonist:** maraviroc (Selzentry) **HIV integrase strand transfer inhibitors:** raltegravir (Isentress), delavirdine (Rescriptor), nelfinavir (Viracept), ritonavir (Norvir) |

*Continued*

# Master the Essentials: Immunological System Medications—cont'd

| Class | Indications for Use | Side Effects | Contraindications and Precautions | Interactions | Examples |
|---|---|---|---|---|---|
| Antimalarials | Prevention and treatment of malaria | Visual disturbances, hearing changes, nausea, vomiting, diarrhea, anorexia, muscle weakness, rash | Known hypersensitivity, pregnancy, breastfeeding, kidney disease, liver disease, uncontrolled vomiting or diarrhea | Cimetidine, kaolin, magnesium trisilicate | Atovaquone/proguanil (Malarone), chloroquine (Aralen), mefloquine (Lariam), primaquine |
| Antiprotozoal drugs | Treatment of protozoal infection | Altered blood glucose levels both high and low; taste changes, diarrhea, nausea, vomiting | Diabetes, heart problems, kidney disease, pancreatic disease, asthma, recent radiation or chemotherapy, caution with pregnancy, breastfeeding | Azathioprine, carbamazepine, antibiotics, NSAIDs, chemotherapy, birth control pills, antihypertensives, antidiabetics, metoclopramide | Metronidazole (Flagyl, Metro I.V.), pentamidine (Nebupent, Pentam 300), trimethoprimsulfamethoxazole (Bactrim, Septra, Sulfatrim) |
| Anthelmintics | Treatment of tapeworms, roundworms, hookworms, pinworms, and flukes | Headache, dizziness, nausea, mild fever, skin rash, fatigue | Known sensitivity, caution with pregnancy and breastfeeding, patients less than 2 years of age | Cimetidine, chloroquine, itraconazole, ketoconazole, dexamethasone, erythromycin, barbiturates, HIV medications, antiseizure medications | Albendazole (Albenza), praziquantel (Biltricide), ivermectin (Stromectol), mebendazole (Vermox), pyrantel (Antiminth, Ascarel, Pin-X), praziquantel (Biltricide) |
| Pediculicides | Lice treatment | Allergic reactions, stinging or skin irritation, dizziness, drowsiness | Known hypersensitivity, nonintact skin, HIV/AIDS, risk factors for seizures | None reported | Permethrin (Acticin, Elimite, and Nix), piperonyl butoxide/pyrethrins (Licide, RID), spinosad (Natroba), malathion (Ovide), benzyl alcohol lotion (Ulesfia), lindane |

| Category | Uses | Side Effects | Contraindications | Drug Interactions | Medications |
|---|---|---|---|---|---|
| Scabicides | Scabies treatment | Mild itching, burning or skin | Known hypersensitivity, caution with pregnancy and breastfeeding, HIV/AIDS, risk factors for seizures | None reported | Crotamiton (Eurax), lindane, permethrin (Acticin, Elimite) |
| Alkylating agents | Leukemia, solid tumors | Allergic reactions, nausea, vomiting, diarrhea, bone marrow suppression, pulmonary fibrosis, hepatotoxicity | Known hypersensitivity, pregnancy, breastfeeding | Anticoagulants, phenobarbital, digoxin | Bendamustine (Treanda), busulfan (Busulfex, Myleran), carboplatin (Paraplatin), carmustin (BiCNU, Gliadel), chlorambucil (Leukeran), cisplatin (Platinol), cyclophosphamide (Cytoxan, Neosar), dacarbazine (DTIC-Dome), ifosfamide (Ifex), lomustine (CeeNU), mechlorethamine (Mustargen), melphalan (Alkeran), oxaliplatin (Eloxatin), streptozocin (Zanosar), temozolomide (Temodar), thiotepa (Thioplex) |
| Antimetabolites | Lung, metastatic breast, pancreatic, and ovarian cancer, GI tumors | Alopecia, bone marrow depression, diarrhea, nausea, neurotoxicity, rash, reproductive ability loss, pulmonary fibrosis, vomiting | Pregnancy, breastfeeding, hepatic impairment | Probenecid, NSAIDs, alcohol, salicylates | 6-Mercaptopurine, cladribine (Cladribine NovaPulse, Leustatin), cytarabine (Cytosar-U, Tarabine PFS), fluorouracil (Efudex, Adrucil), leucovorin (Wellcovorin), methotrexate (Rheumatrex, Trexall), thioguanine (Tabloid) |
| Antitumor antibiotics | Testicular tumors, Hodgkin's lymphoma, tumors of kidney, uterine, bone, muscle, soft tissue cancers | Alopecia, anorexia, bone marrow suppression, cardiotoxicity, nausea, pneumonitis, rash and scaly skin, ulceration of the skin and mouth, vomiting | Known hypersensitivity, pregnancy, renal impairment, heart disease, breastfeeding | Cyclophosphamide, myelosuppressive drugs, hepatotoxic medications, digoxin, phenytoin, oxygen, vitamin E, NSAIDs, warfarin, clopidogrel, ticlopidine | Bleomycin (Blenoxane), dactinomycin (Cosmegen) |
| Plant alkaloids | Soft tissue tumors, Wilms tumor, leukemia, Hodgkin's disease, non-Hodgkin's lymphoma | Alopecia, constipation, diarrhea, nausea, necrosis, neurotoxicity, rash, sensitivity to light, ulcers in the mouth or GI system, vomiting, white blood cell deficiency | Pregnancy, breastfeeding, bacterial infection, severe granulocytopenia, liver impairment | Mitomycin, phenytoin, erythromycin, digoxin | Docetaxel (Docefrez, Taxotere), etoposide (VePesid, Toposar), irinotecan (Camptosar), paclitaxel (Onxol, Taxol), teniposide (Vumon), topotecan (Hycamtin), vinblastine (Velban), vincristine (Oncovin, Vincasar PFS), vinorelbine (Navelbine) |

Continued

## Master the Essentials: Immunological System Medications—cont'd

| Class | Indications for Use | Side Effects | Contraindications and Precautions | Interactions | Examples |
|---|---|---|---|---|---|
| Hormones | Breast, ovarian, testicular, prostate cancer | Hot flashes, decreased sex drive, nausea, vomiting, headache, dizziness, depression | Pregnancy, thromboembolic disorders, breastfeeding, undiagnosed vaginal bleeding | Warfarin, bromocriptine, insulin, corticosteroids, Parlodel, cimetidine, rifampin, heart, hypertension medications, HIV/AIDS medicine, psychiatric medications, migraine medications, narcotics | Aminoglutethimide (Cytadren), anastrazole (Arimidex), bicalutamide (Casodex), estradiol (Estrace, Femtrace, Gynodiol), estramustine (Emcyt), estrogen (Cenestin, Enjuvia, Premarin), exemestane (Aromasin), flutamide (Eulexin), fluoxymesterone (Androxy, Halotestin), goserelin acetate (Zoladex), hydroxyprogesterone caproate (Delta-Lutin, Duralutin, Hylutin, Hyprogesterone, Makena, Prodrox), letrozole (Femara), leuprolide acetate (Eligard, Lupron, Viadur), medroxyprogesterone acetate (Provera), megestrol (Megace), mitotane (Lysodren), nilutamide (Nilandron), raloxifene (Evista), tamoxifen (Soltamox), testolactone (Teslac), testosterone (Andro LA 200, Delatestryl, DepAndro 100, Depo-Testosterone), toremifene (Fareston), triptorelin (Trelstar) |
| Biological response modifiers | Leukemia, malignant melanoma, AIDS-related Kaposi's sarcoma hepatitis B and C | Anemia, bleeding, difficulty breathing, fever, muscle aches and pain, infection, mouth infection, nausea, vomiting, diarrhea, malnutrition, anorexia, alopecia, damage to ear and peripheral nervous system, kidney and heart disease, tingling, loss of reflexes, confusion, personality changes, bone marrow suppression, GI upset | Known hypersensitivity, pregnancy; because of intense side effects, antiemetics may be needed to prevent vomiting | Protease inhibitors, antihypertensives, corticosteroids | Interferon alfa-2a (Roferon-A), interferon alfa-2b (Intron A) |

| | Uses | Adverse Reactions | Contraindications | Drug Interactions | Examples |
|---|---|---|---|---|---|
| **Monoclonal antibodies** | Colon, lung, head, neck, and breast cancer, leukemia, non-Hodgkin's lymphoma | Infusion reactions, arrhythmias, angina, renal failure, bleeding, nausea, thrombocytopenia, rash, abdominal pain, malaise | Known hypersensitivity, pregnancy, breastfeeding | Anticoagulants | Alemtuzumab (Campath), bevacizumab (Avastin), cetuximab (Erbitux), gemtuzumab (Mylotarg), ibritumomab (Zevalin), panitumumab (Vectibix), rituximab (Rituxan), tositumomab (Bexxar), trastuzumab (Herceptin) |
| **Immunomodulators** | Multiple myeloma | Headache, fever, nausea, vomiting, fatigue, myalgia, depression | Known hypersensitivity, depression, kidney or liver disease, autoimmune disorders | Theophylline; neurotoxic, hematotoxic, or cardiotoxic drugs | Lenalidomide (Revlimid), thalidomide (Thalomid) |
| **Radioactive isotopes** | Prostate, lung, cervical, endometrial, bile duct cancer | Radiation sickness, nausea, vomiting, rash, fatigue, low blood counts, difficulty swallowing, changes in taste, anorexia | Pregnancy, breastfeeding | None reported | **Brachytherapy seeds:** iodine-125, iridium-194, palladium-103, thulium-170 |

ACE, angiotensin-converting enzyme; CNS, central nervous system; GI, gastrointestinal; INH, isoniazid; MAO, monoamine oxidase; NSAIDs, nonsteroidal anti-inflammatory drugs.

Signs and symptoms of a mild allergy such as allergic rhinitis are sneezing, nasal congestion, and watery eyes. Patients who have serious reactions, such as anaphylactic shock (the most serious reaction), may experience urticaria (hives), swelling, itching, or difficulty breathing, all of which can be fatal if the patient is not given immediate, proper treatment. Medications used to treat allergic reactions include antihistamines, glucocorticoids, nasal decongestants, nonsteroidal anti-inflammatory drugs (NSAIDs), and immunosuppressants.

### Antihistamines

Antihistamines, such as diphenhydramine (Benadryl), loratadine (Claritin, Tavist), and cetirizine (Zyrtec), as the name suggests, block the histamine response (allergy symptoms) and thereby decrease swelling, itching, and congestion. All these medications are routinely taken by mouth for allergy symptoms associated with seasonal and environmental allergies. In addition, diphenhydramine can be administered by the intravenous (IV) route for severe allergic reactions. These medications are also referred to as $H_1$-receptor antagonists. The effects include relaxation of the respiratory, vascular, and gastrointestinal (GI) smooth muscle.

### Glucocorticoids

Glucocorticoids are steroid-like compounds that suppress the body's inflammatory response. Glucocorticoids such as beclomethasone (Beclovent), budesonide (Entocort), and fluticasone (Flovent) are administered intranasally to combat allergic rhinitis. Medications such as hydrocortisone (Cortef) are administered topically for minor inflammation. Methylprednisolone is a medication that is given systemically, usually in IV form, for acute or severe inflammation such as in spinal cord injury. Because of the serious side effects and danger of long-term suppression of the immune system, glucocorticoids must be used only as prescribed and discontinued gradually. (For a more complete list of glucocorticoids commonly used, please refer to the Master the Essentials table.)

### Nasal decongestants

Nasal decongestants such as naphazoline drops (Privine) and tetrahydrozoline nasal (Tyzine Nasal) can alleviate nasal congestion intranasally by drying secretions. Nasal decongestants such as phenyl-propanolamine (Rhindecon) are taken orally to produce the desired effects. They cause vasoconstriction on the adrenergic receptors in the nose by affecting the sympathetic tone of the blood vessels. The mucous membranes shrink as a result, thereby promoting drainage. These medications are typically used for only 3 to 5 days; otherwise, "rebound" nasal congestion occurs, and the patient continues to suffer.

### Nonsteroidal anti-inflammatory drugs

NSAIDs are, by definition, medications that reduce inflammation and do not contain steroids. They are the most common treatments for inflammation. In addition, NSAIDs also have antipyretic (reduce fever) and analgesic (reduce pain) properties. They accomplish these effects by inhibiting prostaglandin synthesis. Prostaglandins are substances responsible for producing inflammation, fever, and pain. NSAIDs such as ibuprofen (Advil, Motrin) and naproxen (Aleve, Naprosyn) can be purchased over the counter (OTC) and are taken by mouth. Other oral NSAIDs such as diclofenac (Voltaren) and cele-coxib (Celebrex) are available by prescription only for the treatment of conditions such as arthritis. Ketorolac (Toradol) is an NSAID that is given by the IV route for moderate to severe pain. As with all medications, NSAIDs must be taken as directed. Many medications in this class have similar mechanisms, but the patient's response varies. A patient may respond poorly to one NSAID but report great relief from another.

### Immunosuppressants

Immunosuppressants are typically used for long-term therapy of inflammatory diseases, such as rheumatoid arthritis, psoriasis, and Crohn's disease. Rheumatoid arthritis is treated with immunosuppressants such as azathioprine (Imuran, Azasan) and cyclosporine (Neoral, Sandimmune, and Gengraf). Psoriasis (see Chapter 11) is treated with cyclosporine and sirolimus (Rapamune) for a short time (up to several months), alternating with other therapies. Crohn's disease is treated with oral doses of azathioprine (Imuran, Azasan). Corticosteroids are sometimes prescribed for short periods of time to speed up the suppression of the immune system and thus the healing process in inflammatory diseases.

Because long-term suppression of the immune system renders the body vulnerable to infection and certain cancers, the immunosuppressants listed here are used on a long-term basis only to prevent or treat rejection in relation to organ transplants.

## Anti-infective medications

Anti-infective medications are classified by their mechanisms of action or chemical structure. They target the processes of the invading microorganism. Some medications target protein synthesis, others inhibit DNA or RNA synthesis, and still others destroy the cell wall. Anti-infective medications include antibiotics, antitoxins, and antifungal, antiviral, and antiparasitic medications. These medications are discussed in the following subsections.

### Antibiotics

Bacterial organisms have special characteristics: they do not require a **host** (e.g., person or animal) to reproduce, they can change or mutate, and all are potentially vulnerable to antibiotics. Bacteria are named based on their shapes and ability to retain stains, either gram negative or gram positive. Common antibiotic categories include penicillins, cephalosporins, tetracyclines, macrolides, and aminoglycosides. A broad-spectrum antibiotic, one that is effective against many types of bacteria, is prescribed if the bacteria have not yet been identified (A Closer Look 17.1).

---

## A CLOSER LOOK 17.1: **Drug-Resistant Bacteria**

Sometimes a specific bacterium is resistant to antibiotics and is therefore difficult to treat. Resistance to antibiotics occurs when a bacterium becomes weakened, but does not die. The bacterium may then develop an ability to resist this antibiotic the next time it is given. This situation occurs when a medication is not taken for the full time it is ordered. An example of a bacterium-caused disease is otitis media (middle ear infection).

---

Because of the wide range of bacteria, it is vital to prescribe the correct antibiotic. A **culture and sensitivity (C & S)** test can help determine which microorganism is present and which antibiotic would be most effective against it (Fig. 17-2).

Once the bacterium is specifically identified and the laboratory has determined to which antibiotics the microorganism is most vulnerable, the broad-spectrum antibiotic may be changed to one that is more suitable.

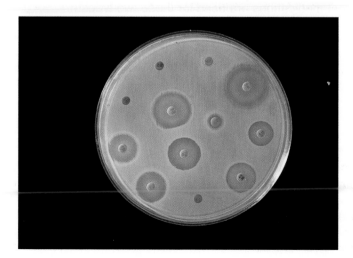

**FIGURE 17-2:** Disk diffusion method. Disks infused with antibiotics are placed on the culture plate to determine which antibiotic will be most effective in killing the bacteria. Clear spaces around the disk represent those antibiotics that are effective against growth of the microorganism.

*Penicillin Medications*

Penicillins such as ampicillin (Omnipen, Principen), amoxicillin (Amoxil), and penicillin (Pen VK) are among the oldest antibiotics, They have been used in various forms since World War II. These medications are used orally, topically, and via injection to treat many common infections, such as strep throat and otitis media. They kill gram-positive and gram-negative bacteria by destroying cell walls (A Closer Look 17.2). Because of the length of time they have been in use, they tend to be the least expensive antibiotics available. Unfortunately, many people are allergic to the penicillins, so other, more expensive antibiotics are needed. (For a more extensive list of penicillin medications, please see the Master the Essentials table.)

### A CLOSER LOOK 17.2: All About Bacteria

Bacteria are characterized by their shape, how they stain, and whether they need oxygen to survive.

*Shape.* Bacteria shaped like rods are called bacilli. An example of a rod-shaped bacterium is gonorrhea. Bacteria shaped like spheres are called cocci. Strep throat is caused by streptococci. Spiral-shaped bacteria are called spirilla. Syphilis and Lyme disease are illnesses caused by spirilla.

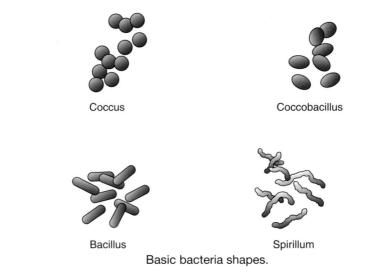

Coccus

Coccobacillus

Bacillus

Spirillum

Basic bacteria shapes.

*Staining.* When stained with violet dye in the laboratory, some bacteria hold onto the purple color in their thick cell walls. They are known as gram-positive bacteria. Those with thinner walls do not retain the stain and so are called gram-negative bacteria. Different medications are used for these two types.

Gram +      Gram -

Gram stain.

*Oxygen.* Some bacteria like to live in oxygen-rich environments (e.g., the lungs), and others do not. Oxygen-loving microbes are known as **aerobes.** Those that prefer to live without oxygen are **anaerobes.** They inhabit other parts of the body (e.g., gastrointestinal tract), where oxygen is not as prevalent as it is in the lungs.

### Cephalosporin medications

Cephalosporins are similar to penicillins. They are more expensive but are useful for people who cannot tolerate penicillins. Cephalosporins are organized into four generations, based on their activity: First generation cephalosporins such as cefazolin (Ancef, Kefzol) and cefadroxil (Duricef) are used mainly for patients who are allergic to penicillin. They act against gram-positive bacteria such as group B streptococci, which can cause pneumonia. Second generation cephalosporins such as cefprozil (Cefzil) and cefuroxime (Zinacef) are commonly used to treat **nosocomial** (infection acquired in a health-care facility) pneumonia and pelvic or intra-abdominal infections. Third generation cephalosporins such as ceftriaxone (Rocephin) and ceftizoxime (Cefizox) act against gram-negative bacteria such as *Escherichia coli (E. coli),* a common cause of intestinal illnesses. Fourth generation cephalosporins such as cefepime (Maxipime) are given by the IV route for severe nosocomial surgical infections.

This group of medications is used to both treat and prevent infections in many patients. The use of alcohol or alcohol-containing substances should be avoided during treatment because of associated abdominal side effects.

### Tetracycline medications

Tetracyclines were commonly used during the 1950s and 1960s, but many bacteria have since found ways to become resistant to them. The main function of this class of medication is to prevent bacteria from making protein (protein synthesis), to interrupt the reproduction of bacteria. Tetracyclines such as doxycycline (Vibramycin), minocycline (Solodyn), and tetracycline (Sumycin) are useful against both gram-negative and gram-positive microbes that cause bacterial infections such as gonorrhea, chlamydia, anthrax, and urinary tract infections. These medications are not used in children or pregnant women because permanent staining occurs on the teeth of the child or fetus.

### Macrolide medications

Macrolides such as erythromycin (E.E.S. Granules, Ery-Tab, Erythrocin Stearate Filmtab), clarithromycin (Biaxin), and azithromycin (Zithromax, Zithromax Z-Pak) are prescribed both orally and by injection for infections that are resistant to penicillins. These drugs function by inhibiting the RNA-dependent protein synthesis to inhibit the reproduction of invading microorganisms, and they may be either **bactericidal** (kill bacteria) or **bacteriostatic** (inhibit growth). These classes of medications are used for upper and lower respiratory tract infections, skin infections, pertussis, diphtheria, pelvic inflammatory disease, syphilis, Legionnaires' disease, strep throat, sinus infections, chronic bronchitis, pneumonia, and otitis media.

### Aminoglycoside medications

Aminoglycosides such as amikacin (Amikin), gentamicin (Cidomycin, Garamycin, Septopal), kanamycin (Kantrex), neomycin (Mycifradin, Neo-Fradin, Neo-Tab), paromomycin (Humatin, Paromycin), and tobramycin (Nebcin, Tobi) are more toxic than other antibiotics. They are ideal against **aerobic** gram-negative bacteria such as *Pseudomonas,* which require oxygen to grow, mycobacteria (tuberculosis), and some protozoans, which are one-celled organisms. Aminoglycosides are administered topically via ointments, eye or ear drops, or as an IV injection. Patients taking aminoglycosides systemically should have blood levels of the antibiotic monitored periodically for efficacy and toxicity. These medications are used only when no other suitable anti-infective is available, because of the risks for damage to the patient's hearing and kidney function.

### Quinolone medications

Quinolones such as ciprofloxacin (Cipro) and ofloxacin (Floxin) are bacteriostatic, which means they prevent bacteria from growing (Drug Spotlight 17.1). Quinolone medications are considered broad-spectrum antibiotics because they are effective against a wide variety of microorganisms. In view of some very serious, although rare, side effects such as ruptured tendons, these medications tend to be reserved for more antibiotic resistant strains of bacteria. These drugs can be given by the IV route, ophthalmically, or orally. Oral quinolones are very useful in the treatment of chronic urinary tract infections. (Refer to the Master the Essentials table for a more complete list of quinolone medications.)

### Sulfonamide medications

Sulfonamides are among the earliest classes of antibiotics. Drugs such as sulfadiazine, sulfamethizole (Thiosulfil Forte), sulfamethoxazole (Gantanol), sulfasalazine (Azulfidine), and sulfisoxazole (Gantrisin), as well as combination sulfonamide medications such as trimethoprim-sulfamethoxazole

**Drug Spotlight 17.1** *Cipro (ciprofloxacin hydrochloride)*

| | |
|---|---|
| Definition | Anti-infective used for bacterial infections; approved for use in patients exposed to the inhaled form of anthrax; used by thousands because of the anthrax by letter attacks in Washington, DC, Florida, and New York in 2001 |
| Side effects | CNS effects: dizziness, confusion, tremors, hallucinations, depression; allergic reactions; pain or rupture of tendon; severe inflammation of the colon; increased sensitivity to sunlight |
| Special considerations | FDA discourages widespread use because of the risk of the development of drug-resistant microorganisms |

CNS, central nervous system; FDA, Food and Drug Administration.
Information on Cipro (Ciprofloxacin Hydrochloride) for Inhalation Anthrax for Consumers: Questions and Answers (11/14/2001). U.S. Department of Health and Human Services, Washington, DC; 2001.

(Septra, Bactrim) and erythromycin-sulfisoxazole (Pediazole), are used to kill bacteria by interrupting their metabolism. Because these "sulfa drugs" tend to collect in the bladder before they are excreted, they are very effective in treating urinary tract infections. Many patients are allergic to sulfonamides and develop various severities of skin reactions, liver and kidney injuries, breathing difficulties, and decreased levels of red blood cells, white blood cells, and platelets. For this reason, it is important to pay close attention to any history of a sulfonamide antibiotic allergy when administering medications.

One drawback of antibiotics is that as they kill the **pathogenic** (disease-causing) bacteria, they also kill healthy or normal flora that are usually present in the human body and are beneficial in helping us fight off infection and in aiding digestion. When these healthy bacteria are destroyed, a **superinfection** can arise. In other words, the normal flora that helps us fight off infection is destroyed, and a new infection occurs. One of the most common examples of this is when a woman is taking antibiotics and the normal flora in the vagina is destroyed, allowing a yeast infection to occur. Thus, not only does she have the original infection to treat, but also the yeast infection, which requires a different antifungal medication.

### Antituberculosis agents

Tuberculosis agents are antibiotics that treat the disease caused by *Mycobacterium tuberculosis,* which mainly affects the lungs. This disease was very well controlled until the 1980s, when the appearance of acquired immunodeficiency syndrome (AIDS) preceded a resurgence of the disease related to the increased numbers of patients with compromised immune systems. Tuberculosis is treated with a mixture of two to four daily medications simultaneously for up to 1 year. Each drug eradicates the mycobacterium in a different way. One of the medications is cycloserine (Seromycin), which prevents the tuberculosis bacteria from growing in the body. Rifampin (Rifadin, Rimactane) is another antibiotic commonly used to treat or prevent tuberculosis. This medication has one unique side effect of which patients and health-care workers must be aware: it turns body secretions, including sweat, tears, urine, feces, and saliva, red orange. If the patient wears contact lenses, this drug will permanently stain them. In addition, rifampin may render hormonally based birth control ineffective. (For a more complete list of antituberculosis agents please see the Master the Essentials table.)

### Antitoxins

Antitoxins are antibodies that are created in response to specific toxins and are able to counteract that toxin in a person at high risk for the disease or condition. An antitoxin is given to a person who has been exposed to a toxin such as diphtheria, tetanus, or botulism but who does not have adequate immunity to combat the invader. An example is a landscaper who received a puncture wound while mowing lawns. Because tetanus microorganisms live in soil and a puncture wound could conceivably allow the tetanus-containing soil deep into his body, he is at risk of developing a life-threatening tetanus infection. He should be administered the tetanus vaccine booster, but this will not provide immediate protection against the invasion. For that, he may receive a tetanus immune globulin (Baytet, HyperTET

S/D) injection to provide immediate neutralization of the tetanus toxoid in his system with antibodies specific to the tetanus toxin.

## Antifungal medications

Antifungal medications treat fungal infections such as tinea pedis (commonly known as athlete's foot) or candidiasis (yeast infection). Fungi can live on the skin or inside the body. Unlike bacteria, fungi can be single-celled organisms or multicellular organisms with a complex structure. The human body can usually fight off fungal infections unless the immune system is compromised by the human immunodeficiency virus (HIV) or other microbes.

Topical antifungal medications such as ketoconazole (Extina, Nizoral) and miconazole (Desenex, Micatin) can treat fungal infections on the skin such as athlete's foot. If the infection is in the oral and GI mucosa (a condition known as thrush), the medication nystatin (Mycostatin) is used because it is not absorbed but coats the mouth and stomach. If the fungi are growing in the body, or if skin infections are worsening, systemic antifungal medications such as fluconazole (Diflucan), itraconazole (Sporanox), and ketoconazole (Nizoral) are given to combat the infection. These systemic medications can be given orally or as an injection. Amphotericin B (Fungizone) is an IV medication reserved for potentially life-threatening fungal infections such as histoplasmosis, which can affect the lungs and other organs. The side effects of Fungizone are very serious and can affect the kidney, liver, blood counts, and electrolytes.

## Medications that fight viruses

Viruses are microorganisms that require a host to reproduce themselves. Hosts can be humans, plants, or animals. Viruses, which are smaller than other microorganisms, insert their genetic material into this host and take over the host's cells to use them as a breeding facility. AIDS, cytomegalovirus (CMV) infection, rabies, smallpox, chickenpox, shingles, influenza, the common cold, and herpes are all caused by viruses. Even some types of cancer have been linked to viruses. The human body reacts to most viruses by developing antibodies to fight the invading microorganisms naturally. In those instances, when the body needs help to fight off a viral infection, antiviral and antiretroviral medications are used. The choice is based on the type of virus infecting the patient.

■ **Antiviral medications.** Antiviral therapy is the use of medications to inhibit the reproduction of a virus. Antiviral therapy is difficult because viruses replicate (reproduce) and mutate rapidly. Unlike antibiotics that kill the invader, antiviral drugs eliminate the materials that the virus needs to reproduce and flourish. This can be done in several ways. The virus can be blocked from entering the host cell, thus preventing the implantation of the virus DNA. Some antiviral medications target the enzymes and proteins the virus needs to replicate and function properly. Another way the virus is stopped is by strengthening the host's ability to fight the infections. Antiviral medications such as acyclovir (Acivir, Acivirax, Cyclovir, Herpex, Zovirax, and Zovir) are used to treat the viruses that cause herpes, chickenpox, and shingles. Zanamivir (Relenza) and oseltamivir (Tamiflu) are used to treat influenza type A and B. Also used to treat influenza type A is amantadine (Symmetrel). Relenza is an inhaled medication, whereas Tamiflu is an oral medication. CMV infection of the eye associated with AIDS and the smallpox virus can be treated with cidofovir (Vistide). Ribavirin (Virazole) is use in fighting the hepatitis C virus and respiratory syncytial virus (RSV). Most other viruses have not yet been conquered.

■ **Antiretroviral medications.** Antiretroviral medications refer specifically to a group of medications used to fight retroviruses such as HIV. Retroviruses are different in that they have an RNA blueprint. The name implies that they use RNA to synthesize DNA, which is the opposite of the normal process. This allows genetic material from a retrovirus to become a permanent part of the genes of an infected cell. This embedding of the retrovirus into the genetic material makes it difficult to combat. HIV specifically attacks the assembling T4, or CD4, cells. Because these cells are the body's defensive soldiers, the host is rendered powerless to fight reproduction of the HIV virus. HIV is simply the virus and its presence in the body. When the virus grows stronger and lowers T4 cell levels significantly, the patient develops AIDS. At this point, the patient begins to suffer from many viral, bacterial, and fungal infections. Therefore, the key is to prevent or delay this development as long as possible with the use of antiretroviral medications. Because HIV mutates easily, it is imperative that patients with AIDS take several medications according to a specific regimen to fight the retrovirus, prevent its reproduction, and protect their own immune system. These medications are classified according to where in the reproduction process they are effective and include the following: nucleoside reverse transcriptase inhibitors (NRTIs), nonnucleoside reverse transcriptase inhibitors (NNRTIs), protease inhibitors (PIs), fusion inhibitors, entry inhibitors, and HIV integrase strand transfer inhibitors. (The Master the Essentials table includes more detail on these medications.)

### Virtual Field Trip

Using your favorite search engine, research medications currently used for patients with AIDS. Discover the average number of pills these patients must take in a day, and develop a schedule to assist a patient in implementing this regimen.

### Antiparasitic medications

Parasites are organisms that live on or in another organism (host) and that often cause diseases. Common parasitic diseases include malaria, worms, lice, and scabies. Although most parasitic diseases (e.g., malaria) are not common in North America because of the cold winters, purified drinking water, and advanced septic systems, knowing the types of medications used to treat them is important because you may encounter a patient who, for instance, develops a parasitic disease after traveling abroad. The following classes of medications are used to treat parasitic infections and disease.

■ Antimalarials: Antimalarial medications such as atovaquone/proguanil (Malarone), chloroquine (Aralen), mefloquine (Lariam), and primaquine are taken to prevent a patient from contracting malaria as well as to treat the disease. These medications work by inhibiting the growth of the malaria parasite in the red blood cells of the body. To prevent malaria, these medications should be combined with the use of personal protection, such as long sleeves and pants and insect repellent.

■ Antiprotozoals: Protozoan microorganisms differ from bacteria and fungi in that they do not have a cell wall. Therefore, the antibiotics effective against bacteria have very little effect on protozoans. Medications such as metronidazole (Flagyl, Metro I.V.) and trimethoprim-sulfamethoxazole (Bactrim, Septra, Sulfatrim) are given orally or by the IV route to combat vaginal infections such as trichomonas, giardiasis (infection of the intestines), and *Pneumocystis carinii* (causes pulmonary disease). These medications disrupt the strands of DNA and thus prevent the reproduction of this infection. Metronidazole is also the drug of choice in giardiasis (infection of the intestines).

■ Anthelmintics: Tapeworms, roundworms, and flukes are all treated with anthelmintics, which affect the nervous system of the worm and paralyze it or prevent the worm from absorbing glucose. Tapeworms do not enter the tissue of their host and are treated with albendazole (Albenza) and praziquantel (Biltricide) orally. Roundworms enter the tissue and thus are more difficult to kill. Ivermectin (Stromectol) is prescribed for the treatment of roundworms. Mebendazole (Vermox), pyrantel (Antiminth, Ascarel, Pin-X), and praziquantel (Biltricide) are given orally for the treatment of hookworms, whipworms, pinworms, and flukes.

■ Pediculicides: Lice are parasites that live on the blood found on the body, scalp, and pubic area. Head lice spread easily among children who are in close proximity during play. Body lice is the only type known to spread disease, and this type is spread through close contact in crowded conditions, such as seen with homeless people. Pubic lice are spread through sexual contact. Treatment consists of shampoos and lotions that either attack the nervous system of the louse or suffocate them. These medications containing permethrin (Acticin, Elimite, and Nix), piperonyl butoxide/pyrethrins (Licide, RID), and spinosa (Natroba) can be purchased OTC without a prescription. Prescription lotions and shampoos include malathion (Ovide), benzyl alcohol lotion (Ulesfia), and lindane. All treatment for lice must include treatment of close contacts, as well as cleaning of bedding and any clothing or hair care items used on the patient.

■ Scabicides: Scabies are itch mites that burrow in the webbing of the fingers and toes, as well as the axillary area. They are spread by skin-to-skin contact, sometimes as brief as a handshake. Medication consists of topical pesticide lotions such as crotamiton (Eurax), lindane, and permethrin (Acticin, Elimite). It is again important to clean the bedding because scabies can live for a period of time when not on the body.

## Vaccines

Vaccines offer immunity from a disease (Check Up 17.1). The two types of immunity are natural and acquired. Natural immunity is the kind that humans have developed as a whole through evolution, such as the resistance to distemper. Acquired immunity occurs in a variety of ways. **Active natural immunity** is created when a microbe invades the body, and the body learns to fight it, such as the childhood disease chickenpox. Once a child contracts the disease, he or she will develop antibodies to fight it, and those antibodies will remain in the system to guard against any further attacks. This immunity is permanent. **Passive natural immunity** is temporary and occurs when a mother passes her immunity to her fetus through the placenta. This immunity generally lasts for about 3 to 6 months.

**Active artificial immunity** is acquired when a patient is given a vaccination of live, attenuated (weakened) or dead bacteria, viruses, or toxoids, and the patient's body forms antibodies. This protection may be semipermanent (i.e., years) or permanent. **Passive artificial immunity** occurs when antibodies from a donor are directly given to a patient to teach the patient's immune system how to fight. This protection is temporary.

Vaccines act by provoking memory B cells to prepare for a future attack from a similar microbe. Boosters (later doses given for the semipermanent vaccines) are given to boost the immune system into continuing its protection. To see whether the body has produced enough antibodies in response to a vaccination, a blood titer, or level, may be determined.

Some vaccines have side effects, including fever and redness and pain at the injection site. Severe reactions, called anaphylaxis, are possible, and patients must always be observed for at least 15 minutes after a vaccination. Assess the patient for rash or difficulty breathing. Document your observations even if the patient tolerated the procedure well.

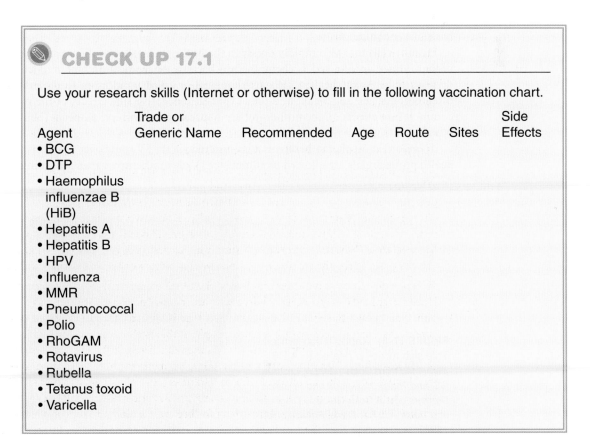

### CHECK UP 17.1

Use your research skills (Internet or otherwise) to fill in the following vaccination chart.

| Agent | Trade or Generic Name | Recommended | Age | Route | Sites | Side Effects |
|---|---|---|---|---|---|---|
| • BCG | | | | | | |
| • DTP | | | | | | |
| • Haemophilus influenzae B (HiB) | | | | | | |
| • Hepatitis A | | | | | | |
| • Hepatitis B | | | | | | |
| • HPV | | | | | | |
| • Influenza | | | | | | |
| • MMR | | | | | | |
| • Pneumococcal | | | | | | |
| • Polio | | | | | | |
| • RhoGAM | | | | | | |
| • Rotavirus | | | | | | |
| • Rubella | | | | | | |
| • Tetanus toxoid | | | | | | |
| • Varicella | | | | | | |

## Antineoplastic medications (chemotherapy)

Cancer is a disease caused by a disorderly and uncontrolled division of cells. Many chemicals, such as nicotine and alcohol, can trigger a cell to begin dividing abnormally. Although in most cases, the body can spot an abnormal cell and eliminate it, in some individuals, the body cannot make that identification, so the abnormal cell remains, and cancer results.

Cancer cells typically divide much more rapidly than normal, healthy cells and can spread to surrounding or distant body areas, a process called **metastasis.** For instance, cancers of the breast frequently metastasize to the brain, bones, or liver (A Closer Look 17.3).

---

### A CLOSER LOOK 17.3: Types of Tumors

Tumors are classified as benign or malignant. Tumors that are not fatal are called **benign.** Benign tumors grow slowly and do not metastasize. They may be removed if they impede the function of surrounding tissues; they do not usually grow back when removed.

**Malignant** tumors are cancerous. They must be treated, or the patient will die. They spread as nonfunctional tissues that compete with healthy tissue for the blood and nutrient supply. Malignant cancers are treated with surgery, radiation, and/or chemotherapy unless the patient decides not to be treated.

---

Sarcomas (Fig. 17-3), carcinomas, and other malignant cancers must be completely eliminated, or they can return. For this reason, a powerful treatment, chemotherapy, is often prescribed. **Chemotherapy,** usually a combination of several antineoplastic (anticancer) and cytotoxic (destruction to cells) medications, is frequently given in several doses for maximum effectiveness. These medications act as toxins, or poisons, to the malignant cells. Each patient receives a highly individualized combination of medications because no two cancers or persons are identical. In addition, the drugs are given on an intermittent basis, never continuously.

Healthy cells that also rapidly divide in the body, such as hair follicles and the mucous membranes of the GI tract, are affected by chemotherapy because the medication's main function is to target rapidly dividing cells. As the healthy cells are damaged or killed in addition to the malignant cells, patients often become sick and weak, and they experience negative side effects of the medications. The most common side effects of chemotherapy are nausea and vomiting, alopecia (hair loss), and decreased blood counts.

Therefore, most chemotherapy is administered via the IV route over a period of time. Whether allied health professionals are allowed to administer IV chemotherapy varies according to state, facility, and

**FIGURE 17-3:** Kaposi's sarcoma. This skin tumor is related to AIDS. *(Reprinted from Goldsmith, LA, Lazarus, GS, and Tharp, MD: Adult and Pediatric Dermatology: A Color Guide to Diagnosis and Treatment. F.A. Davis, Philadelphia; 1997.)*

level of training. Because chemotherapy is usually a long process, patient education regarding IV therapy, care of venous lines, and recognition of signs and symptoms of infection is vital. Infiltration, or accidental leakage of medication into surrounding tissue, is always a risk with IV therapy. These substances are particularly toxic if they infiltrate tissues. Always assess the IV site for swelling or coolness. The potential for infiltration increases when the rate of the IV infusion is increased too quickly or when pressure is put on the vein. If infiltration occurs, the IV catheter must be removed, and a new IV line must be started in a different location.

If the patient complains of burning pain or aching in the vein, the chemotherapy may have irritated or damaged the vein wall, with resulting phlebitis and thrombosis. You may need to obtain an order to dilute the strength of the medication, lower the infusion rate, or change the site.

Because of the caustic nature of these medications, it is common practice to insert a central line or port (see Chapter 10) to administer chemotherapeutic agents into a larger vein, with less risk to surrounding tissues.

Other complications result from the destruction of hematopoietic cells. The first is a suppressed immune system, leading to infections that quickly become overwhelming because of the patient's inability to fight the invading microorganisms. In addition, patients may have difficulty with bleeding as a result of low platelet counts and anemia from low red blood cell counts. For these reasons, patients must be protected from injury and infectious visitors or health-care workers who may endanger their health.

Major organ damage can result from the toxic effects of these drugs. Therefore, the patient must be closely observed for any signs of organ compromise, such as decreased urine output, change in skin color, or change in blood test results.

Antineoplastic agents are toxic to cells, but they can also be dangerous or even fatal to persons who administer them and thus require special handling. Exposure to chemotherapy poses risks to reproductive health in men and women, as well as other problems. For that reason, gloves should be worn while administering, handling, or transporting antineoplastic agents, so that agents are not absorbed through the skin. Ensure that packages of hazardous drugs are well labeled and secured properly. Although protocols vary by location, follow all safety measures, and do not perform any task outside your scope of practice. All staff members handling these drugs should be required to complete specialized training to protect themselves, their patients, and the patients' families. Regulations always include wearing protective clothing, strictly following safety measures, and rigidly observing protocols for drug preparation and delivery (Box 17.1).

Among the antineoplastic medications available for treating cancer are alkylating agents, antimetabolites, antitumor antibodies, plant extracts, hormones, biological response modifiers, monoclonal antibodies, immunomodulators, and radioactive isotopes. These agents are usually given parenterally: by the intramuscular (IM), subcutaneous (SC), IV, or intrathecal route. In some instances, creams and gels are administered topically for mild forms of skin cancer.

## Virtual Field Trip

Using your favorite search engine:
Download a patient teaching aid for cancer.
Print a list of common side effects of cancer medications

### Alkylating agents

Alkylating agents are among the oldest categories of antineoplastic medications. They work by attaching to DNA and altering its shape, thus preventing it from reproducing normally. Alkylating agents are effective during all phases of the cell cycle, and because blood and bone marrow cells are especially sensitive to them, these medications are ideal for treating leukemia. Examples of oral and IV alkylating agents are chlorambucil (Leukeran), cisplatin (Platinol), cyclophosphamide (Cytoxan, Neosar), dacarbazine (DTIC-Dome), mechlorethamine (Mustargen) (Drug Spotlight 17-2), oxaliplatin (Eloxatin), stretozocin (Zanosar), and thiotepa (Thioplex). (For a more complete list, please see the Master the Essentials table.) An effect of these drugs is the possibility of permanent infertility in both male and female patients.

## BOX 17.1 Special Handling of Chemotherapeutic Drugs

Always give as ordered, and have another colleague double-check the order.

Frequently assess the IV site.

Help the patient with oral hygiene as needed.

Assess for malnutrition related to nausea, vomiting, and diarrhea.

Administer an antiemetic, as ordered.

Encourage soft, mild foods.

Offer cool liquids.

Measure input and output.

Inquire about pregnancy, and perform a test as ordered before administering to women.

Assess for complications.

Use standard precautions to decrease infection in the patient, and protect yourself.

Assess vital signs, as ordered.

Educate the patient about the effects of the therapy.

Dispose of chemotherapeutic products according to facility standards.

### Drug Spotlight 17.2 *Mustargen (mechlorethamine hydrochloride)*

| | |
|---|---|
| Definition | Commonly known as nitrogen mustard; one of the first chemotherapeutic agents; some originally produced as chemical weapons in the early part of the 20th century; these agents blister the skin |
| Uses | Used to treat cancers such as Hodgkin's disease and some blood and lung cancers |
| Side effects | These most common side effects are temporary:<br>• Nausea and vomiting<br>• Hair loss<br>• Mouth sores<br>• Discoloration of infusion veins<br>Infertility may be permanent |
| Route of administration | Given via IV route; very damaging to tissue, thus given with extreme care |
| Special considerations | No antidote exists for this drug, which is considered a poison; if exposed:<br>• Contact poison control<br>• Remove clothing, cutting off any clothes that must be removed over head<br>• Place all clothes in plastic bag<br>• Wash off skin |

### Antimetabolite medications

Antimetabolites disrupt critical cell pathways. When cancer cells try to construct DNA or proteins, these cells inadvertently use antimetabolites, which kill the cells. These drugs are used to treat ovarian, breast, and GI tumors. They can also be used to treat some cases of leukemia. Antimetabolite medications include 6-mercaptopurine, cladribine (Cladribine NovaPulse, Leustatin), cytarabine (Cytosar-U, Tarabine PFS), fluorouracil (Efudex, Adrucil), leucovorin (Wellcovorin), methotrexate (Rheumatrex, Trexall), and thioguanine (Tabloid). They can be administered orally, topically, or through an IV line.

### Antitumor antibiotics

Bacteria found in soil are used to create antibiotics that can kill cancer cells. Many of these agents cause cell death by altering the DNA molecules and breaking the actual DNA strands. Although these medications have properties of antibiotics, they are used for their cytotoxic effects. Bleomycin (Blenoxane) is an example of an antitumor antibiotic that is used primarily in combination with other antineoplastic medications to treat Hodgkin's lymphoma and testicular cancer. Another antitumor antibiotic is dactinomycin (Cosmegen) which is used to treat cancers of the kidneys, uterus, testicles, bones, muscles, joints, and soft tissues. The factor that limits the use of this class of medications is that in damaging the cancer cells, lung cells are also injured.

### Plant extracts (alkaloids)

Plant extracts, or alkaloids, called mitotic inhibitors, prevent cell division. Plants used for this purpose include periwinkle, the mandrake plant, the Pacific yew, and a shrub called *Camptotheca acuminata*. These drugs are called mitotic inhibitors because they prevent formation of the mitotic spindle, and the cells cannot complete mitosis. This causes cell death. Cancers treated with plant alkaloids include soft tissue, breast, ovarian, testicular, stomach, prostate, head, neck, and lung cancers, Wilms' tumor, leukemia, Hodgkin's disease, and non-Hodgkin's lymphoma. Examples include docetaxel (Docefrez, Taxotere), etoposide (VePesid, Toposar), irinotecan (Camptosar), paclitaxel (Onxol, Taxol), teniposide (Vumon), topotecan (Hycamtin), vinblastine (Velban), vincristine (Oncovin, Vincasar PFS), and vinorelbine (Navelbine).

### Hormones

Hormones can help the brain communicate with other organs in the body (see Chapter 15) and can tell them when to grow and how to function. Some hormones such as testosterone, estrogen, and luteinizing hormone are powerful and can significantly impair the growth of some tumors. Tumors that depend on hormones for growth can be eradicated by large amounts of an opposing hormone. For example, tumors that thrive under the effects of estrogen, such as breast cancer, can be killed by injections of fluoxymesterone (Androxy, Halotestin), testolactone (Teslac), or testosterone (Andro LA 200, Delatestryl, DepAndro 100, and Depo-Testosterone). Conversely, a patient with prostate or testicular cancer may be treated with oral doses of antiandrogens such as bicalutamide (Casodex), flutamide (Eulexin), or nilutamide (Nilandron), which block testosterone production, or with estrogen, such as or Cenestin, Enjuvia, Premarin, or estradiol (Estrace, Femtrace, Gynodiol), which makes the environment unfavorable for tumor growth. (Please see the Master the Essentials table for a more complete list of hormonal medications used as antineoplastic agents.)

### Biological therapy

Biological therapy involves boosting the body's immune system, rather than destroying the cancer cells as do the previous medications discussed. However, biological therapy also alters the nature of the response and often produces severe side effects. Three drug classes fall under this heading: biological response modifiers, monoclonal antibodies, and immunomodulators.

One type of biological therapy is the biological response modifier, which boosts the immune system. The exact mechanisms by which these medications exhibit antitumor effects are not clear. Biological response modifiers include the interleukins, which stimulate the growth of blood cells important to the immune system. Interferon alfa-2a (Roferon-A) is used to treat leukemia and AIDS-related Kaposi's sarcoma. Interferon alfa-2b (Intron A) is used to treat leukemia, malignant melanoma, AIDS-related Kaposi's sarcoma, and hepatitis B and C.

Monoclonal antibodies are substances that specifically target tumor cells. Whereas toxic substances are nonselective and kill any rapidly growing cells (both diseased and healthy), monoclonal antibodies attack cancer cells only. They attach themselves to the tumor antigens and make them easily recognizable to the body's immune system. Monoclonal antibody medications such as alemtuzumab (Campath), bevacizumab (Avastin), cetuximab (Erbitux), gemtuzumab (Mylotarg), ibritumomab (Zevalin), panitumumab (Vectibix), rituximab (Rituxan), tositumomab (Bexxar), and trastuzumab (Herceptin) are used in the treatment of colon, lung, head, neck, and breast cancers, as well as leukemia and non-Hodgkin's lymphoma.

A third form of biological therapy uses immunomodulatory cytokines, which are messenger proteins that deliver messages within the cells. In some patients with cancer, these cytokines are not functional.

Immunomodulators such as lenalidomide (Revlimid) and thalidomide (Thalomid) stimulate the immune system in patients with multiple myeloma. The use of thalidomide carries a high risk of birth defects, as was seen in the 1950s and 1960s. Those patients prescribed thalidomide are encouraged to use multiple methods of birth control to prevent pregnancy.

### Radioactive isotopes

Radiation can also be used to kill cancer cells. Radiation in some form is used to treat roughly half of all patients with cancer patients. Tumors are the target of radiation therapy. In addition to external irradiation, radioactive isotopes can be swallowed as capsules or solutions, or they can be implanted. Iodine-125, iridium-194, palladium-103, and thulium-170 are radioactive isotopes implanted in the form of seeds. This procedure is called brachytherapy, and the seeds emit radiation to shrink the tumor. Always be extremely careful when handling these substances because they are dangerous. Follow your facility's policy about isolating the patient and the patient's body fluids after administering radioactive isotopes because they will emit radiation for a period of time after implantation.

### SUMMARY

The immune system functions to maintain health by blocking or fighting foreign invaders. When the immune system is overstimulated by conditions such as allergies or autoimmune disorders, anti-inflammatory medications are used to suppress the immune system. When the immune system is weakened by bacteria, viruses, parasites, or other microorganisms, medications are available to help restore function. The classifications of anti-infective medications include antibiotics, antitoxins, antifungals, antivirals, and antiparasitics. Anti-infective agents assist in fighting infections, and vaccines assist in preventing infections.

Antineoplastic agents are those used to treat cancer. These agents must be carefully handled, administered, and disposed of because of their toxicity and hazards to the health professional and to all persons coming into contact with the patient or their secretions or waste.

Educating patients and their families about these medications and their possible complications will ensure safety for all: the health professional, the patient, and the family.

## Activities

To make sure that you have learned the key points covered in this chapter, complete the following activities.

### True or False
Write true if the statement is true. Beside the false statements, write false, and correct the statement to make it true.

Bacteria are identified by their shape and ability to retain a dye. _____

Anticancer drugs work against slowly dividing cells. _____

Tetracycline is the antibiotic of choice for pregnant women and small children. _____

Antiretrovirals are given to fight HIV infections. _____

Only the person actually administering chemotherapy must follow safety rules. _____

Some antituberculosis agents turn body secretions red/brown. _____

Malaria is caused by a parasite. _____

Anti-inflammatory medications are used when the immune system is not active enough. _____

C cells are the part of the immune system, which is known as memory cells recording attacks of microorganisms. _____

Antibiotics are considered anti-infective medications. _____

### Multiple Choice
Choose the best answer for each question.

**1. Which class of medications treats worms?**
   A. Antimalarials
   B. Anthelmintics
   C. Antiprotozoals
   D. Pediculicides

**2. Which is NOT a side effect of Cipro?**
   A. Severe inflammation of the colon
   B. Increased sensitivity to sunlight
   C. CNS effects: dizziness, confusion, hallucinations
   D. Nasal congestion

**3. Which vaccine is given for rubella?**
   A. Varicella
   B. MMR
   C. DTP
   D. Pneumococcus
   E. HiB

**4. Which immunity provides immunity to a fetus?**

A. Active natural immunity

B. Active artificial immunity

C. Passive natural immunity

D. Passive artificial immunity

**5. Which of the following healthy cells are harmed along with cancer cells by chemotherapy?**

A. Hair follicles

B. Hematopoietic cells

C. Mucous membranes

D. All of the above

**6. Which of the following antineoplastic medications was developed after its use in World War I?**

A. Mustargen

B. Cisplatin

C. Methotrexate

D. Leucovorin

**7. Tinea pedis is more commonly known as _____.**

A. Ringworm

B. Yeast infection

C. Athlete's foot

D. None of the above

**8. The class of drugs used to treat HIV infections is _____.**

A. Antivirals

B. Antiretrovirals

C. Antifungals

D. Antibiotics

**9. Which of the following are types of worms?**

A. Round

B. Tape

C. Pin

D. All of the above

**10. What is an example of an active natural immunity?**

A. Patient has the measles

B. Patient is given antibodies

C. Patient is given a live attenuated vaccine

D. Mother passes immunity to infant

Respond to the following situations on a separate sheet.

1. Harvey has injured his foot on a dirty nail. What vaccine will most likely be ordered? Why?

2. Beth has been prescribed an antibiotic for 10 days and calls to say that she is feeling better and is discontinuing it because it gives her an upset stomach. Explain to her why she should continue her medication despite feeling better and having side effects.

3. Holly brings her baby in for vaccinations. She is concerned that her baby needs so many shots and asks whether it is really necessary. How do you respond?

4. Beverly has cervical cancer and is to begin treatment with a radioactive isotope implant. What teaching should be done before beginning therapy?

5. Larry has come in because the antifungal spray is not working on his athletes' foot, and now a few of his toenails are becoming thick and painful, signs indicating that the infection is worsening. What will the prescriber order for him?

# Essentials Review

For further study and practice with drug classifications learned in this chapter, complete the following table to the best of your ability. Use resources such as the *PDR,* the Internet, or printed drug guides for help.

| Trade Name | Generic Name | Classification | Purpose | Side Effects | Contraindications and Precautions | Examples | Patient Education |
|---|---|---|---|---|---|---|---|
| Bicillin | | | | | | | |
| Nydrazid | | | | | | | |
| Flagyl | | | | | | | |
| Zovirax | | | | | | | |
| Platinol | | | | | | | |
| Blenoxane | | | | | | | |

# 18

# Pulmonary System Medications

*The body depends on the respiratory, or pulmonary, system to bring oxygen to the cells and dispose of carbon dioxide. If this system works improperly, immediate medication may be needed. The fastest method for conveying medication to the lungs is through inhalation.*

## LEARNING OUTCOMES

At the end of this chapter, the student will be able to:

18.1  Define all key terms.

18.2  Describe how the respiratory system functions to exchange oxygen and carbon dioxide.

18.3  Discuss the actions of mast cell stabilizers, bronchodilators, anticholinergics, xanthines, and beta-adrenergic agonists used in the treatment of asthma and other respiratory disorders.

18.4  Describe two medications that may be used to treat a viral respiratory illness.

18.5  Compare and contrast antitussive and expectorant medications and when each is appropriate to use.

18.6  Discuss tuberculosis, how it is treated, and why its occurrence has increased.

---

### KEY TERMS

Alveoli
Apnea
Chronic obstructive
  pulmonary disease
  (COPD)

Dyspnea
Expiration
Hypoxia
Inspiration
Latent tuberculosis (TB)

Purified protein derivative
  (PPD)
Respiration
Respiratory syncytial virus
  (RSV)

---

## ◼ THE PULMONARY SYSTEM

The pulmonary system is responsible for **respiration**—the process of inhaling oxygen ($O_2$) into the bloodstream and exhaling the waste in the form of carbon dioxide ($CO_2$). It works with the musculoskeletal systems during this process. To survive, the muscles need $O_2$ supplied and $CO_2$ removed. The diaphragm, the large muscle under the stomach, facilitates breathing. When the diaphragm contracts, the lungs are compressed, and $CO_2$ is expelled up through the bronchial tubes and trachea, out of the mouth, and into the air. This outward movement of air is known as **expiration.** The now mostly empty lungs inhale $O_2$ from the air; the inward movement of air is called **inspiration.** Both require energy (Fig. 18-1).

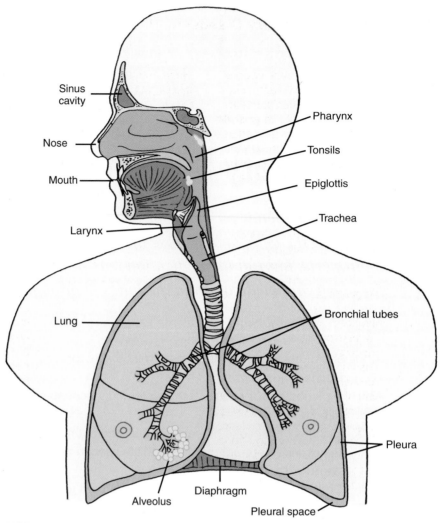

FIGURE 18-1: Respiratory system.

The brain regulates the rate and depth of breathing, depending on the needs of the body. For example, when you exercise, your body requires more $O_2$, and therefore you breathe more rapidly.

The exchange of $CO_2$ and $O_2$ occurs at the level of the **alveoli** (tiny air sacs in the lungs). Any time alveolar function is impaired, $CO_2$ builds up, and oxygenation declines. Changes in alveolar function occur with smoking and in diseases such as asthma.

$O_2$ is vital to every cell in the body. Even 4 to 6 minutes without breathing can cause death because the lack of $O_2$ can cause the heart to stop beating and can have serious implications for other systems to fail, given that the brain also needs $O_2$ to function. Often, it is a medical emergency when someone either stops breathing or presents with **dyspnea** (trouble breathing) (Fast Tip 18.1).

Diseases such as asthma, **chronic obstructive pulmonary disease (COPD),** and tuberculosis (TB) can cause dyspnea or impair the lung's ability to function. Pulmonary medications can improve pulmonary function in these patients (Table 18.1).

---

● *Fast Tip 18.1*   Fast Relief for Dyspnea

Pulmonary medications are usually administered via inhalation for quick action. Examples of this route are the nebulizer and the inhaler.

## TABLE 18.1 Common Pulmonary Diseases

| Pulmonary Disease | Overview | Symptoms | Medications |
|---|---|---|---|
| Asthma | Asthma is a disease caused by an increased reaction of the tracheobronchial tree to stimuli that results in episodic narrowing and inflammation of the airways. Although the cause is not always known, the airways are chronically inflamed. | Breathlessness, air hunger (pursing of lips, gasping for air), coughing, and dyspnea are common symptoms. If asthma continues for a long time, status asthmaticus, or an asthma attack that does not stop, becomes a medical emergency. | Antiasthmatic medications target both the bronchoconstriction and the inflammation. |
| COPD | The main diseases included under COPD are chronic bronchitis and emphysema. Chronic bronchitis is an inflammation of the bronchial tree. In response to irritation, mucus floods the bronchi and impairs breathing. Emphysema occurs after years of chronic inflammation, when the bronchioles lose elasticity and the alveoli dilate beyond effectiveness. COPD is usually caused by tobacco smoking, both direct and second-hand. Irritants and pollutants in the air can also cause COPD. There is no cure for COPD. | Dyspnea and coughing occur, particularly a cough that is productive (one that brings up mucus). | A patient with COPD needs a variety of drugs to treat infections because the lungs, the first line of defense, have been damaged. The patient also needs drugs to decrease the bronchospasm that is created by the chemical irritation and to control the chronic cough that comes from irritating the pharynx. Mucolytics and expectorants are usually indicated, along with oxygen therapy. Oxygen must be given only at low levels (4 L/min maximum). Higher levels may lead to dangerous $CO_2$ levels and cause the patient to stop breathing. |
| Cystic Fibrosis | Cystic fibrosis is a genetic disease that affects the respiratory and digestive systems. In the respiratory system, thick secretions are excreted into the lungs, and patients require vigilant respiratory care to keep the lungs clear and free from infection. | Patients have persistent productive cough, frequent infections in the lungs, wheezing, shortness of breath, failure to gain weight, salty-tasting skin, and GI difficulties. | Mucolytic medications assist in breaking up thick secretions, and antibiotics treat lung infections. |
| Tuberculosis | Tuberculosis (TB) is an infection caused by *Mycobacterium tuberculosis*, a gram-positive bacterium. | Patients have a persistent cough, night sweats, and weight loss. | The TB bacterium is gram-positive but frequently resists treatment with traditional antibiotics. Consequently, it is often treated with a combination of drugs. Treatment must continue for as long as 6 to 12 months. |

COPD, chronic obstructive pulmonary disease; GI, gastrointestinal.

## ■ PULMONARY MEDICATIONS

The medications used to treat pulmonary infections or disease are determined by the part of the pulmonary system that is affected. Some medications liquefy secretions, and others dry them up. Some medications act locally, whereas others act systemically (see the Master the Essentials table for descriptions of the most common pulmonary system drugs).

## Master the Essentials: Respiratory Medications

This table shows the various classes of respiratory medications and key side effects, contraindications and precautions, interactions, and examples of each class.

| Class | Indications for Use | Side Effects | Contraindications and Precautions | Interactions | Examples |
|-------|---------------------|--------------|-----------------------------------|--------------|----------|
| Mast cell stabilizers | Prevention of asthma attacks | Throat irritation, bad taste, wheezing, cough | Hypersensitivity | None reported | Cromolyn sodium (Intal), nedocromil (Tilade aerosol) |
| Anti-influenza agents | Reduction of influenza symptoms | Anorexia, bronchitis, diarrhea, dizziness, dry mouth, headache, insomnia, nervousness, urinary retention | Hypersensitivity, kidney or liver impairment, pregnancy, breastfeeding, underlying respiratory disease | Acetaminophen, aspirin, cimetidine | Zanamivir (Relenza), oseltamivir (Tamiflu) |
| Antitussives | Coughing cessation | Constipation, dizziness, respiratory depression, sedation, urinary retention | Asthma, COPD, addiction-prone patients, hypersensitivity | MAO inhibitors, other CNS depressants | Dextromethorphan (Robitussin Cough, Vicks 44 Cough and Cold, Triaminic Cough and Cold), codeine |
| Expectorants | Achievement of a more productive cough | Vomiting, diarrhea, abdominal pain | Hypersensitivity | None reported | Guaifenesin (Duratuss, Mucinex, Robitussin) |
| Anticholinergics | Dilation of the bronchi | Agitation, confusion, dizziness, drowsiness, headache, increased heart rate, thickened secretions, bronchitis | Hypersensitivity, cardiac instability, glaucoma, prostatic hypertrophy | Use with other anticholinergics not recommended | Ipratropium (Atrovent), tiotropium (Spiriva) |
| Xanthines (methylxanthines) | Relief of asthma symptoms | Dysrhythmias, CNS stimulation, GI distress, increased blood glucose and heart rate, urinary frequency | Diabetes mellitus, glaucoma, peptic ulcer, pregnancy, hypersensitivity | Barbiturates, hydantoins, ketoconazole, loop diuretics, beta blockers, calcium channel blockers, oral contraceptives | Aminophylline (Phyllocontin, Truphylline), theophylline (Elixophyllin, TheoCap, Slo-Bid, Theo-Dur Sprinkles) |

| | Action | Side effects | Conditions | Drug interactions | Drugs |
|---|---|---|---|---|---|
| **Beta-adrenergic agonists** | Dilation of the bronchi | CNS stimulation; increased appetite, blood glucose, and blood pressure | CV disorders, diabetes mellitus, hyperthyroidism, kidney problems, seizure disorders | MAO inhibitors, tricyclic antidepressants, cardiac glycosides, beta blockers | Albuterol (Proventil, Ventolin), bitolterol (Tornalate), epinephrine (Adrenalin), formoterol (Foradil), levalbuterol (Xopenex), isoproterenol (Isuprel), metaproterenol (Alupent, Metaprel), pirbuterol (Maxair), salmeterol (Serevent), terbutaline (Brethaire, Brethine, Bricanyl) |
| **Decongestants** | Removal of fluid buildup in the respiratory passages | Hypersensitivity reactions, anxiety, decreased cardiac output, decreased urine output, electrolyte imbalances, headaches, nervousness, racing heart rate, seizures, tremor | CV disorders, diabetes mellitus, hyperthyroidism, lactation, pregnancy, hypersensitivity | Other sympathomimetics, MAO inhibitors, beta blockers, methyldopa | Phenylephrine (Dimetapp, Neo-Synephrine, PediaCare, Sudafed PE Quick Dissolve, Triaminic), pseudoephedrine (Chlor-Trimeton, Contac Cold, Drixoral, Triaminic) |
| **Glucocorticoids** | Decrease of inflammation | Cough, dry mouth, hoarseness, oral fungal infection, throat irritation, headache, dizziness | Viral, bacterial, or fungal infections, heart failure, cirrhosis, diabetes mellitus, hypertension, hypothyroidism, renal failure | Barbiturates, phenytoin, oral contraceptives | Beclomethasone (Vanceril, Beclovent), budesonide (Pulmicort), dexamethasone sodium phosphate (Decadron, Dexone), flunisolide (Aerobid), fluticasone (Flovent), methylprednisolone (Medrol, Solu-Medrol), mometasone furoate (Asmanex), triamcinolone (Azmacort), prednisone (Deltasone, Orasone, Prednicot), prednisolone (Orapred) |
| **Mucolytics** | Loosening or breaking up of thick mucus | Drowsiness, mouth inflammation, runny nose, bronchospasm, nausea, vomiting | CV disease, diabetes mellitus, ineffective cough, lactation, pregnancy, thyroid abnormalities | Activated charcoal | Acetylcysteine (Mucomyst) |

*Continued*

**Master the Essentials: Respiratory Medications—cont'd**

| Class | Indications for Use | Side Effects | Contraindications and Precautions | Interactions | Examples |
|---|---|---|---|---|---|
| Oxygen | Provision of additional needed oxygen to the lungs | Alveolar changes, blindness in premature infants, confusion, hypoventilation | Avoidance of high doses in patients with COPD | None reported | Oxygen |
| Respiratory stimulants | Treatment of apnea | Abdominal pain, blood in stools, seizure, fever, bradycardia or tachycardia, sleep problems, fussiness, loss of appetite | Hypersensitivity, seizure disorders, heart, kidney or liver disease, hyperglycemia or hypoglycemia | Caffeine-containing foods (chocolate, cola) | Theophylline, caffeine citrate (Cafcit) |
| Smoking cessation aids | Smoking cessation; decrease in symptoms of nicotine withdrawal such as a tight chest | **Nicotine:** cardiac irritability, local irritation, headache **Bupropion:** nausea, vomiting, constipation, appetite changes, headache, insomnia **Varenicline:** nausea, constipation, unusual dreams | Hypersensitivity, pregnancy, breast-feeding, epilepsy, anorexia, bulimia | Alcohol, benzodiazepines, beta blockers, insulin, MAO inhibitors | Bupropion (Budeprion, Wellbutrin, Zyban), nicotine (Nicorette, NicoDerm, Nicotrol), varenicline (Chantix) |

CNS, central nervous system; COPD, chronic obstructive pulmonary disease; CV, cardiovascular; GI, gastrointestinal; MAO, monoamine oxidase.

## Mast cell stabilizers

Mast cell stabilizers inhibit allergy cells called mast cells from bursting open and releasing substances that cause inflammation. These medications are used to prevent or decrease the occurrence of asthma attacks. They do not cure the disease or help during an acute attack, but rather they decrease the body's reaction to asthma triggers, such as air pollutants, respiratory infections, chemicals, food allergies, pollen, dust, mold, animal dander, and stress.

Cromolyn sodium (Intal) and nedocromil sodium (Tilade) are examples of mast cell stabilizers. These medications should not be used for acute asthma attacks, but as a preventive measure. They take 2 to 6 weeks to start working. They are administered via a nebulizer or metered-dose inhaler most commonly, but they also come in an intranasal form for seasonal allergies.

## Anti-influenza agents

Medications can ease the signs and symptoms of influenza. These medications are usually taken for 2 to 5 days. Although prevention of influenza through vaccination is preferred, anti-influenza agents can reduce the duration of the illness. Examples of drugs used to treat influenza include zanmivir (Relenza) and oseltamivir phosphate (Tamiflu). Relenza is a powder that is delivered via an inhaler, and Tamiflu is taken by mouth as a capsule or liquid. These medications do not cure influenza or prevent patients from spreading it to others. They reduce the severity of influenza symptoms and shorten the duration of the illness.

## Antitussives and expectorants

Antitussives stop coughs by blocking the cough reflex. If a cough is dry and thus not productive, an antitussive may be prescribed to allow the patient to rest, especially at night. Some narcotic analgesics, such as codeine, are effective antitussives in low dosages.

When secretions are present, expectorants are used to increase the body's ability to clear the lungs and upper airway by thinning the secretions. Expectorants such as guaifenesin (Duratess, Mucinex, Robitussin) can also soothe respiratory tract mucous membranes. These medications are given by mouth as a syrup, tablet, or capsule.

## Antibiotics

Many respiratory illnesses either are caused by or are accompanied by bacterial infections, and antibiotics are therefore prescribed to combat or prevent the infections as appropriate (see Chapter 17). Intravenous antibiotics may be administered for serious infections requiring hospitalization, such as pneumonia. The usual treatment for most other respiratory infections consists of oral antibiotics for a period of 10 to 14 days. Occasionally, a patient is given an injection of an antibiotic, followed by an oral medication course. This injection jump starts the healing process without the need for IV infusions and hospitalization.

One bacterium in particular, *Mycobacterium tuberculosis,* causes a highly contagious infection, TB. Tubercles remain in a patient's body for a lifetime and can be reactivated if the infection is not treated. For this reason, many patients with immunologic disorders such as acquired immunodeficiency syndrome (AIDS) can die of TB. Pharmacological treatment of TB requires exact adherence to a regimen of several drugs over 6 to 12 months because TB heals very slowly. These medications can also be given to close companions of infected patients to prevent infection. The most common combination of drugs consists of INH (isoniazid) and Rifadin (rifampin), but usually a combination of up to four antibiotics is used. In addition, those patients with **latent tuberculosis (TB)** (infected with TB, but without the disease) are treated with one antibiotic for 6 to 12 months to prevent them from developing the disease at some point later in life. Patients with latent TB are not contagious. Rifampin has a unique side effect of which patients must be made aware. Tears, urine, perspiration, and other body fluids will turn orange yellow. This can be scary for a patient who is unaware of this side effect (A Closer Look: Tuberculosis Diagnosis).

---

### A CLOSER LOOK: Tuberculosis Diagnosis

What is the difference between having the disease and having latent TB? When a person is given a TB test **(purified protein derivative [PPD]),** the skin test result is positive in both TB disease and latent TB. The difference is that those patients with latent TB do not have any signs of active disease such as changes to their chest radiographs. They have been exposed to the disease and the tubercles are in their bodies but are not making them sick. Prophylactic administration of antibiotics helps to keep the disease from becoming active.

---

### Antiviral medications

As discussed in Chapter 17, antiviral medications are used to prevent the growth of a virus. Antibiotics cannot kill a virus and may actually cause harm by increasing the patient's risk of developing an infection resistant to antibiotic treatment. Although a virus cannot be killed, its replication can be inhibited. Antiviral medications are usually administered to decrease the duration of a viral illness and/or minimize the symptoms. For example, **respiratory syncytial virus (RSV)** is a common virus that affects premature and other small infants adversely because of the extremely thick secretions associated with this viral illness. Small infants who have another risk factor such as being immunocompromised or those with congenital birth defects may be at risk of developing complications such as pneumonia or bronchiolitis. These infants are therefore given an antiviral drug called ribavirin (Virazole) (Drug Spotlight 18.1). This drug is given as an aerosol treatment continuously for approximately 3 to 5 days. Exposure to these medications has serious side effects, so visitors and health-care workers must be educated and monitored closely during administration of this medication.

### Bronchodilator medications

Bronchodilators relieve acute bronchospasm and include anticholinergics, xanthines (methylxanthines), and beta-adrenergic agonists. They relax the smooth muscle of the bronchi and allow the patient to breathe more easily. When inhaled, these drugs work immediately on the pulmonary system. When they are taken orally, it takes longer for the patient to feel the effect, but the action is of longer duration, and side effects may be felt for longer as well.

---

### Drug Spotlight 18.1 *Virazole (ribavirin)*

| | |
|---|---|
| Definition | Antiviral medication used for respiratory syncytial virus (RSV) |
| Patient profile | Used primarily in infants and children at risk for developing complications such as pneumonia from underlying chronic illness or prematurity |
| Side effects | Thickened sections leading to potential respiratory distress, rash, eye irritation |
| Risk factors | Possible risk to developing fetus, so women who are possibly pregnant or trying to become pregnant (including parents and health-care workers) should avoid being in room where drug is administered |
| Special instructions | Removal of contact lenses before entrance into the room because of the possibility of damage to the contacts and increased eye irritation |
| Route of administration | Aerosol treatment administered via a tent for 3 to 5 days |

### Anticholinergics

Parasympatholytics or anticholinergics dilate bronchi by blocking the action of acetylcholine, which causes bronchospasm. These medications are used to prevent bronchospasms, not to treat those already in progress.

Because these drugs stimulate the sympathetic nervous system, you can expect a fight or flight response, including increased heart rate and blood pressure. This effect also dries up lung secretions and thereby decreases congestion and improves pulmonary function. Examples of anticholinergic bronchodilators include ipratropium bromide (Atrovent) and tiotropium (Spiriva). Both these medications are administered via inhalation and are prescribed for patients with bronchitis, emphysema, or COPD. Atrovent is inhaled as a mist, and Spiriva is inhaled in powder form.

### Xanthines (methylxanthines)

Xanthines, also called methylxanthines, include theophylline and aminophylline. These medications relax smooth muscle and relieve bronchospasm. Asthma is the most common illness for which these medications are used. Because patients metabolize them at different rates, the dosage must be carefully adjusted based on the patient's reaction. These medications have a narrow safety margin, so careful monitoring is essential. In other words, there is a small difference between the amount of medication needed to be effective and the amount that produces toxic effects in the patient. IV aminophylline may be given as a continuous infusion for serious asthma attacks when the patient is hospitalized. Oral forms such as aminophylline (Phyllocontin, Truphylline) and theophylline (Elixophyllin, TheoCap, Slo-Bid, Theo-Dur Sprinkles) should be taken on an empty stomach with a full glass of water, for faster absorption. However, taking this medication on a full stomach decreases gastric upset.

### Beta-adrenergic agonists

Beta-adrenergic agonists are bronchodilators that are commonly used for treating asthma (Fig. 18-2). They stimulate beta-2 receptor sites in the sympathetic nervous system and result in bronchial dilation. Short-acting agents include albuterol (Proventil, Ventolin), bitolterol (Tornalate), levalbuterol (Xopenex), isoproterenol (Isuprel), metaproterenol (Alupent, Metaprel), pirbuterol (Maxair), and terbutaline (Brethaire, Brethine, Bricanyl); they are mainly used as needed. A long-acting agent, such as formoterol (Foradil) or salmeterol (Serevent), is used to control asthma.

Additionally, a drug called epinephrine (Adrenalin) is given as a subcutaneous injection in episodes of severe dyspnea associated with asthma. This acts as a bronchodilator and opens up the airways when other drugs do not create the desired response in an emergency situation. Other forms are found in multidose inhalers (MDIs) as a part of a combination of drugs to help with milder asthma attacks.

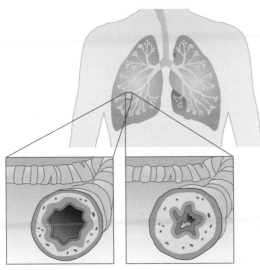

Normal bronchiole    Asthmatic bronchiole    **FIGURE 18-2:** Asthma.

## Decongestants

Decongestants cause the blood vessels in the nasal mucous membranes to constrict, thus reducing nasal passage drainage. They are available as nasal sprays and oral medications that are combined with different medications to treat cold and allergy symptoms. The main decongestant medications include phenylephrine (Dimetapp, Neo-Synephrine, PediaCare, Sudafed PE Quick Dissolve, Triaminic) and pseudoephedrine (Chlor-Trimeton, Contac Cold, Drixoral, Triaminic). Use of the topical form provides immediate relief of nasal mucosal swelling and congestion. These medications must be used on a short-term basis only, to avoid rebound congestion problems. They should never be given to children younger than 2 years old. In addition, because many of these medications are mixed with antipyretics and analgesics in cold and allergy remedies, dosages of medications such as acetaminophen and ibuprofen need to be monitored closely, to avoid overdose situations.

## Glucocorticoids

Glucocorticoids suppress the immune system, which means inflammation is decreased. When the risk of asthma exacerbation increases (e.g., pollen counts are high), medications such as beclomethasone (Vanceril, Beclovent), budesonide (Pulmicort), flunisolide (Aerobid), fluticasone (Flovent), mometasone furoate (Asmanex), and triamcinolone (Azmacort) are usually taken daily in an oral or inhaled form as prophylaxis, but they are not used for acute episodes. To treat acute asthma episodes or other respiratory illnesses such as croup, short periods of oral steroids such as dexamethasone sodium phosphate (Decadron, Dexone), prednisone (Deltasone, Orasone, Prednicot), prednisolone (Orapred), and methylprednisolone (Medrol) may be prescribed in an oral form. In severe acute episodes, medications such as methylprednisolone (Solu-Medrol) may be used in an intravenous form in much higher doses, to dilate the airways and allow respirations to ease.

As discussed previously (see Chapter 17), glucocorticoids should be taken only in the short term. If taken for more than 10 days, oral glucocorticoids may have severe adverse effects resulting from immune system suppression. Medications in this class should be taken at the lowest effective dose for the least amount of time as possible.

## Mucolytics

Mucolytics liquefy very thick lung secretions so the secretions can be excreted through coughing. These drugs do this by changing the composition of the mucus. Combined with expectorants, mucolytic agents help remove irritating substances from the lungs. Acetylcysteine (Mucomyst) is an example of a mucolytic. This type of drug is most commonly used as an aerosol treatment in patients with cystic fibrosis. This genetic disease causes the respiratory secretions to be extremely thick and difficult to cough up. With frequent daily mucolytics as part of their respiratory care, these patients are able to remove the secretions through coughing and thus decrease the occurrence of lung infections.

## Oxygen

$O_2$ is used as therapy for low oxygenation, or **hypoxia.** Long-term use includes management of COPD; acute use is needed to treat dyspnea and carbon monoxide poisoning. $O_2$ can be delivered by nasal cannula, mask, endotracheal tube, hood, or tent.

$O_2$ is considered a drug and must have an order to administer it. It is important not to give more $O_2$ than ordered. For instance, patients with COPD tend to retain $CO_2$. This leads to higher than normal levels of $CO_2$ and lower than normal levels of $O_2$ in the blood (Fig. 18-3). Normally, the body reacts to higher levels of $CO_2$ by prompting the lungs to breathe more deeply and rapidly to exhale the excess $CO_2$. In patients with COPD, however, the body has adapted to the long-term higher levels of $CO_2$, so these patients have lowered $O_2$ levels as the trigger to breathe. Giving a patient with COPD more $O_2$ than is prescribed can actually shut off this adaptive mechanism and cause the patient's breathing to stop or slow markedly, thus further lowering the $O_2$ level in the blood.

Additionally, too much $O_2$ can damage the eyes, especially those of premature infants. Therefore, we give the lowest levels of $O_2$ that produce the results that the prescriber desires.

## Respiratory stimulants

For patients who have problems with **apnea** (periods of breathing cessation), medications to stimulate the respiratory center of the brain may be prescribed. The most common patient is the premature infant whose brain is not developed to the degree of a normal newborn. These infants require a nudge to breathe, and that is done with medications such as caffeine citrate (Cafcit) or theophylline. Many

**FIGURE 18-3:** Chronic obstructive pulmonary disease (COPD). (A) Normal alveoli. (B) Destructive changes of COPD.

premature infants take these medications for many months after release from the neonatal intensive care unit. In the adult patient, the reason for sleep apnea is usually a structural problem causing an obstruction. Medication has not been proven to help with this situation. Surgery, lifestyle change such as weight loss, or an assistive breathing apparatus is used to open the obstructed airway.

## Smoking cessation

Because tobacco smoking is addictive and causes so many illnesses (e.g., emphysema, lung cancer, and bronchitis) in both smokers and those around them, medications have been developed to facilitate smoking cessation. Combined with hypnosis and behavioral therapy, these medications can be extremely effective. Because it is very difficult to quit completely and suddenly ("cold turkey"), smoking cessation aids, which contain the drug nicotine, deliver small, consistent doses of nicotine to help the individual gradually withdraw from nicotine use. This treatment is usually administered via a transdermal patch (NicoDerm) or in gum (Nicorette). Be sure to educate patients and enforce for them that they cannot smoke while using nicotine patches, to avoid a nicotine overdose. In addition, patients should not wear nicotine patches when they are inside magnetic resonance imaging (MRI) equipment because patients have been reported to suffer burns at the site of the patch. Other routes for nicotine include inhalation (Nicotrol) and nasal spray (Nicotrol).

Another drug that may be prescribed as an oral medication is bupropion hydrochloride (Budeprion, Wellbutrin, Zyban). This drug was originally developed as an antidepressant, but it has been found to have significant benefit in the battle to stop smoking. However, it has serious risks of suicidal ideation and completion. The potential benefits of this medication should therefore be weighed heavily against the risks when this drug is considered. Patient education must be thorough with each prescription of this drug.

A newer oral medication used with behavior modification that works to convince your brain that smoking is not pleasurable is varenicline (Chantix). The patient may smoke during treatment but slowly loses the desire to do so.

### Virtual Field Trip

Visit the American Lung Association's Web site, and find tips for smoking cessation to create a teaching plan for patients.

## ●●● SUMMARY

The pulmonary system must function properly to maintain health. Many medications exist to help heal a malfunctioning system and work by opening the bronchi, drying secretions, decreasing the histamine response, treating infections, conveying $O_2$ to the lungs, stopping coughs, loosening mucus, and forcing out secretions. Smoking cessation drugs help patients stop a habit that could lead to significant complications, as well as death.

---

**KEY TERMS**

| | | |
|---|---|---|
| Alimentary canal | Flatulence | Morbidly obese |
| Calculus | Gastroesophageal reflux | Nausea |
| Cathartic | disease (GERD) | Peristalsis |
| Constipation | *H. pylori* | Reflux |
| Diarrhea | Halitosis | Stomatitis |
| Digestion | Heartburn | Thrush |
| Emesis | Hemorrhoid | Ulcer |
| Fissure | Hydrochloric acid (HCl) | |

---

## ■ GASTROINTESTINAL SYSTEM

The gastrointestinal (GI), or digestive, system consists of a long tube called the **alimentary canal** that begins at the mouth and ends at the anus, with accessory organs attached (Fig. 19-1). The alimentary canal is responsible for the four major functions of the digestive system: ingestion, digestion, absorption, and excretion. The goal of each function is to allow nutrients from food to be used as cellular energy.

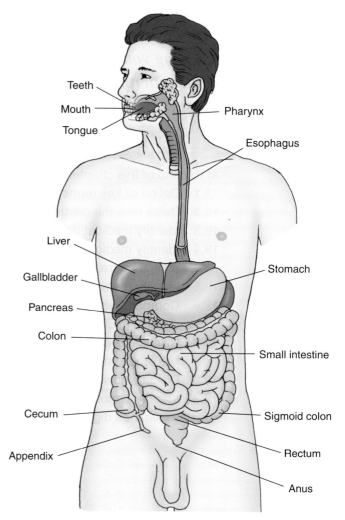

**FIGURE 19-1:** The gastrointestinal system.

Digestion begins in the mouth, where food is consumed and broken down into a usable form first by mechanical digestion (chewing) and then by chemical digestion (enzymes). Certain enzymes perform specific functions with respect to digesting the three complex organic molecules found in food: fats, proteins, and carbohydrates. These enzymes work at various sites along the GI tract. Food particles are chewed in the mouth and then swallowed, move through the oropharynx, then the esophagus, into the stomach, and are then pushed through the small intestine and large intestine via **peristalsis** (wavelike movements). If this process is impeded, toxic substances can build up. Infection can develop when the normal flora living in the alimentary canal is disturbed.

Review Table 19.1 to understand the role of the major digestive organs more clearly.

The stomach's environment is high in **hydrochloric acid (HCl),** which helps it break down food for absorption. **Reflux** or backflow of HCl into the esophagus can lead to ulcers, or mucosal breakdown. When the mucosa is penetrated, it creates a prime environment for infection to spread because food moving through the digestive tract comes from outside sources that may carry harmful microorganisms. Although the HCl and normal flora of the digestive tract kill some organisms, the GI system can still be a major site of infection.

**Digestion** is the process of converting food into chemical substances used by the body. However, depending on our food choices, we can damage our GI system. Bad or "junk" food can damage the system by overworking the pancreas, liver, and gallbladder. Extreme undereating can lead to anorexia nervosa, and extreme overeating can cause obesity. Other ways to damage the GI system include using medications that change the acidity of the stomach and eating food or other substances that contain harmful microbes, such as worms, viruses, or bacteria.

## ■ GASTROINTESTINAL MEDICATIONS

GI medications are used to treat specific disorders of the GI system or to control certain signs and symptoms, such as abdominal pain, change in bowel habits, heartburn, gas, weight loss, nausea, vomiting, difficulty swallowing, loss of appetite, and blood or mucus in the feces (see the Master the Essentials table for descriptions of the most common GI system drugs).

GI drugs work to increase or decrease function by changing the muscle tone, replacing deficient enzymes, or increasing or decreasing the emptying time or rate of passage through the system. Some drugs such as Reglan serve to move food through the system at a more rapid rate when a patient is having difficulty with reflux or heartburn. Other medications such as pancreatic enzymes are given to patients with cystic fibrosis to aid in the process of digestion.

Timing of GI medication administration is important as well. Some medications are taken to coat the stomach lining or to reduce gastric acidity and must be ingested on an empty stomach. Other medications must be taken with food so they can be absorbed properly. Some foods such as grapefruit can affect the absorption of certain medications if they are eaten at the same time the medicine is taken. It is important to understand the effect of food and medications on the GI system.

The following sections detail the most common complaints and disorders of the GI system and the medications used to manage them.

---

### TABLE 19.1  Functions of the Major Digestive Organs

| Stomach | • Stores food<br>• Mixes food with hydrochloric acid<br>• Passes this mixture, called **chyme**, into the small intestine |
|---|---|
| Small Intestine | • Carbohydrates, fats, and proteins broken down here<br>• Pancreatic enzymes and bile from the liver aid digestion<br>• End products of digestion absorbed into the bloodstream through mucous membranes |
| Large Intestine | • Absorbs extra water and electrolytes<br>• Eliminates waste products (feces) |

## Master the Essentials: Gastrointestinal Medications

This table shows the various classes of gastrointestinal medications and key side effects, contraindications and precautions, and interactions for each class.

| Class | Side Effects | Indications for Use | Contraindications/ Precautions | Interactions | Examples |
|---|---|---|---|---|---|
| Antacids | Constipation, diarrhea (especially with magnesium compounds), electrolyte imbalances, flatulence, kidney stones, osteoporosis | Peptic ulcers, GERD, acid indigestion | Heart failure, dehydration, kidney or liver disease | Antibiotics, salicylates | Magnesium hydroxide (Dulcolax, Phillips Milk of Magnesia), magnesium oxide (Mag-ox 400, Uro-Mag), aluminum hydroxide gel (Alterna gel), calcium carbonate (Tums), aluminum-magnesium combinations (Maalox, Mylanta) |
| Anorexiants | Palpitations, arrhythmias, dry mouth, hair loss, blurred vision, hypotension, dizziness, drowsiness | Obesity | Arteriosclerosis, heart disease, hypertension, glaucoma, pregnancy | MAO inhibitors, SSRIs, TCAs, alcohol, other diet medications | Phentermine (Adipex-P, Oby-Cap, T-Diet, Zantryl) |
| Antidiarrheals | Nausea, vomiting, drowsiness; constipations (kaolin and pectin) | Diarrhea | Hypersensitivity, bloody diarrhea | Alcohol, opiates, barbiturates, sedatives, metoclopramide; digoxin, allopurinol (kaolin and pectin) | Bismuth subsalicylate (Pepto-Bismol), diphenoxylate with atropine (Lomotil), loperamide (Imodium), kaolin and pectin (Kaopectate), *Lactobacillus acidophilus* (Lactinex, Bacid) |
| Antiemetics | Drowsiness, agitation, confusion, constipation, dry mouth, nausea, anorexia | Nausea, vomiting, motion sickness prophylaxis | Sensitivity, severe emesis, seizure disorder, pregnancy, prolonged QTc interval (5-HT$_3$ receptor antagonists) | Anticholinergics, lithium, CNS depressants | Chlorpromazine (Thorazine), prochlorperazine (Compazine, Compro), dolasetron (Anzemet), ondansetron (Zofran), granisetron (Kytril), palonosetron (Aloxi), dimenhydrinate (Dramamine), diphenhydramine (Benadryl), meclizine (Antivert, Bonine), promethazine (Adgan, Phenergan, Promethacon), trimethobenzamide (Benzacot, Tigan, Ticon), scopolamine (Scopace, Transderm-Scop), nabilone (Cesamet), phosphorated carbohydrate solution (Emetrol), metoclopramide (Reglan) |

## Master the Essentials: Gastrointestinal Medications—cont'd

| Class | Side Effects | Indications for Use | Contraindications/ Precautions | Interactions | Examples |
|---|---|---|---|---|---|
| Antiflatulents | None reported | Excessive intestinal gas | None reported | None reported | Simethicone (Alka-Seltzer Anti-Gas, Bicarsim, Equalize Gas Relief Drops, Flatulex, Gas Aid, Gas Free, Gas-X, Genasyme, Gerber Gas Relief Infantaire Gas Relief, Little Tummys, Maalox Anti-Gas, Mi-Acid Gas Relief, Mylanta Gas, Mylicon, Mytab Gas, Phazyme, SimePed) |
| Antifungals | Nausea, vomiting, diarrhea | Thrush | Hypersensitivity, pregnancy | None reported | Nystatin (Bio-Statin, Mycostatin, Nilstat) |
| Anthelmintics | Abdominal pain, diarrhea | Parasitic infection of GI tract | Hypersensitivity, pregnancy | Carbamazepine, hydantoins | Albendazole (Albenza), praziquantel (Biltricide), ivermectin (Stromectol), mebendazole (Vermox), pyrantel (Antiminth, Ascarel, Pin-X) |
| Antispasmodics | Palpitations, vision disturbances, headache, nervousness | Irritable bowel syndrome, diverticulitis, peptic ulcer | Hypersensitivity, glaucoma, bowel obstruction, urinary retention | Digoxin, phenothiazines, TCAs | Dicyclomine (Bentyl), glycopyrrolate (Robinul) |
| Bowel evacuants | Nausea, abdominal fullness, bloating, cramping | Preparation for GI procedures (surgical and radiological) such as endoscopy, colonoscopy, sigmoidoscopy | GI obstruction, ileus, gastric retention, bowel perforation, pregnancy | Administration of oral drugs within 1 hour may be flushed from GI tract | Polyethylene glycol electrolyte solution (Colyte, GoLYTELY, MoviPrep, NuLYTELY, PEG-3350 with Electrolytes, TriLyte), polyethylene glycol 3350 (GlycoLax, MiraLax) |
| Gallstone solubilizing agents | Headache, abdominal pain, diarrhea, dyspepsia, nausea | Gallstones | Hypersensitivity, intermittent acute cholecystitis, gallstone pancreatitis | Antacids, bile acid sequestrants, oral contraceptives | Ursodiol (Actigall, Urso) |
| GI stimulants (prokinetic agents) | Extrapyramidal symptoms, dizziness, drowsiness, fatigue, headache, insomnia, restlessness | GERD | GI hemorrhage, pheochromocytoma, sensitivity | Alcohol, cimetidine, cyclosporine, digoxin, levodopa, MAO inhibitors, anticholinergics | Metoclopramide (Reglan, Metozolv ODT), cisapride (Propulsid) |

*Continued*

## Master the Essentials: Gastrointestinal Medications—cont'd

| Class | Side Effects | Indications for Use | Contraindications/ Precautions | Interactions | Examples |
|---|---|---|---|---|---|
| *H. pylori* agents | Diarrhea, tinnitus, infection, mild GI problems | Peptic ulcer | Kidney or liver insufficiency | Salicylates, digoxin, anticoagulants | Amoxicillin (Amoxil, Trimox), clarithromycin (Biaxin), metronidazole (Flagyl), tetracycline |
| $H_2$-receptor antagonists | Constipation, diarrhea, nausea, headache, malaise, rash | Duodenal ulcer, gastric ulcer, GERD | Hypersensitivity, liver impairment | Antacids, benzodiazepines, opioids, phenytoin, beta blockers, calcium channel blockers, cyclosporine | Cimetidine (Tagamet), famotidine (Pepcid), nizatidine (Axid), ranitidine (Zantac) |
| Laxatives and stool softeners | Diarrhea, nausea, vomiting, cramping, bloating, flatulence | Constipation | Hypersensitivity, nausea, vomiting, fecal impaction, intestinal obstruction | Antacids, $H_2$ antagonists, proton pump inhibitors | Psyllium (Metamucil, Citrucel), mineral oil (Fleet Mineral Oil), magnesium hydroxide (MOM), docusate (Colace), senna with docusate bisacodyl (Peri-Colace, Dulcolax, Fleet), glycerine (Colace suppository), polyethylene glycol solution (MiraLax) |
| Lipase inhibitors | Flatulence, fecal urgency, oily stool, incontinence, abdominal pain | Obesity | Hypersensitivity, malabsorption syndrome cholestasis | Prevastatin, warfarin | Orlistat (alli, Xenical) |
| Prostaglandins | Diarrhea, abdominal pain | Duodenal or gastric ulcer | Pregnancy, history of allergy to prostaglandins, heart disease | Antacids | Misoprostol (Cytotec) |
| Proton pump inhibitors | Headache, abdominal pain, nausea, constipation, diarrhea | Active duodenal ulcers, GERD, benign gastric ulcers | Hypersensitivity, liver disease | Clarithromycin, sucralfate, benzodiazepines, azole antifungals, digoxin, hydantoins | Esomeprazole (Nexium), lansoprazole (Prevacid), omeprazole (Prilosec), pantoprazole (Protonix), rabeprazole (Aciphex) |
| Mucosal protectant | Constipation, diarrhea, nausea, vomiting, flatulence, rash | Ulcers | Renal failure | Antacids, anticoagulants, digoxin, $H_2$ antagonists, hydantoins | Sucralfate (Carafate) |

CNS, central nervous system; GERD, gastroesophageal reflux disease; GI, gastrointestinal; 5-$HT_3$, serotonin; MAO, monoamine oxidase; SSRIs, selective serotonin reuptake inhibitors; TCAs, tricyclic antidepressants.

## Medications to treat constipation

Many of the medications discussed in the previous chapters have a systemic effect and an effect on body systems other than the one for which the medication is prescribed. For example, medications that change smooth muscle tone to open up the respiratory tract in an asthmatic patient or that decrease the blood pressure in a cardiac patient can also affect the rate at which food moves through the body. When peristalsis slows, **constipation** or infrequent, hard stools can result. Some medications that contribute to constipation are diuretics, which remove fluid from the body and thereby cause hard stools. One such medication is furosemide (Lasix). As a result, the colon reabsorbs too much fluid, the feces become hard, and the alimentary canal does not clear. One class of medications that can help relieve constipation consists of laxatives. Laxatives help promote bowel movements and are classified as bulk-forming agents, osmotics, stimulants, or stool softeners. Laxatives can help diagnose GI disorders by cleansing the bowels to allow observation of the intestinal walls during examinations. These medications should not be used for losing weight because they could lead to a dependency on them to have a bowel movement and may also cause electrolyte imbalances. A **cathartic** is a stronger medication that facilitates fast emptying of the colon.

- **Bulk-forming laxatives.** Bulk-forming laxatives such as psyllium (Metamucil) increase bulk and water content of the stool as they resemble dietary fiber. This medication is available as a powder that can be added to liquid, as a capsule, and as a wafer to be eaten. Prunes and bran have the same effects. Bulk-forming laxatives are the best laxatives to take during pregnancy and if needed on a routine basis; they absorb water and create larger, softer stools. These larger stools stimulate peristalsis and thus purge the body of feces. These laxatives take 12 hours to 3 days to work.

- **Lubricant laxatives.** Lubricant laxatives such as mineral oil increase the water-to-fecal mass to ease the passage of stool and are usually taken as suppositories. Lubricant laxatives are typically oily. They take 6 to 8 hours to work.

- **Osmotic laxatives.** Osmotic laxatives, given rectally, such as glycerin or sorbitol exert an immediate action that draws water into the stool and irritates the bowel to increase peristalsis. The result is evacuation of stool, sometimes in the form of diarrhea, within 15 to 60 minutes. These laxatives are contraindicated in patients with hypertension, edema, or congestive heart failure because of the stress on the cardiovascular system caused by this rapid action. Milk of Magnesia is a mild osmotic laxative sometimes called a saline laxative. It increases the amount of water in the large intestines and usually works within 2 to 12 hours, depending on the dose. Salt ions can suck water toward themselves and thus lubricate the GI tract. Milk of Magnesia is therefore a safe option for those patients with hypertension, edema, or congestive heart failure.

- **Stimulant laxatives.** Stimulant laxatives stimulate peristalsis because they act directly on the intestinal mucosa and irritate the bowel. They are typically effective within 6 to 8 hours. Some examples include bisacodyl, senna, aloe, cascara sagrada, and castor oil. Side effects include cramping, diarrhea, flatulence, and nausea. Senna, aloe, and cascara sagrada discolor urine. Castor oil should not be used during pregnancy because of the risk of premature labor or during lactation because it may cause diarrhea in the infant.

- **Stool softeners.** Stool softeners decrease the consistency of stool by reducing surface tension and attracting water and fat to the stool to soften it and improve its passage through the colon. Docusate (Colace) is a detergent stool softener. This type of laxative is typically used routinely in patients with limited mobility resulting from injury or chronic illness.

- **Bowel evacuators.** Bowel evacuators are cleansing solutions that are used to remove stool before diagnostic tests, such as colonoscopy. They are made as mixes similar to body fluids, so material held in the bowel is rejected. Typically, the patient is asked to drink 1 gallon of fluid mixed with a bowel evacuator within a 2- to 3-hour time frame. Side effects can include bloating, nausea, and fullness. Examples of bowel evacuants include polyethylene glycol electrolyte solution (Colyte, GoLYTELY, MoviPrep, NuLYTELY, PEG-3350 with Electrolytes, TriLyte) and polyethylene glycol 3350 (GlycoLax, MiraLax).

In addition to the previously mentioned pharmacological medications to treat constipation, some nonpharmacological treatments for constipation include exercising, laughing (because it massages the intestines and thus encourages peristalsis), increasing dietary fiber, drinking more fluids, decreasing consumption of dairy products, and drinking warmed prune juice.

### ✳ CRITICAL THINKING

Patients can become dependent on laxatives. Why is this problematic? What are some nonpharmacological treatments for constipation?

## Medications to treat diarrhea

The opposite of constipation is **diarrhea,** which is an increase in the frequency and fluidity of bowel movements. Almost all individuals have diarrhea at one time or another, but if it occurs over several days, the body can lose too much fluid and too many electrolytes. This loss can occur within several hours in small children and infants.

Diarrhea is a symptom, not a disease. Certain chemicals, inflammation, infections, and other medications can cause diarrhea. Anti-infective therapy frequently causes diarrhea. Anxiety and circulatory disorders can cause diarrhea as well.

Stools of excessive volume and fluidity are more than just a bother. The cramping that frequently accompanies diarrhea can be very painful. Diarrhea can signal that the person has eaten spoiled or contaminated food and has an intestinal infection. In small children and the elderly, diarrhea can cause life-threatening loss of valuable fluid and electrolytes. Fortunately, several available medications, such as opioid-related antidiarrheals and absorbents, can help treat diarrhea.

Opioid-related antidiarrheal medications are highly effective and are used for the most serious cases of diarrhea. They work by inhibiting GI motility, decreasing peristalsis, and slowing the function of the GI system, thus allowing more time for water to be reabsorbed through the intestinal wall. An example is loperamide (Imodium), which is taken orally and is available over the counter (OTC), as well as by prescription. Another example is diphenoxylate with atropine (Lomotil), which comes in tablet form and is available only by prescription because of the addictive qualities of this drug. Side effects include dizziness, dry mouth, agitation, numbness, drowsiness, and tachycardia.

### Absorbents

Absorbents, such as bismuth (Pepto-Bismol) (Drug Spotlight 19.1) or kaolin and pectin (Kaopectate), are taken after every bowel movement to absorb toxins or bacteria and to coat the walls of the GI tract. Because the treatment focuses on the cause of the diarrhea, medications may also include antibiotics, anti-inflammatories, or antiparasitics. The most common use of antibiotics for diarrhea occurs with "traveler's diarrhea." Exposure to the water or contaminated food in foreign countries leads to bacterial, viral, or parasitic infections. Ciprofloxacin (Cipro), ofloxacin (Floxin), and azithromycin (Zithromax Z-Pak) are commonly used antibiotics, depending on the destination of the traveler. Ulcerative colitis is an example of inflammation that causes diarrhea and is treated with anti-inflammatory drugs such as sulfasalazine (Azulfidine), mesalamine rectal (Canasa, Rowasa), balsalazide (Colazal), and olsalazine (Dipentum). Antiparasitic medications are discussed later in this chapter (also see Chapter 17 for more information).

## Medications to treat nausea and vomiting (antiemetics)

**Nausea,** although an uncomfortable feeling that vomiting is imminent, is not dangerous. Sometimes nausea is caused by unusual smells, pregnancy hormones, or emptiness of the stomach. **Emesis,** or vomiting, occurs when the patient ejects the contents of the stomach.

Antiemetics decrease nausea and vomiting and are also used to treat motion sickness. Examples of antiemetics include phenothiazines such as prochlorperazine (Compazine), antihistamines such as diphenhydramine (Benadryl) and meclizine (Antivert, Bonine), trimethobenzamide (Benzacot, Tigan, Ticon), cannabinoids, phosphorated carbohydrate solution (Emetrol), and 5-hydroxytryptamine-3 (5-HT$_3$, serotonin) receptor antagonists such as ondansetron (Zofran).

■ **Phenothiazines.** Phenothiazines block dopamine receptors in the area of the brain that stimulates vomiting. Two examples, chlorpromazine (Thorazine) and prochlorperazine (Compazine,

**Drug Spotlight 19.1** *Pepto-Bismol (bismuth subsalicylate)*

| | |
|---|---|
| Definition | The pink medicine that relieves five different gastrointestinal symptoms: heartburn, nausea, indigestion, upset stomach, and diarrhea |
| Form | Available as suspension, tablets, and chewable tablets |
| Contraindications | • Salicylate in this medication may make gout symptoms worse<br>• May make ulcer symptoms worse<br>• May make bleeding problems worse<br>• Taking other salicylate medications with this drug may lead to overdose<br>• Mothers should not breastfeed while taking this medication |
| Special concerns | • This drug used only in teenagers 12 years and older and adults; younger children usually not given medication for diarrhea, but managed with fluid replacement therapy only; in addition, this drug should never be used in a child or teenager with a viral illness because of the unknown association between salicylates and Reye's syndrome<br>• Elderly patients should check with their physician before using this medication |
| Side effects | • Tongue may turn black: normal, secondary to interaction of bismuth and the sulfides found in the digestive tract; subsides after discontinuation of medication<br>• Stools turn black: same reason as tongue |

Compro), are used to control the nausea and vomiting that occur with chemotherapy and can be administered orally, by injection, or by the intravenous (IV) route. In addition, prochlorperazine may be given as a rectal suppository. These drugs tend to produce sedation while treating the nausea and vomiting. These medications are available by prescription only.

■ **5-Hydroxytryptamine-3 receptor antagonists.** 5-HT$_3$ is more commonly known as serotonin. Therefore, these medications are known as serotonin antagonists and are also commonly used to prevent and treat the nausea and vomiting associated with chemotherapy. They block the chemical serotonin, which is produced in the brain and in the stomach. Examples of this class of medications include dolasetron (Anzemet), ondansetron (Zofran), granisetron (Kytril), and palonosetron (Aloxi). These medications are all administered either orally or by the IV route. Additionally, Zofran may be given as an injection. These medications are available by prescription only.

■ **Antihistamines.** The action of antihistamines in decreasing nausea and vomiting is unclear. It is believed that these medications block signals to the brain's movement center. Therefore, they tend to work best on the nausea associated with motion sickness. Dramamine (dimenhydrinate), diphenhydramine (Benadryl), meclizine (Antivert, Bonine), and promethazine (Adgan, Phenergan, Promethacon) are examples of this class of drugs used for nausea and vomiting. All these medications are available to be taken orally, and dimenhydrinate, diphenhydramine, and meclizine may be purchased OTC. Dimenhydrinate, diphenhydramine, and promethazine may also be administered by injection or by the IV route. Promethazine may also be given by rectal suppository.

■ **Anticholinergic medications.** As discussed in Chapter 13, anticholinergic medications block the effects of the neurotransmitter acetylcholine. It is thought to act on the chemoreceptor trigger zone, which is an area of the medulla in the brain that can be stimulated by blood-borne medications or hormones and that initiates vomiting. Trimethobenzamide (Benzacot, Tigan, Ticon) is an anticholinergic that can be given orally, rectally, or by intramuscular injection and is available by prescription only. Another prescription anticholinergic medication is scopolamine (Scopace, Transderm-Scop) which can be given by the IV, IM, or subcutaneous route for nausea and vomiting. In addition, scopolamine can be used as a transdermal disc placed behind the ear before exposure to a motion sickness–causing event.

- **Cannabinoids.** These are manufactured forms of cannabis. Marijuana is the herbal form of cannabis. An example of a cannabinoid is nabilone (Cesamet), and it works by affecting the area of the brain that controls the nausea and vomiting impulses. This medication has a high level of addiction possibility and therefore should be prescribed only when other antiemetics are unsuccessful for the patient receiving chemotherapy. In addition, the patient may suffer from altered thinking and thus should take this medication with care. Cesamet is taken orally before the start of chemotherapy and for a period of time during and after each chemotherapy dose. This drug and marijuana are controlled substances, and marijuana is legal for medical use only in approximately a dozen states in the United States.

- **Phosphorated carbohydrate solution.** The trade name of phosphorated carbohydrate solution is Emetrol, and it contains dextrose, fructose (a type of sugar), and phosphoric acid. It decreases the hyperactivity of the smooth muscle of the gastric mucosa. This medication is contraindicated in patients with diabetes mellitus because of the fructose content. It is available OTC and is taken by mouth. It is thought to be safe to use during pregnancy, but, as always, the physician's advice should be sought before any medication is taken at this time.

## Medications used to treat gastroesophageal reflux disease

If the cardiac sphincter is loose, stomach acid can move upward into the esophagus, thus causing irritation and damage to the mucosa. This can result in **gastroesophageal reflux disease (GERD)** (Fig. 19-2). The burning sensation that the patient feels when acid damages the esophagus is **heartburn.** Heartburn does not actually involve the heart, but pain is localized near the heart, and patients often report that it feels like their heart is burning. Several medications are available to alleviate the symptoms of GERD and also promote healing.

### Antacids

Antacids, as the name implies, decrease the amount of hydrochloric acid (HCl) in the stomach. Antacids create a more alkaline environment, which neutralizes the acid and protects the vulnerable mucosa, thereby relieving the pain and destruction associated with GERD. Except for sodium bicarbonate (baking soda), antacids are not readily absorbed and do not alter the pH of the entire body. These medications contain aluminum, calcium, magnesium, sodium, or a combination of these active ingredients. Thus, the prescriber will choose an antacid based on which of these substances the patient would benefit from best and which should be avoided. For example, a woman with osteoporosis would benefit from a calcium-based antacid. Conversely, a patient suffering from calcium-based kidney stones should avoid dietary calcium, so another medication would be chosen.

Some antacids may need to be taken regularly to condition the stomach to decrease acid production. Timing of these medications is critical; they must be taken before food. Sometimes antacids are given

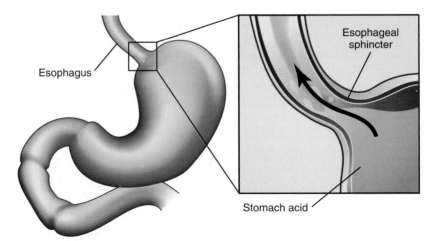

**FIGURE 19-2:** Gastroesophageal reflux disease.

in suspensions, which must be shaken, or chewable tablets. Chewable tablets are usually taken with a glass of water or milk. Action occurs within 30 minutes to 3 hours. $H_2$-receptor blockers are given 1 hour before or 3 hours after meals. Long-term use of antacids can increase acid secretion. Patients should be cautioned not to overuse sodium bicarbonate because of its systemic effect, and they should be told that changing gastric acid pH may affect absorption of other medications.

Antacids are also used to lower elevated acid levels resulting from spicy foods and to decrease the nausea related to pregnancy hormones. Many mild antacids, such as Tums and Rolaids, are available OTC.

### Proton pump inhibitor drugs

Proton pump inhibitors reduce the acidity of the stomach by binding to stomach enzymes. Because they act on enzymes that cause increased acidity, these medications tend to protect the stomach for a time. They inhibit hydrogen and potassium ions and are used as short-term treatment for GERD and benign peptic ulcers. Side effects include abdominal pain, headache, constipation, diarrhea, and nausea. Examples of proton pump inhibitors are esomeprazole (Nexium), lansoprazole (Prevacid), omeprazole (Prilosec), pantoprazole (Protonix), and rabeprazole (Aciphex). These medications are given by mouth and are mostly available by prescription, although some are beginning to be available in low doses OTC. In addition, all these medications except pantoprazole may be given by the IV route when the patient is unable to tolerate the oral form.

### Gastric stimulants

Gastric stimulants or prokinetic agents stimulate gastric activity in the patient with decreased peptic activity. They decrease esophageal sphincter pressure and increase gastric emptying, which improves peristalsis. If a patient is at risk for aspiration of stomach contents, this drug may be given to decrease the amount of time the food is in the stomach and thus reduce the risk of aspiration pneumonia or choking. This quick emptying of the stomach has the added benefit of working as an antiemetic. An example of a GI stimulant is metoclopramide (Reglan). Reglan is given primarily by the IV route in the hospital setting, but it may also be given by intramuscularly or by mouth. Side effects include drowsiness, restlessness, headache, dry mouth, menstrual period changes, and diarrhea.

## Medications used to treat peptic ulcers

The stomach secretes HCl to break down food into amounts small enough to allow easy absorption. However, the stomach can create too much acid, which erodes the mucosal layer and can lead to a peptic **ulcer** (perforation of the mucosa) (Fig. 19-3). Acid from the stomach can spill into the duodenum and erode the mucosa there as well.

Patients at high risk for ulcers are those with type O blood, cigarette smokers, those infected with *Helicobacter pylori (H. pylori),* and those who do not cope well with stress. Alcohol, caffeinated foods and beverages, and certain drugs (corticosteroids, aspirin, nonsteroidal anti-inflammatory drugs [NSAIDs]) can also increase the risk of a peptic ulcer.

In the past, patients with peptic ulcers were encouraged to drink lots of milk because it was thought that ulcers were related to the acidity of the stomach, and milk is alkaline. Now it is known that *H. pylori* grows very well in milk, and milk was perhaps one of the worst treatments to recommend. This is why it is important for allied health professionals to keep current on treatments supported by research. Some medications used to treat peptic ulcers include mucosal protectants, prostaglandins, antispasmodics, $H_2$-receptor antagonists, antibiotics, and proton pump inhibitors. Each is described in more detail here.

■ **Mucosal protectants.** Mucosal protectants such as sucralfate (Carafate), which is aluminum hydroxide and sulfated sucrose, are used to treat ulcers. This oral medication works to cover and protect the ulcer to promote healing, but it must be taken on an empty stomach. Mucosal protectants are like a bandage protecting a wound from dirt and injury and allowing it to heal. Side effects include constipation and vitamin deficiency.

■ **Prostaglandins.** Prostaglandins are hormone-like substances with a wide range of effects on the body, such as contraction and relaxation of smooth muscle, moderation of inflammation, and control of blood pressure. In the case of peptic ulcers, misoprostol (Cytotec) is a

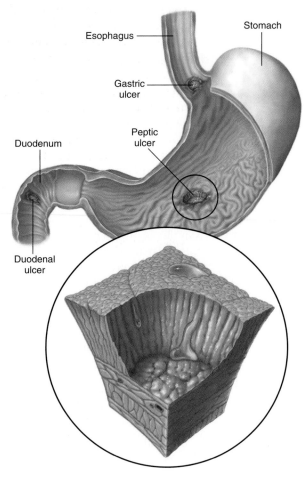

**FIGURE 19-3:** Peptic ulcer.

prostaglandin that inhibits gastric acid secretion and thus decreases the amount of acid in the stomach and protects the lining of the stomach. It is used to reduce the risk of NSAID-induced ulcers. This medication is taken orally, and side effects may include diarrhea, stomach cramps, and nausea during the first weeks of treatment; these side effects can be reduced by taking the medication with food. This drug must not be used during pregnancy because of the risk of miscarriage, premature labor, or possible birth defects.

■ **Antispasmodics.** Antispasmodics (anticholinergics) decrease secretions and gastric mobility, reduce gastric spasm, and slow gastric motility. These effects decrease the exposure of the fragile gastric mucosa to HCl by keeping food in the stomach and reducing the amount of stomach acids produced. These medications are also used to treat GERD, ulcerative colitis, diverticulitis, biliary spasm, and irritable bowel syndrome. Examples include dicyclomine (Bentyl) and glycopyrrolate (Robinul). These are both available by prescription only. They may be administered orally but if needed can be given as an intramuscular injection and, in the case of glycopyrrolate, as an IV dose.

■ **$H_2$-receptor antagonists.** $H_2$-receptor antagonists are a group of drugs that block histamine from binding to parietal cells and prevent the parietal cells from secreting the gastric acid HCl. $H_2$-receptor antagonists include the drugs cimetidine (Tagamet), famotidine (Pepcid), nizatidine (Axid), and ranitidine (Taladine, Zantac). All these medications are available both by prescription and in other forms OTC. Initial treatment of ulcers with cimetidine, famotidine, and ranitidine may be accomplished via IV therapy. Then, once the acute phase is treated, oral forms of the medications are begun. Nizatidine is only administered orally. In addition, ranitidine may be given as an intramuscular injection. $H_2$-receptor antagonists can be taken with or without meals, but they should be given approximately 30 minutes before meals so that medications levels are at the optimum levels when acid is actively being produced. In addition, they should not be given within 1 hour of an antacid because the antacid may inhibit the absorption of the H$_2$-receptor antagonist. Side effects may include nausea, vomiting, diarrhea, dry mouth, dizziness, weakness, headache, and muscle cramps.

■ **Antibiotics.** Antibiotics fight *H. pylori,* which is a bacterium that can damage the GI tract. It is associated with 75% of gastric ulcers with 90% of duodenal ulcers. When the *H. pylori* is killed, the ulcer has a chance to heal. Antibiotics used to treat *H. pylori* include amoxicillin (Amoxil, Trimox), clarithromycin (Biaxin), metronidazole (Flagyl), and tetracycline. These agents are never used alone but in a combination of two antibiotics. This approach helps to avoid failure of treatment as well as antibiotic resistance. It is important that patients complete the entire 7- to 14-day regimen, even if they feel better, to remove the bacterium completely. Bismuth compounds can also be prescribed because they are bacteriostatic and stop *H. pylori* from sticking to the mucosa.

■ **Proton pump inhibitors.** As discussed earlier in relation to GERD, these drugs reduce the acidity of the stomach and thus decrease exposure of the ulceration to acid. They are frequently combined with antibiotics to act against *H. pylori.*

Antacids and GI stimulants are also often used in the treatment of ulcers.

### CRITICAL THINKING

What risks for peptic ulcers involve lifestyle, not genetics? What lifestyle changes should a patient with a peptic ulcer make?

## Medications to treat gallstones

Cholelithiasis, or the abnormal condition of having stones in the gallbladder, is caused when cholesterol or calcium forms a **calculus** (stone) (Fig. 19-4). Cholesterol cannot be seen on radiographs, but calcium stones can. Symptoms of gallstones are bloating, gas, and nausea. Most symptomatic patients undergo surgical removal of the stones and/or gallbladder. For those patients who cannot tolerate surgery, medication such as ursodiol (Actigall, Urso) may be prescribed in an oral form. Ursodiol is a naturally occurring bile acid that decreases the production of cholesterol and inhibits absorption of cholesterol by the intestines. Therapy can take up to 2 years, but if partial dissolution of the gallstones is not seen within 12 months, this treatment is likely to be unsuccessful. Side effects include flulike symptoms, stomach pain, dizziness, back pain, and headache.

## Medications to treat obesity

Obesity rates in North America are increasing and are prompting many physicians to prescribe medications to decrease appetite. Many factors cause obesity: metabolic abnormalities, overeating, insulin resistance, and a sedentary lifestyle. A person is considered **morbidly obese** when he or she is 20% above ideal body weight. Obesity increases the workload of the pancreas, which helps digest carbohydrates,

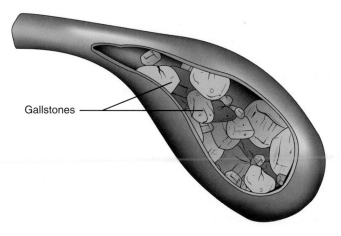

Gallstones

**FIGURE 19-4:** Cholelithiasis.

and the liver, which helps digest fats. It also causes increased workload on the circulatory system. Lifestyle changes are the best way to reduce obesity, but anorexiants (appetite suppressants) are sometimes necessary.

### Appetite suppressants

Appetite suppressants, also known as anorexiants, which give a feeling of fullness and sometimes create nausea, can be used (with caution) to decrease food intake and thus decrease obesity potential. They mimic the sympathetic system, so most are controlled substances. They are oral medications intended for short-term use only. Examples of these drugs include phentermine (Adipex-P, Oby-Cap, T-Diet, Zantryl). Taking phentermine concurrently with other diet medications can cause pulmonary hypertension, which can be fatal. In addition, phentermine can be habit-forming and affects cognitive function, so patients must be extremely cautious when taking this medication.

### Lipase inhibitors

Lipase inhibitors such as orlistat (Alli, Xenical) can also be used to manage obesity. These drugs bind to the enzyme lipase, so the intestines cannot break down dietary fat. Instead, fats are eliminated in the feces. This reduces the amount of fat absorbed into the body and thereby reduces serum lipids. These medications are given by mouth and should not be taken by children or patients with chronic health problems without close supervision by their physician. Xenical is available by prescription only, whereas alli is the OTC version of this drug. Medication should not be taken more than three times a day or with a meal that does not contain fat. Meals with a high fat content will result in unpleasant GI side effects. Vitamin supplements may be suggested by the physician to compensate for any losses anticipated through use of this medication.

---

### Virtual Field Trip

Using your favorite search engine:
1. Find an article on obesity, and download it.
2. Find a body mass index calculator, and figure out yours.
3. Download some weight loss tips to help make a teaching plan for your clients.

---

 *CRITICAL THINKING*

What are some lifestyle changes that can lead to reduced weight?

## Medications to treat hemorrhoids

**Hemorrhoids** are swollen varicose veins, and they usually occur if the anus, a sphincter at the end of the rectum, becomes irritated. **Fissures** are cracks in the same area. For these irritants, an anorectal preparation is often used to decrease swelling and soothe cracks. An example of a hemorrhoid cream is a combination of pramoxine, phenylephrine, glycerin, and petrolatum (Preparation H), which is applied topically to the hemorrhoids to shrink the swelling. Another medicated cream used for hemorrhoid treatment is pramoxine combined with zinc oxide (Anusol, Tronolane, Tucks). Pramoxine is an anesthetic to numb the pain and itching, whereas zinc oxide is a mineral that promotes healing. Some of these preparations contain lanolin or mineral oil, which act as an emollient to lubricate the anus and makes the passage of stool less traumatic. Anal fissures and hemorrhoids can be treated with rectal suppositories such as hydrocortisone acetate (Anusol-HC). This medication works by suppressing inflammation.

## Medications to treat flatulence

**Flatulence** is gas released by the GI tract. Often, flatulence is caused by foods rather than by disease. Patients who complain of flatulence should be cautioned to decrease consumption of cabbage, onions, and beans and to use straws for drinking. Flatulence is more common in patients with air swallowing, diverticulitis, peptic ulcer, irritable bowel syndrome, and dyspepsia. Antiflatulents may also be used with gastroscopy and bowel radiography. The main drug in this class is simethicone (Flatulex, Gas-X, Genasyme, Mylicon). Many of these medications are available OTC, and all are oral medications. (See the Master the Essentials table for a more complete list of antiflatulent medication.) There are no reported adverse effects for this medication.

## Medications to treat fungal infections of the gastrointestinal tract

Oral candidiasis, **thrush,** is a fungal infection of the mucous membranes of the mouth (Fig. 19-5). Commonly, the only symptom is the presence of thick, white patches on the tongue and cheeks. These patches may extend into the esophagus and become painful and bleed if untreated. Nystatin (Bio-Statin, Mycostatin, Nilstat) is the main drug used to treat thrush. It is available as a suspension or a troche (lozenge). Regardless of the form used, it should be kept in the mouth as long as possible to coat the affected area. Troches should not be chewed or swallowed whole. Intestinal candidiasis is also treated with nystatin, but in tablet form. In this instance, the drugs should be swallowed whole. Because these medications are essentially topical applications and are not absorbed systematically, side effects are not expected to occur.

## Medications to treat intestinal parasites

Anthelmintics kill intestinal parasites, such as roundworms, tapeworms, and pinworms, by affecting the nervous system of the worm, paralyzing them, or preventing the worm from absorbing glucose. Roundworms do not enter the tissue of their host and are treated with albendazole (Albenza) and praziquantel (Biltricide) orally. Roundworms enter the tissue and thus are more difficult to kill. Ivermectin (Stromectol) is prescribed for the treatment of roundworms. Mebendazole (Vermox), pyrantel (Antiminth, Ascarel, Pin-X), and praziquantel (Biltricide) are given orally for the treatment of hookworms, whipworms, pinworms, and flukes. Laxatives may also be given at the same time to expel the dead parasites. Side effects are abdominal cramps, headaches, anorexia, nausea, and vomiting.

### CRITICAL THINKING

Why is it important to cook chicken, beef, pork, and fish thoroughly?

## Medications to induce vomiting and treat drug overdose

Some medications are used to induce vomiting to rid the body of a harmful substance or toxin. Vomiting may or may not be beneficial, depending on the circumstance. If caused by food poisoning, vomiting is therapeutic because it helps rid the body of toxins. Antiemetics stop vomiting, and emetics promote it. Emetics, such as syrup of ipecac, induce vomiting in 80% to 90% of patients within 20 to 30 minutes. Syrup of ipecac has been widely used to induce vomiting in poisoning incidents outside the hospital. Now, however, parents are advised to destroy any syrup of ipecac that they have in the home because the benefits are inconclusive, and it may be dangerous. For instance, if it

**FIGURE 19-5:** Oral candidiasis (thrush).

is given when a corrosive substance has been ingested, the substance will cause further damage when it is brought back up. Most poisonings are treated with activated charcoal. Charcoal attracts the toxin and inactivates the poison as it travels the length of the GI tract in most instances. The poison is then excreted in the stool. Always call poison control anywhere in the United States at 1-800-222-1222 to receive the most current recommendations before acting to prevent further injury to a patient.

### Nutritional supplements

Poor nutrition can result in poor health. Malnutrition can be caused by lack of availability of food, excessive dieting, poor dietary choices, or illnesses that reduce appetite. Medications that reduce nausea and vomiting can improve nutritional status. Furthermore, nutritional supplements such as a multivitamin can compensate for a lack of vitamins in food.

Nutritional supplements may not sound like drugs, but they are frequently prescribed to improve nutrition in patients who are malnourished. These supplements are more easily tolerated in a patient who is weak and possibly has a compromised immune system. Liquid nutritional supplements can help improve health. Examples include Boost and Ensure. Store brands are available, but be sure to ask the prescriber whether substitutions are allowed. Some prescribers want specific nutrients found only in certain supplements. The patient can usually choose the flavor of the supplement, however.

### Digestants

In some instances, patients have difficulty in digesting the food that they eat, most commonly because of a food allergy or possibly a genetic disorder such as cystic fibrosis. If a patient has no medical reason to avoid a certain food, medications can be given to assist with the digestion of the meal. One example is Lactaid, which is used in patients who are lactose intolerant to enable them to tolerate milk products. Patients with cystic fibrosis do not produce digestive enzymes in quantities sufficient to digest any food. Therefore, they require digestive enzymes (Enzymatic Digestant Oral) with every meal and snack that they ingest.

### Mouthwashes and other oral treatments

Mouthwashes or mouth rinses are used to decrease **halitosis** (bad breath) or **stomatitis** (inflammation of the mouth). Fluoride preparations can prevent tooth decay by hardening the tooth enamel. They are prescribed in tablets, drops, or mouth rinses. For a patient who does not produce saliva, saliva substitutes are prescribed. Oral topical anesthetics can be used for teething pain and mouth ulcers. Hydrogen peroxide is available OTC and acts as a weak antibacterial agent in the mouth. Dentifrices or toothpastes are used to clean teeth, decrease plaque, and prevent gum disease. Some have whitening elements as well.

 SUMMARY

For the GI system to function optimally, it is important to understand how the food we eat and drink affects it. Sometimes, what we consume can cause illness, pain, or discomfort. When disorders of the GI system occur or when a need exists to control certain signs and symptoms, such as abdominal pain, change in bowel habits, heartburn, gas, weight loss, nausea, vomiting, difficulty swallowing, loss of appetite, obesity, malnutrition, and blood or mucus in the feces, we must turn to medications to alleviate the discomfort.

# Activities

To make sure that you have learned the key points covered in this chapter, complete the following activities.

## True or False
Write true if the statement is true. Beside the false statements, write false, and correct the statement to make it true.

Flatulence is intestinal gas. _____

*H. pylori* is the bacterium responsible for causing GERD. _____

Type AB blood is a risk factor for the development of ulcers. _____

Anthelmintics are used to treat intestinal parasites. _____

Halitosis means bad breath. _____

High-fat meals are allowable when taking lipase inhibitors such as orlistat. _____.

Laxatives may be prescribed when a patient is taking anthelmintic medications. _____.

Cholelithiasis is a condition in which stones are present in the gallbladder. _____.

Medication taken for gallstones is effective within 6 weeks. _____.

Thrush is oral candidiasis. _____.

## Multiple Choice
Choose the best answer for each question.

**1. A crack at the end of the rectum is called a _____.**
- A. Halitosis
- B. Pica
- C. Peristalsis
- D. Fissure

**2. Intestinal gas is called _____.**
- A. GERD
- B. Halitosis
- C. *Helicobacter pylori*
- D. Flatulence

**3. Which of the following is NOT a type of antiemetic?**
- A. Phenothiazines
- B. Antihistamines
- C. Prostaglandins
- D. Cannabinoids

**4. Which medication is used to treat GERD?**

A. Laxatives

B. Proton pump inhibitors

C. Antiemetics

D. Emetics

**5. Which causes a reduction in spasms associated with GI disorders?**

A. Anticholinergics

B. Laxatives

C. Antiemetics

D. Prostaglandins

**6. Inflamed varicose veins located in the rectum are called _____.**

A. Pica

B. Peristalsis

C. Hemorrhoids

D. Fissures

**7. The medication prescribed for oral thrush is _____.**

A. Nystatin

B. Simethicone

C. Amoxicillin

D. Activated charcoal

**8. The medication prescribed for *H. pylori* is _____.**

A. Nystatin

B. Simethicone

C. Amoxicillin

D. Activated charcoal

**9. The medication taken for flatulence is _____.**

A. Nystatin

B. Simethicone

C. Amoxicillin

D. Activated charcoal

**10. A medication administered to treat a drug overdose is _____.**

A. Nystatin

B. Simethicone

C. Amoxicillin

D. Activated charcoal

Respond to the following situations on a separate sheet.

1. Butler is having gastric bypass surgery, and the surgeon is removing most of Mr. Butterworth's stomach. How will that affect the absorption of drugs he takes?

2. Cliff wants to lose weight. He wants to be put on Xenical but continue his lifestyle. What do you teach him?

3. Marilyn takes Dulcolax every night to a have bowel movement. Is this a good practice? Why or why not?

4. Joyce says that her mother always drank milk to treat her stomach ulcer. She does not understand why she is taking antibiotics and told not to use milk to treat the ulcer. What would you say?

# Essentials Review

For further study and practice with drug classifications learned in this chapter, complete the following table to the best of your ability. Use resources such as the *PDR,* the Internet, or printed drug guides for help.

| Trade Name | Generic Name | Classification | Purpose | Side Effects | Contraindications and Precautions | Examples | Patient Education |
|---|---|---|---|---|---|---|---|
| Maalox | | | | | | | |
| Imodium | | | | | | | |
| Mycostatin | | | | | | | |
| Ipecac | | | | | | | |
| Reglan | | | | | | | |
| Biaxin | | | | | | | |
| Pepcid | | | | | | | |
| Cytotec | | | | | | | |
| Prilosec | | | | | | | |

# Reproductive and Urinary System Medications

*T*he reproductive system is responsible for the procreation of our species, whereas the urinary system's main function is to remove toxins from our body while conserving electrolytes. Reproductive disorders can cause pain, infertility, and sometimes death if they are not treated. Most medications used in the reproductive system are hormone based. A prime example is birth control pills, which can not only prevent pregnancy, but also help to manage painful menstruation. Urinary system disorders can cause discomfort and pain, and untreated urinary system failure can lead to death. One of the most common groups of medications used for the urinary system consists of diuretics, which increase the excretion of water and waste products. Another common group of medications comprises those used for benign prostatic hypertrophy (BPH). These medications decrease the size of the prostate gland and allow urine to flow more freely.

## LEARNING OUTCOMES

At the end of this chapter, the student will be able to:

20.1 Define key terms

20.2 List actions of the reproductive hormones FSH, LH, and ICSH.

20.3 Describe how contraceptives work.

20.4 Discuss the relation of diuretics to electrolyte imbalances.

20.5 Describe the effects of estrogens, progestins, agents for cervical ripening, oxytocin, tocolytics, ovulation stimulants, androgens, diuretics, and BPH medications.

## KEY TERMS

Androgen
Benign prostatic
  hypertrophy (BPH)
Enuresis
Estrogen
Follicle-stimulating
  hormone (FSH)

Hormone replacement
  therapy (HRT)
Interstitial cell-stimulating
  hormone (ICSH)
Luteinizing hormone (LH)
Progestin

Sexually transmitted
  disease (STD)
Tocolytic

# ■ THE REPRODUCTIVE SYSTEM

Several hormones, known as gonadotropic hormones, and their interactions are responsible for optimal functioning of the testes and ovaries. These hormones are secreted by the pituitary gland and include **follicle-stimulating hormone (FSH), luteinizing hormone (LH),** and **interstitial cell-stimulating hormone (ICSH).** These hormones are responsible for the production of both the female hormones estrogen and progestin and the **androgen** (male hormone) testosterone. Testosterone, estrogen, and progesterone are hormones that promote the health, growth, and function of the reproductive system. The testes in the male (testicles) produce testosterone (Fig. 20-1A). The ovaries in the female secrete female sex hormones (estrogen and progesterone) (Fig. 20-1B).

As discussed in Chapter 15, FSH regulates sperm and egg production. LH triggers the release of the egg in women and promotes secretion of estrogen and progesterone. In men, LH is called ICSH and regulates testosterone production. Table 20.1 summarizes the reproductive hormones.

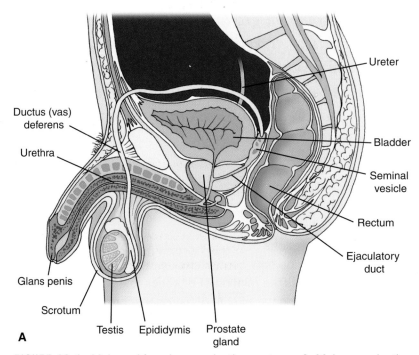

**FIGURE 20-1:** Male and female reproductive systems. **A,** Male reproductive system. Internal and external male reproductive system.

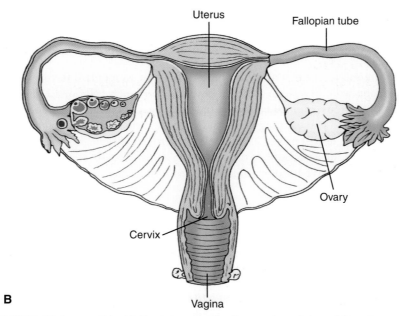

**B**

**FIGURE 20-1—cont'd:  B,** Female reproductive system. Internal female reproductive system.

## TABLE 20.1   Reproductive Hormones

| Hormone | Action | Too Much Causes.... | Too Little Causes... |
|---|---|---|---|
| **Prolactin** | Stimulates milk production in the mammary gland | • Overproduction of breast milk in women<br>• Milk production in non-nursing patient a possible sign of a pituitary tumor<br>• Parlodel used to suppress lactation in women who choose not to breastfeed, but side effect is increased fertility | Underproduction of milk in women; baby has difficulty nursing |
| **Follicle-stimulating hormone (FSH)** | Stimulates sperm production in men and egg production in women | Increased fertility | Men: sterility<br>Women: Irregular or absent menses |
| **Luteinizing hormone (LH)** | Stimulates release of the ripened egg in women (ovulation); also helps in the production of the female hormones (estrogens and progestins) | Multiple gestations (e.g., twins, triplets) | Infertility (woman cannot ovulate, so cannot conceive) |
| **Interstitial cell–stimulating hormone (ICSH)** | Stimulates production of androgens (male hormone testosterone) | Aggressiveness, excessive hair | Feminine attributes in men (e.g., high voice, small muscles) |

# ■ MEDICATIONS FOR DISORDERS RELATED TO FEMALE HORMONES

If the hormone levels are either too high or too low in women, fertility can be affected. Too little progesterone will not sustain a pregnancy, and too much FSH or LH may lead to multiple births. The classifications of medications used include contraceptives such as medroxyprogesterone (Provera), used to prevent pregnancy and stabilize menstrual cycles, and hormone replacement medications such as testosterone (AndroGel) or estrogen (Premarin), used when a normally occurring hormone is lacking as a result of disease or the aging process (see the Master the Essentials table for a more comprehensive list of medications used in treatment of reproductive health and illness).

## Master the Essentials: Reproductive and Urinary Medications

This table shows the various classes of reproductive and urinary medications and key side effects, contraindications and precautions, interactions, and examples for each class.
Reproductive System Medications

| Class | Indications for Use | Side Effects | Contraindications and Precautions | Interactions | Examples |
|---|---|---|---|---|---|
| Androgens | Low testosterone levels, certain breast cancers | Headache, increased or decreased libido, anxiety, depression, acne, hirsutism, nausea, gynecomastia; amenorrhea or virilization in women | Serious heart, kidney, or liver disease; hypersensitivity, pregnancy, male with breast or prostate cancer | Anticoagulants, insulin, propranolol, corticosteroids, cyclosporine | Testosterone (AndroGel) |
| Antispasmodics | Incontinence resulting from overactive bladder | Dry mouth and eyes, blurred vision, constipation, nausea, dizziness, fatigue, flulike symptoms | Known sensitivity, glaucoma, stomach disorders, difficulty urinating, liver or kidney disease, history of long QT syndrome, myasthenia gravis | Arsenic trioxide, chloroquine, halofantrine, droperidol, HIV/AIDS medication, antibiotics, narcotics, psychiatric medications, cardiac medications, alcohol | Darifenacin (Enablex), fesoterodine (Toviaz), oxybutynin (Ditropan, Oxytrol, Urotrol), solifenacin (VESIcare), tolterodine (Detrol), trospium (Sanctura) |
| BPH medications | Enlarged prostate gland | Decreased libido, mild impotence, palpitations, dizziness, somnolence, asthenia, nausea | Hypersensitivity, liver impairment | Alcohol, beta blockers, verapamil | Alfuzosin (Uroxatral), doxazosin (Cardura, Carduran, Cascor, Doxadura), dutasteride (Avodart), finasteride (Propecia, Proscar), tamsulosin (Flomax), terazosin (Hytrin) |

## Master the Essentials: Reproductive and Urinary Medications—cont'd

| Class | Indications for Use | Side Effects | Contraindications and Precautions | Interactions | Examples |
|---|---|---|---|---|---|
| Cervical ripening agent | Inducement of labor | Uterine hyper-stimulation, GI effects, back pain, fetal bradycardia | Prior cesarean section, cephalopelvic disproportion, prior traumatic delivery, ruptured membranes, hypersensitivity, placenta previa | Oxytocics | Dinoprostone (Prepidil) |
| Erectile dysfunction drugs | Erectile dysfunction (impotence) | Fatal cardiovascular events, flushing, headache, abnormal vision, dyspepsia, back pain | Hypersensitivity, heart disease, kidney or liver impairment | Erythromycin, grapefruit, nitrates, alcohol, alpha blockers, amlodipine, angiotensin II receptor blockers, beta blockers, diuretics, enalapril, metoprolol, protease inhibitors | Alprostadil (Caverject, Edex), sildenafil (Revatio, Viagra), vardenafil (Levitra, Staxyn), tadalafil (Adcirca, Cialis) |
| Estrogens | Estrogen replacement | Breast enlargement and tenderness, cardiovascular risk, decreased folic acid, edema, gallbladder disease, GI upset, headache, increased triglycerides, irregular menstrual bleeding, visual disturbances, DVT, PE | Asthma, diabetes, heart problems, lactation, liver dysfunction pregnancy, stroke, seizures, smoking, breast cancer, abnormal uterine bleeding, DVT, PE, MI, hypersensitivity | Anticoagulants, anti-infectives, corticosteroids, oral hypo-glycemic, tricyclic antide-pressants, thyroid hormones, hydantoins, topiramate | Oral: Estrace or Premarin    Cream: Estrace, Dienestrol    Patch: Estraderm Vivelle    Vaginal: Estring, Vagifem |
| Loop diuretics | Congestive heart failure, renal insufficiency | Hyperglycemia, fluid and electrolyte loss, GI problems, headache, hypotension, hearing loss | Children, cirrhosis, diabetes, kidney disease, lactation, pregnancy, anuria, hypersen-sitivity | Blood pressure medications, corticosteroids, lithium, digoxin, aminoglyco-sides, antico-agulants | Furosemide (Lasix), ethacrynic acid (Edecrin), torsemide (Demadex), bumetanide (Bumex) |

*Continued*

## Master the Essentials: Reproductive and Urinary Medications—cont'd

| Class | Indications for Use | Side Effects | Contraindications and Precautions | Interactions | Examples |
|---|---|---|---|---|---|
| Osmotic diuretics | Increased intracranial pressure, increased intraocular pressure | CNS effects, fluid and electrolyte imbalances, hypotension or hypertension, tachycardia, edema, headache, nausea, vomiting, diarrhea | Cardiovascular or kidney failure; pulmonary edema; active intracranial bleeding | Lithium | Mannitol (Osmitrol) |
| Ovulation stimulants | Female infertility | Ovarian hyper-stimulation, headache, gynecomastia, injection site pain, vasomotor flushes | Liver disease, pregnancy, uncontrolled thyroid or adrenal disease, ovarian cysts, abnormal uterine bleeding, hypersensitivity | None reported | Clomiphene (Clomid, Serophene), menotropins (Humegon, Menopur, Repronex), chorionic gonadotropin (Ovidrel, Pregnyl) |
| Oxytocin | Induction of labor | Uterine rupture, embolism, fetal trauma and death, forceful contractions, hemorrhage, tachycardia, nausea, vomiting | Cephalopelvic disproportion, fetal distress, placenta previa, scarred uterus, unfavorable fetal positions, prolonged use in severe toxemia, hypersensitivity | Cyclopropane anesthesia, sympath-omimetics, vasocon-strictors | Oxytocin (Pitocin, Syntocinon) |
| Potassium-sparing diuretics | Congestive heart failure, polycystic ovary syndrome | GI distress, high blood potassium, hypotension, headache, drowsiness | Cirrhosis, lactation, pregnancy, renal impairment, hypersensitivity, serum potassium >5.5 mEq/L | ACE inhibitors, lithium, NSAIDs, potassium supplements, digoxin | Amiloride hydrochloride, spironolactone (Aldactone), triamterene (Dyrenium) |
| Progestins | Birth control | Breast tenderness, decreased bone density, headache, irregular menses, swelling, insomnia, depression, nausea, weight changes | Cardiovascular disease, depression, edema, pregnancy, hypersensitivity, thrombophlebitis, thromboembolic disorder, breast cancer, undiag-nosed vaginal bleeding, missed abortion | Amino-glutethimide, rifampin | Errin, Ovrette, Provera |

**Master the Essentials:** Reproductive and Urinary Medications—cont'd

| Class | Indications for Use | Side Effects | Contraindications and Precautions | Interactions | Examples |
|---|---|---|---|---|---|
| Thiazide diuretics | Hypertension, edema | Hyperglycemia; low chloride, potassium, and blood pressure | Anuria, hypersensitivity, renal decompensation, hepatic coma | Antidiabetic medications, corticosteroids, lithium, NSAIDs, digoxin, anesthetics, anticoagulants, antigout medications | Chlorothiazide (Diuril); chlorthalidone (Hygroton, Thalitone); indapamide (Lozol); hydrochlorothiazide, also known as HCTZ (Aquazide, HydroDIURIL, Microzide); metolazone (Mykrox, Zaroxolyn) |

ACE, angiotensin-converting enzyme; BPH, benign prostatic hypertrophy; CNS, central nervous system; DVT, deep vein thrombosis; GI, gastrointestinal; MI, myocardial infarction; NSAIDs, nonsteroidal anti-inflammatory drugs; PE, pulmonary embolism.

## Contraceptive medications

Some of the most common drugs used for contraception are based on hormones that a woman naturally produces. When administered as a drug, they prevent pregnancy by overriding the body's own mechanism to make **estrogens** and **progestins** (the two main hormones secreted by the ovaries). The body, while receiving hormones from an outside source regularly, stops producing its own estrogens and progestins. Contraceptives contain such low doses of the hormones that they usually inhibit the body's ability to conceive, by inhibiting ovulation (release of an egg from the ovary), inhibiting fertilization (joining of the egg and sperm to form an embryo), preventing implantation (embedding of the embryo into the uterine wall), or preventing growth of the fetus.

One of the most common forms of birth control is the "pill." It is available in formulations that provide differing amounts of estrogen and progestin during the menstrual cycle. Monophasic pills, such as ethinyl estradiol and norgestrel (Cryselle 28, Lo/Ovral 28, Ogestrel-28) or ethinyl estradiol and norethindrone (Aranelle, Modicon, Ortho-Novum), deliver a constant amount of hormone during the first 21 days of the cycle. Biphasic birth control pills, such as ethinyl estradiol and norethindrone (Jenest-28) and ethinyl estradiol and desogestrel (Apri, Desogen, Mircette, Ortho-Cept), contain a constant dose of estrogen but two different doses of progestin in the monthly cycle dosage. This allows the lining of the uterus to develop normally during the menstrual cycle. These differing doses are reflected by pills of different colors. Triphasic birth control pills, such as ethinyl estradiol and norethindrone (Aranelle, Junel FE 1/20, Ortho-Novum 7/7/7) and ethinyl estradiol and levonorgestrel (Alesse, Levlite, Lutera, Portia, Tri-Levlen), contain a varying amount of both estrogen and progestin with three different strengths during the monthly cycle dosage, each denoted with a pill of a different color.

In addition, there is the minipill progestin (Errin, Ovrette, Provera), which contains only progestin and therefore is slightly less effective. Evidence proving that any of the three foregoing types of birth control is superior to the others is lacking. A multitude of manufactured variations exists, and it may take experimentation to determine the best birth control method for an individual woman.

Sometimes patients experience symptoms of pregnancy while taking contraceptive pills or tablets because normal reproductive functioning shuts down, so the body behaves as though it is pregnant (e.g., weight gain, mood swings, and breast tenderness).

If contraception fails or fails to be used properly, a woman can use postcoital high-dose estrogen to prevent pregnancy. The medications prescribed for this postcoital contraception are levonorgestrel emergency contraceptive (Plan B) and ethinyl estradiol and levonorgestrel (Preven).

Contraceptive hormones are also commonly delivered via vaginal ring ethinyl estradiol and etonogestrel (NuvaRing), implants, intrauterine devices (IUDs), and transdermal patches. NuvaRing is a flexible ring containing estrogen and progestin that is inserted into the vagina every month. This prevents ovulation, fertilization, and implantation. This ring is removed after 3 weeks, to allow normal menstruation to occur. A new ring is placed 7 days after removal of the previous ring.

The only available implant currently is etonogestrel (Implanon), which contains a hormone that prevents ovulation, makes it more difficult for sperm to reach the uterus, and prevents implantation of a fertilized egg. The implant is a small plastic rod containing the medication and is placed in the upper arm. This method provides contraception for up to 3 years.

The levonorgestrel intrauterine system Mirena contains the hormone progestin and is placed in the uterus by a physician. This device makes the uterus a very unwelcoming place for sperm, and the lining of the uterus becomes a difficult place in which to implant a fertilized egg. The hormone-based IUD may be left in place for 5 years. Another type of IUD that does not contain hormones is the copper IUD. Copper is naturally toxic to sperm, and the fluids produced in response by the uterus and fallopian tubes are also deadly to sperm. These copper IUDs may be left in place for 10 years.

Transdermal patches such as the Ortho Evra patch contain ethinyl estradiol and norelgestromin, which are forms of estrogen and progestin, to prevent ovulation. A new patch is applied weekly for 3 weeks, and no patch is used for the fourth week, to allow a normal menstrual period to occur.

All these hormone-based contraceptive medications must be taken with care. They have a risk of serious side effects, such as the formation of blood clots, especially in women more than 35 years old. Smoking increases the risk of blood clots. Women with a history of blood clots or diseases involving the vascular system should not be prescribed these medications.

Another common method of birth control is the use of barrier devices such as condoms or diaphragms in combination with spermicides containing nonoxynol-9 such as Encare and Conceptrol. The barrier devices are the only contraceptives effective against sexually transmitted diseases (STDs), as well as preventing pregnancy.

The medication mifepristone (Mifeprex), originally known as RU-486, is used to stop a pregnancy. This medication blocks the hormone progesterone, which is necessary for pregnancy to be successful. The medication is only used during the first 7 weeks since the last menstrual period. Because this medication causes cramping and bleeding, it is not advised in patients taking blood thinners such as Coumadin. This medication is given in an oral form and is taken in the physician's office. If, on rechecking, the patient is still pregnant after 3 days, she will be administered an additional oral dose of mifepristone and rechecked in 2 weeks.

Table 20.2 summarizes the information on contraceptive medications.

## Hormone replacement therapy

Women experiencing menopause (permanent cessation of menses) may choose to take **hormone replacement therapy (HRT).** This term refers to the administration of hormones to replace those that are no longer being naturally produced during and after menopause. If a woman no longer has a uterus, her own estrogen is replaced because there is no build up of the lining of the uterus. If the woman still has a uterus, estrogen is usually combined with a progestin in this therapy, so the endometrial lining is shed in the same way it would be in the presence of natural hormones. If estrogen is taken without the addition of progesterone in these women, the risk of endometrial cancer is higher. Estrogen therapy is taken as a pill such as Estrace or Premarin, a cream such as Estrace or Dienestrol, or a patch such as Estraderm or Vivelle. Combination estrogen-progesterone therapy is prescribed as an oral pill (Prempro) or a patch (Climara-Pro). Women also produce small amounts of testosterone, and when these levels begin to decline, replacing testosterone may help relieve the symptoms of menopause, such as hot flashes and vaginal dryness. A combination of estrogen and testosterone is administered as a tablet in medications such as Covaryx and Estratest. HRT has been shown to decrease bone loss and cardiovascular dysfunction. However, studies have shown that using HRT increases the risk of breast cancer, stroke, and blood clots. Therefore, HRT is an individual decision. If a woman does not elect HRT, alternative treatments to relieve menopausal symptoms should be discussed, and treatment should be reevaluated on an annual basis

### TABLE 20.2  Examples of Contraceptive Medications

| Type | Action | Examples |
| --- | --- | --- |
| Monophasic tablets | Prevent ovulation | Ethinyl estradiol and norgestrel (Cryselle 28, Lo/Ovral 28, Ogestrel-28), ethinyl estradiol and norethindrone (Aranelle, Modicon, Ortho-Novum) |
| Biphasic tablets | Prevent ovulation | Ethinyl estradiol and norethindrone (Jenest-28), ethinyl estradiol and desogestrel (Apri, Desogen, Mircette, Ortho-Cept) |
| Triphasic tablets | Prevent ovulation | Ethinyl estradiol and norethindrone (Aranelle, Junel FE 1/20, Ortho-Novum 7/7/7), ethinyl estradiol and levonorgestrel (Alesse, Levlite, Lutera, Portia, Tri-Levlen) |
| Vaginal ring | Inhibits reproductive function | Ethinyl estradiol and etonogestrel (NuvaRing) |
| Implants | Prevent ovulation, fertilization, and implantation | Etonogestrel (Implanon) |
| Transdermal patches | Prevent ovulation | Ethinyl estradiol and norelgestromin (Ortho Evra patch) |
| IUDs | Prevent implantation, kill sperm | Levonorgestrel intrauterine system (Mirena), copper IUD |
| Spermicides | Kill sperm | Nonoxynol-9 (Encare and Conceptrol) |
| Barrier devices | Prevent fertilization | Diaphragm, male condom, female condom |
| Postcoital contraception | Prevents ovulation, fertilization, and implantation | Levonorgestrel emergency contraceptive (Plan B), ethinyl estradiol and levonorgestrel (Preven) |
| Abortifacient | Kills fetus within 49 days from menstrual period | Mifepristone (Mifeprex) |

IUD, intrauterine device.

HRT can also be used to treat prostate cancer in men because estrogen decreases testosterone levels. In addition, men are believed to endure their own form of menopause in which their testosterone levels diminish. Studies are showing a possible decrease in heart disease, diabetes, and death when androgen replacement therapy is administered. The most common method of administering the androgen testosterone in these patients is through a gel (AndroGel) that is rubbed into the skin on a daily basis.

### Virtual Field Trip

Using your favorite search engine, research one drug from each category of contraceptives in Table 20.2 (monophasics through abortifacients). Create a poster to help teach teenagers about contraceptive options.

## MEDICATIONS FOR ABNORMAL UTERINE BLEEDING

Abnormal uterine bleeding is a condition in which vaginal bleeding occurs irregularly or too heavily. Correcting the hormonal imbalance that typically causes this condition is often indicated. Combination therapy of estrogen and progesterone, as oral contraceptives, can be prescribed. Progestins (progesterone) alone can also be prescribed to regulate the rhythm and amount of menstruation.

The medications leuprolide (Eligard, Lupron) and goserelin (Zoladex) are gonadotropin-releasing hormone agonists. They are frequently used to suppress buildup of the endometrial lining in patients with endometriosis by reducing estrogen levels in women and thus creating an artificial menopause-like condition that allows the endometrial lining to heal. These medications are injected approximately once a month; treatment is short term, lasting no more than 6 months. In some patients, the effects are temporary; in others, symptoms of endometriosis are long term. Side effects mimic those of menopause: hot flashes, bone loss, lack of menstrual periods, mood swings, insomnia, headaches, vaginal dryness and increased cholesterol levels. These symptoms continue through the length of treatment.

# ■ LABOR MEDICATIONS

Labor needs to occur when the baby is fully developed and able to survive outside the mother's womb. Unfortunately, because of unforeseen circumstances, the baby either may be in danger of being born too early to survive or does not seem in any hurry to be born but is developmentally ready. In these instances, medications used for labor include those to hasten labor, which include cervical ripening agents and oxytocin, and those to slow or stop labor, such as tocolytics.

Cervical ripening agents are those that are applied topically to the cervix of the uterus to prepare it for labor, by softening the cervix in the hopes of initiating dilation. Dinoprostone (Prepidil) is a prostaglandin used for cervical ripening. The gel form is inserted into the cervix; the vaginal insert is placed in the posterior fornix of the vagina. The cervix is then allowed time to soften gently. If labor does not begin in approximately 6 hours, a second dose may be administered, or the patient may be started on oxytocin (Pitocin, Syntocinon), which is the pituitary hormone that causes the uterus to contract. Both medications should not be used simultaneously because this may cause a much stronger effect than with either drug alone. If labor fails to progress, synthetic oxytocin (Pitocin) can be given by the intravenous (IV) route over time to encourage the uterus gently to contract (however, women in labor may argue that there is nothing gentle about this drug). This medication is administered only in a controlled setting in which the mother is closely monitored for complications such as developing hypertension. It may also be given after the baby is born to contract the uterus and thus help control postpartum bleeding.

Labor **tocolytics** have an effect opposite that of oxytocin. They slow or stop uterine contractions and are indicated to prevent premature birth and allow the baby to mature, especially its lungs. Terbutaline, magnesium sulfate, calcium channel blockers, and nonsteroidal anti-inflammatory drugs (NSAIDs) are agents used as tocolytics. These medications are labeled for other uses, but they are commonly used to stop labor. Terbutaline (Brethine) is labeled as a bronchodilator used to treat asthma, but as a beta blocker, one of its effects is to decrease uterine contractions. Terbutaline is commonly the first drug given to treat preterm labor. It is administered as an IV drip, and the mother is monitored to watch for any complications because beta blockers affect the cardiac system by increasing the heart rate and lowering blood pressure. This medication should only be used on a short-term basis (for 24 to 48 hours) under close supervision in a hospital setting.

Magnesium sulfate is not proven to stop preterm labor, but it is commonly used to treat preeclampsia (pregnancy-related condition) and premature labor. It may be given by the IV route for a short time (24 to 48 hours) and is thought to act as a calcium channel blocker, by keeping the calcium from the muscles, where it is needed for the uterus to contract. There is some belief that if other tocolytics are ineffective and premature birth is imminent, magnesium sulfate may reduce the possibility of cerebral palsy in the preterm infant. Side effects include hypotension, cardiac arrhythmias, and weakness.

A medication that can be taken orally for preterm labor is nifedipine (Adalat CC, Procardia). This medication is a calcium channel blocker, which relaxes smooth muscles such as the uterus. This medication is used when the cervix is minimally dilated, the amniotic sac remains intact, and other tocolytic medications have not been successful. Again, this medication is preferably used on a short-term basis (for 24 to 48 hours).

Indomethacin (Indocin) is a strong NSAID that is administered by the IV route, orally, or as a rectal suppository. This drug is commonly used as an anti-inflammatory drug for joint conditions. Indocin has a strong antiprostaglandin effect, which is necessary for uterine contractions. Use should be limited to less than 7 days, to minimize effects on the developing fetus. This medication should not be used during the last 2 months of pregnancy because of the effects on fetal cardiac development.

# ■ INFERTILITY MEDICATIONS

Medications can also help women increase their fertility. Some medications are used to help ovaries release multiple eggs, to increase the chance that one will be fertilized and grow into a fetus. These drugs are referred to as ovulation stimulants. Clomiphene (Clomid, Serophene) is an example of a drug that increases the hormones FSH and LH, which initiate ovulation. This is the drug of choice when infertility has no obvious cause, and the medication is taken orally with minimal side effects. Menotropins (Humegon, Menopur, Repronex) are given as an injection that stimulates follicle ripening and release. This treatment is indicated in women who have functional ovaries but in whom hormonal stimulation is lacking. Chorionic gonadotropin (Ovidrel, Pregnyl) is given as an injection in combination with clomiphene to stimulate the release of a mature egg. The patient should be prepared for the possibility of not becoming pregnant or becoming pregnant with multiple fetuses when fertility drugs are used.

# ■ MEDICATIONS FOR OTHER FEMALE HORMONE DISORDERS

Premenstrual dysphoric disorder (formerly premenstrual syndrome or PMS) is frequently treated with selective serotonin reuptake inhibitors (SSRIs). Serotonin levels are increased with the use of SSRIs, and this leads to alleviation of many symptoms of PMS such as hot flashes, depressions, anxiety, and pain.

Medications are also used to treat infections of the female reproductive tract. Some infections are caused by **sexually transmitted diseases (STDs)** such as syphilis. Among the more popular drugs for vaginal infections are as follows: antibacterials such as metronidazole (Flagyl), used orally or by the IV route to treat trichomonas infections; antivirals such as acyclovir (Zovirax), used orally and intravenously to treat herpes infections; and antifungals such as miconazole (Monistat), used topically or orally to treat vaginal yeast infections (see Chapter 17 for a review of immune system medications such as antibacterials, antivirals, and antifungals).

# ■ MEDICATIONS FOR MALE HORMONE DISORDERS

Androgens are male sex hormones that promote maturation of the male sexual organs and male sexual characteristics. Men who have low androgen levels may need testosterone to increase their masculine traits. Testosterone can also be used to lower estrogen levels in women with breast cancer, just as estrogen is used to lower testosterone levels in men who have prostate cancer.

# ■ MEDICATIONS TO TREAT ERECTILE DYSFUNCTION, DECREASED LIBIDO, AND INFERTILITY

Erectile dysfunction, or impotence, is a fairly common disorder, frequently related to atherosclerosis, diabetes, stroke, and hypertension. This disorder may also have psychological roots, such as guilt, fatigue, depression, and fear of failure to perform adequately.

Erectile dysfunction drugs such as phosphodiesterase type 5 inhibitors usually work by dilating the arteries leading to the penis and constricting the veins and thereby holding the blood in the penis and sustaining an erection. If erectile dysfunction is associated with physiological decline, it is vitally important that the patient give a complete history to the prescriber. Medications such as sildenafil (Revatio, Viagra), vardenafil (Levitra, Staxyn), and tadalafil (Adcirca, Cialis) can be dangerous for patients with a history of cardiovascular disease, stroke, and sickle cell anemia or eye problems. Sildenafil, vardenafil, and tadalafil are taken by mouth approximately 30 minutes to 1 hour before sexual activity and no more often than one dose per day. Cialis may also be prescribed to be taken orally on a daily basis to provide more flexibility in sexual readiness.

Another medication for erectile dysfunction is alprostadil (Caverject, Edex), which is either injected into the penis or inserted as a urethral pellet. This medication begins to work within 5 to 20 minutes and lasts approximately 1 hour. It should be administered no more than once a day and three times a week. The most common side effects are minor and include mild pain at the site of administration.

## ❓ CRITICAL THINKING

**Why may erectile dysfunction drugs affect the entire cardiovascular system and not act just on the penis?**

Reduced libido can occur in both men and women as a result of either emotional or physiological changes, such as depression, or the physical changes of aging, which include gaining or losing weight and the development of wrinkled and sagging skin, thus leading to a general feeling of decreased attractiveness. Many medications decrease libido in men and women. Among them are Benadryl, Aldactone, Aldomet, Catapres, Chlor-Trimeton, Valium, alcohol, Zantac, Tagamet, Dopar, and Inderal. Amphetamines increase libido.

A variety of drugs can be used to treat male infertility, including human chorionic gonadotropin (hCG), a substance naturally present in pregnant women. When hCG is administered as an injection in a male patient, it increases the testosterone levels, which, in turn, increase sperm production.

## ■ THE URINARY SYSTEM

The urinary system's main functions are filtration of the blood and removal of the waste products that the kidneys have filtered out as unnecessary or dangerous (Fig. 20-2). This system consists of the kidneys, ureters, bladder, and urethra. The kidneys act as the filters for our blood. The ureters transfer the filtered waste products in water to the bladder, where they are stored until removal from the body via the urethra. This system is closely linked to the reproductive system, especially in men, because the urethra is encased in the penis and acts as a conduit to transfer sperm from the man to the woman during sexual intercourse. The most commonly used medications for treatment of disorders and diseases of the urinary system are diuretics.

### Diuretics

Diuretics, commonly referred to as water pills, increase excretion of body fluids from the kidneys. This is necessary in certain medical conditions. The most common conditions for which diuretics are used are hypertension (high blood pressure) and heart failure. If the circulating pressure is too high and/or the heart muscle is not pumping with adequate strength, consequences will include lack of adequate blood flow, damage to tissue, and possible death if these situations remain untreated. Decreasing the amount of circulating volume lessens pressure on the blood vessels. Think of a garden hose. When there is a rapid flow of water (high volume), the pressure is high, but if you turn the hose down (lower the volume), the pressure is reduced to a gentle stream. In addition, if the heart is not pumping adequately, lowering the amount of liquid that it is required to push throughout the body will decrease the effort the heart must exert.

Other medical conditions requiring diuretics include kidney failure when hypertension and edema are present. Kidney stones can be minimized or prevented through the use of diuretics, which limit the amount of calcium excreted in the urine. In addition, glaucoma treatment may include diuretics to decrease the circulating fluid in the body, including the eyes. Diuretics can be categorized into four main areas: loop, thiazide, potassium-sparing, and osmotic.

#### Loop diuretics

The most effective diuretics work in the loop of Henle, located in the nephron (A Closer Look: The Nephron...Building Block of the Kidney). Not surprisingly, they are called loop diuretics. They mainly are used to treat congestive heart failure by decreasing the volume of blood that the heart must circulate through the body. This effect also decreases the amount of fluid in the lungs and makes

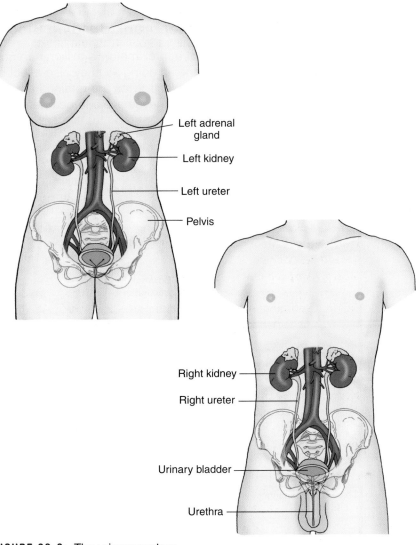

**FIGURE 20-2:** The urinary system.

breathing easier. In renal insufficiency, it helps the kidneys to produce more urine and thus rids the body of toxins. One problem with this type of diuretic is that a vital electrolyte is lost along with the sodium and water. This electrolyte is potassium, which plays a major role in maintaining a proper heart rhythm. Many patients taking diuretics must have their potassium levels monitored and possibly take potassium supplements. Examples of these drugs include furosemide (Lasix), ethacrynic acid (Edecrin), torsemide (Demadex), and bumetanide (Bumex). These medications are commonly taken orally, but they are also administered by the IV route. Furosemide and bumetanide may be given as an intramuscular injection.

### Thiazide diuretics

Thiazides, which block sodium reabsorption and increase water excretion, are used to treat moderate hypertension. They are less effective than loop diuretics and also deplete potassium from the body, just as do loop diuretics. Many of these patients take potassium supplements to prevent potassium depletion or are prescribed a potassium-sparing diuretic instead. Examples are as follows: chlorothiazide (Diuril); chlorthalidone (Hygroton, Thalitone); indapamide (Lozol); hydrochlorothiazide, also known as HCTZ (Aquazide, HydroDIURIL, Microzide); and metolazone (Mykrox, Zaroxolyn). These medications are all taken orally. Chlorothiazide may also be administered by the IV route.

## A CLOSER LOOK: The Nephron...Building Block of the Kidney

Each kidney is made up of approximately a million nephrons. The kidneys regulate volume and content of urine. In doing so, they also affect blood pressure. Each nephron determines which electrolytes are retained and which are disposed of outside the body. Thus, the kidneys have a large role in maintaining the acid-base balance in the body.

The kidney and the nephron.

### Potassium-sparing diuretics

Potassium-sparing diuretics are frequently prescribed instead of or in combination with loop or thiazide diuretics to minimize the risk of potassium imbalances. These drugs block the reabsorption of water and sodium back into the bloodstream, but they allow potassium to be reabsorbed. Examples include amiloride hydrochloride, spironolactone (Aldactone), and triamterene (Dyrenium), which are all given orally.

### Osmotic diuretics

Osmotic diuretics such as mannitol are used for patients who have increased intracranial pressure as a result of head trauma, a brain tumor, or other illness affecting the brain, to lower the pressure exerted on the brain by swelling. In addition, this medication may be given to those patients suffering from high intraocular pressure and those who are in the anuric (no urine output) stage of acute renal failure, to lower the amount of edema. These diuretics may also be administered in cases of toxic overdose, to flush the toxins from the body more rapidly. Osmotic diuretics function by pulling more fluid out of the body tissues and into the circulation, where it is then filtered through the kidneys and excreted. Osmotic diuretics such as mannitol (Osmitrol) are given by the IV route only in a controlled setting because the patient must be closely monitored during the administration. Side effects include dizziness, eye pain, anorexia, confusion, and dehydration.

### Electrolyte imbalances and diuretics

Although diuretics may relieve congestion by removing excess fluid from the body, they can have a devastating effect on the patient's electrolyte balance. To function properly, the body needs electrolytes: sodium (Na), potassium (K), calcium (Ca), and magnesium (Mg). IV infusion therapy may be needed to replenish lost electrolytes; alternatively, electrolytes can be taken orally in supplements or through dietary changes to prevent imbalances. Any time a diuretic is prescribed, the patient must be monitored to make sure that it is not adversely affecting the electrolyte levels.

## Other medications for urinary disorders

Other common disorders of the urinary system include **benign prostatic hypertrophy (BPH)**, infection, gout, and urinary incontinence.

Many older men suffer from **BPH.** This nonmalignant growth of the prostate gland constricts the urethra and impedes the outflow of urine (Fig. 20-3). During its early stages, BPH can be treated with alpha-adrenergic blockers, such as alfuzosin (Uroxatral), doxazosin (Cardura, Carduran, Cascor, Doxadura), dutasteride (Avodart), finasteride (Propecia, Proscar), tamsulosin (Flomax), or terazosin (Hytrin). These drugs relax smooth muscle in the prostate gland and decrease blockage of the urethra, thus allowing urination to occur. For a close look at Avodart, see Drug Spotlight 20.1.

Urinary tract infections can cause frequency, urgency, pain, and blood in the urine. They are usually treated with broad-spectrum antibiotics (Bactrim, Augmentin), analgesics (Pyridium), and antispasmodics (methenamine, flavoxate).

Although gout affects the musculoskeletal system, it is caused by the inability of the kidneys to clear uric acid from the bloodstream. Antigout medications can cause rashes in hypersensitive individuals (see Chapter 12 for further information on medications to treat gout).

Certain antispasmodics such as darifenacin (Enablex), fesoterodine (Toviaz), oxybutynin (Ditropan, Oxytrol, Urotrol) solifenacin (VESIcare), tolterodine (Detrol), or trospium (Sanctura) can effectively treat urinary incontinence by decreasing the contractions of the bladder and thus eliminating urgency symptoms that lead to wetting accidents. These medications are taken by mouth, and a few are additionally available as a transdermal patch.

**Enuresis** (bedwetting) can be treated effectively with desmopressin (DDAVP) (nasally or orally) and oral imipramine (Tofranil). DDAVP is a manufactured form of the naturally occurring hormone found in the pituitary gland that is responsible for how the body uses water. You should also advise patients not to drink caffeinated drinks after 6 p.m. because these drinks can irritate the bladder and cause enuresis.

dangerous if taken in the wrong quantities or when they interact with certain medications. For example, St. John's wort can lower cyclosporine levels, an effect that can ultimately lead to rejection of a transplanted organ.

For the foregoing reasons, it is essential that patients discuss with their physician the herbal remedies they are using, to avoid any detrimental effects from interactions. In addition, because self-medication occurs routinely, patients may fail to seek a physician's assistance for many serious health issues. An open, accepting attitude by the office staff is critical in successful discussions of these treatments.

If you visit any herbal store, you may be surprised to see the variety of herbal and/or natural products and the routes by which they can be administered. Most are swallowed as tablets, but others can be brewed as teas, chewed on as a root, or rubbed on the skin. Furthermore, some herbs (e.g., eucalyptus for asthma) are used as **aromatherapy,** in which they are burned and their aroma inhaled. Herbs are also just one type of plant substance used in homeopathy.

---

### A CLOSER LOOK: Homeopathy

**Homeopathy** is a type of complementary and alternative medicine based on the principle that "like cures like" with highly diluted preparations. This means that a patient may take a substance similar to the one that is harming his or her body, thereby training the body to fight the dangerous substance with a small amount of a similar substance. For example, a patient who experiences symptoms similar to someone allergic to cat dander would be exposed to an extremely dilute (1:1,000) mixture of water and cat dander.

A German physician, Samuel Hahnemann (1755–1843), developed homeopathy and homeopathic remedies. In the 1800s, physicians would often cut people open to bleed them because they believed that bleeding purged the body of evil disease. Physicians also administered harsh enemas to force the body to purge disease. Not surprisingly, these drastic measures failed to work and often, in fact, killed patients, so Dr. Hahnemann developed homeopathy.

Three laws support homeopathy and how it should work:

• A remedy starts healing from the top of the body and works downward.
• A remedy starts from within the body, working outward, and from major to minor organs.
• Symptoms clear in reverse order to their manner of appearance.

More than 2,000 homeopathic remedies are available from animal, vegetable, and mineral sources. You can find them by doing an Internet search on homeopathy or by visiting the National Homeopathy Center (www.homeopathic.org).

Homeopaths are practitioners who are skilled in homeopathy and who advise patients on the selection and dosing of homeopathic preparations. Homeopaths are usually not regulated by any medical board or governmental agency.

---

The most common herbs are listed in Table 21.1. Some sources of information on herbs may not contain data about safety, efficacy, and dosing. Furthermore, because herbs are not regulated as are most pharmaceutical preparations, there may be inconsistent amounts of an herb in different manufacturers' products. In addition, herbs are not regulated by the Food and Drug Administration (FDA).

Herbs are sometimes considered **complementary and alternative medicine (CAM).** CAM therapies include treatments such as massage therapy, aromatherapy, acupuncture, acupressure, and medications such as herbs, minerals, and vitamins used to complement or as an alternative to conventional medical therapy. Sometimes the patient believes that conventional treatment does not or cannot eliminate the disease. Other patients may consider modern medical treatment dangerous. Most herbs have had less

## TABLE 21.1   Examples of Herbs and Possible Benefits

| Herb | Purpose |
|---|---|
| Aloe vera | Treats acne, astringent, blood cleanser, treats burns, seals cuts, helps with shingles, tonic |
| Angelica | Diaphoretic, tonic, antispasmodic, expectorant; induces fetal abortion |
| Barberry | Respiratory aid, anti-infective |
| Camphor | Bronchodilator |
| Caraway | Antispasmodic |
| Cayenne pepper | Decongestant, expectorant, emetic |
| Chamomile | Calming, digestive aid, anti-infective, antiseptic, antispasmodic |
| Cedar | Decreases oily skin, treats dandruff, tonic |
| Celery seed | Expectorant, lithotrophic (expels stones) |
| Cumin | Boosts immune system, sexual stimulant |
| Echinacea | Boosts immune system |
| Evening primrose | Decreases scaling and redness, prevents multiple sclerosis, decreases liver damage from alcohol, maintains hormonal balance, decreases inflammation, acts as an immunosuppressant |
| Feverfew | Antispasmodic, decreases migraines |
| Garlic | Stimulant, carminative, expectorant, fungicide, antibiotic, antispasmodic; decreases blood pressure and cholesterol |
| Ginger | Digestive aid |
| Ginkgo biloba | Increases blood flow, anti-infective |
| Ginseng | Energizer, boosts immune system, increases concentration |
| Green tea | Prevents cancer |
| Horehound | Respiratory problems |
| Hyssop | Antiretroviral |
| Kava kava | Improves mood |
| Licorice | Antiulcer, heals rashes, aids respiration |
| Melatonin | Sleep |
| Mustard | Digestive aid, anti-infective, emetic, laxative |
| Myrrh | Analgesic, antispasmodic, anti-infective |
| Nutmeg | Calming; hallucinogen in high doses |
| Onion | Stimulant, expectorant, rejuvenates |
| Peppermint | Digestive aid, stimulant, antispasmodic |
| Rosemary | Improves hair, decreases muscle tension |
| Saffron | Stimulant, expectorant |
| Saw palmetto | Tonic, urinary antiseptic, increases sex drive |
| Senna | Cathartic, antispasmodic, antiseptic |
| Skullcap | Antianxiety, antispasmodic |
| St. John's wort | Antidepressant, diuretic, antiviral, analgesic |
| Turmeric | Digestive aid |
| Valerian | Sedative |
| Witch hazel | Astringent, anti-inflammatory |
| Yams | Anti-infective, antispasmodic |
| Yarrow | Aids in blood clotting, diaphoretic, anti-inflammatory, antiseptic, tonic, antispasmodic |

scientific testing than modern drugs. This is the main reason that insurance companies refuse to pay for many alternative therapies, including herbal remedies. These companies believe that the evidence supporting CAM effectiveness is insufficient.

### Virtual Field Trip

Using your preferred search engine, research one form of alternative medicine. Find a few specific herbs that are used in that therapy, and share this information with the class.

Many CAM therapies emphasize an Eastern philosophy rather than a Western philosophy of healing (Fast Tip 21.1). Eastern philosophy focuses on the body's ability to heal itself and uses herbs to promote self-healing. Practitioners of Eastern medicine believe that disease is a result of imbalance within the body and that health returns once balance is restored. Some examples of CAM include acupuncture, acupressure, and reflexology.

Western philosophy focuses on medications to target specific problems. Practitioners of Western medicine believe that disease is caused by physiological disorders and that health is the absence of disease.

Eastern and Western philosophies are meeting halfway as integrative therapy, combining conventional medical treatment with CAM therapies.

### CRITICAL THINKING

If a placebo (inactive medication) works almost 60% of the time, what does this say about the role of faith in healing?

### Vitamins, minerals, amino acids, and lipids

Vitamins are **organic** (containing carbon) nutrients that are essential to regulate the chemical processes in the body. These nutrients work to maintain strong bones, release energy from food, and control hormonal activity. The FDA has established recommended daily allowances (RDAs) for vitamins and minerals. Vitamin and mineral deficiencies can lead to illness, but overdoses can also cause illness or death. Although a small amount of a vitamin is good, **megadoses** (larger than the FDA recommendations) are not usually better. The **recommended daily allowance (RDA)** for each vitamin varies for women, men, pregnant women, infants, children, and adolescents. It is common to see changes in the urine with vitamin supplements. The urine may become bright yellow and have a strong odor. If the supplement dosages are within the recommended range, it is usually not a concern. However, if the doses are too large for long periods of time, serious health issues may arise, such as the following: kidney, liver, and heart and nerve damage; kidney and bladder stones; and an increased risk of diabetes and gout.

■ **Fat-soluble vitamins:** Fat-soluble vitamins are not excreted from the body. They are stored when they are not currently needed and can build up to toxic levels if more than the recommended intake is ingested. Vitamins A, D, E, and K are fat-soluble vitamins. Vitamins A, D, and K are stored in the liver, and vitamin E is spread throughout the fatty tissue of the body (Table 21.2). Vitamin A is a requirement for healthy skin, teeth, bone, and soft tissue such as mucous membranes. It also is essential for vision, reproductive, and immune system health. Vitamin D plays a key role in the healthy development of bone and the retention and absorption of calcium and phosphorus in the body. Vitamin E is thought to have a role in the formation of red blood cells and muscles, as well as the support of the immune system. Vitamin K is important in the clotting processes of the human body, and without it, bleeding abnormalities may occur.

■ **Water-soluble vitamins:** Water-soluble vitamins are vitamins that are not stored and are excreted by the body. These vitamins include vitamins B and C and must be ingested daily (see Table 21.2). Vitamin B includes $B_1$ (thiamine), $B_2$ (riboflavin), $B_3$ (niacin), $B_5$ (pantothenic acid),

---

**Fast Tip 21.1**  Eastern and Western Healing Philosophies

It is important to understand the different philosophies that patients and health-care providers may have toward healing. If, for example, a patient who values Eastern philosophy visits a provider who values Western philosophy, conflicts in the choice of treatment may result.

## TABLE 21.2   Fat and Water-Soluble Vitamins

| Vitamin | Function | Deficiency | Excess |
|---|---|---|---|
| **Fat-Soluble** | | | |
| **Vitamin A** | Anticarcinogenic; heals skin disorders; improves vision; determines growth of bones, hair, teeth, skin, and gums | Susceptibility to vision problems, immunodeficiency | Birth defects, death |
| **Vitamin D** | Prevents osteoporosis, treats psoriasis, boosts immune systems, decreases cancer, makes strong bones and teeth | Tooth and bone deformation and fractures, rickets (children) osteomalacia, osteoporosis, tetany | Nausea, vomiting, diarrhea, kidney stones, dizziness, redness of skin, muscle and bone pain, cardiac arrhythmias, vertigo, tinnitus |
| **Vitamin E** | Acts as an antioxidant and diuretic, decreases PMS and miscarriage, increases immunity, decreases fatigue, treats skin problems and baldness, heals burns and wounds, improves neurological functioning | Rare because most adults have large vitamin E stores in adipose tissue; may contribute to retinopathy in prematurity and early childhood | Muscle weakness, fatigue, nausea, abnormal blood cell counts; in large doses significantly decreases clotting time |
| **Vitamin K** | Clots blood | Increased clotting time, blood in urine, petechiae, bruising, blood in stool | No known reaction |
| **Water-Soluble** | | | |
| **Vitamin B$_1$ (thiamine)** | Protects against imbalances caused by alcohol consumption; decreases heart disease, neurological diseases, anemia, herpes, and other infections; treats diabetes mellitus; helps convert sugar into energy | Emaciation, constipation, anorexia, nausea, GI upset, neuritis, pain, tingling in the extremities, loss of reflexes, muscle weakness, fatigue, ataxia, confusion, memory loss | Rare except when given by IV route: feeling of warmth, sweating, weakness, nausea, restless, symptoms of anaphylactic shock |
| **Vitamin B$_2$ (riboflavin)** | Works with enzymes to metabolize fats, proteins, and carbohydrates; aids vision; improves growth and reproductive system; helps skin, hair, and nails grow; can improve athletic performance; decreases cancer; improves anemias | Glossitis, cheilosis, dermatitis | Rare: burning or prickling sensations, hypersensitivity reaction |
| **Vitamin B$_3$ (niacin)** | Prevents and treats schizophrenia; aids in cell respiration; decreases cholesterol; cures migraines; decreases blood pressure; alleviates arthritis, acts as an antioxidant; produces energy from food; improves skin, nerves, and tongue | Peripheral vascular damage, dermatitis, diarrhea | Headache, flushing, burning sensation, postural hypotension, jaundice |

*Continued*

## TABLE 21.2  Fat and Water-Soluble Vitamins—cont'd

| Vitamin | Function | Deficiency | Excess |
| --- | --- | --- | --- |
| **Water-Soluble** | | | |
| **Vitamin B$_5$ (pantothenic acid)** | Encourages wound healing, produces energy, decreases stress on the body, improves metabolism, decreases fatigue, boosts the immune system | Extremely rare because available in diet and also produced by intestinal bacteria; fatigue | None known |
| **Vitamin B$_6$ (pyridoxine)** | Boosts the immune system, decreases diabetes mellitus, assimilates proteins and fats, decreases skin and nervous system disorders, improves nausea, decreases PMS and menopausal symptoms, stops muscle cramps and spasms; decreases cancers, acts as a natural diuretic | Dermatitis, glossitis, depression, confusion, anemia, convulsions | Nerve damage to the arms and legs |
| **Vitamin B$_7$ (biotin, also known as vitamin H)** | Decreases graying of hair, eases muscular aches and pains, treats eczema and dermatitis, decreases baldness | Hair loss, rash around face and genitals, neurological symptoms | None known |
| **Vitamin B$_9$ (folic acid)** | Improves lactations, decreases cancers, improves skin and appetite, acts as an analgesic, decreases infection, metabolizes RNA and DNA, forms blood, decreases spina bifida in fetuses | Anorexia, diarrhea, decreased weight, weakness, sore mouth, irritability | Hypersensitivity reaction |
| **Vitamin B$_{12}$ (cobalamin)** | Improves memory and concentration, uses food for energy, increases growth, decreases cancer, acts as an antiallergen | Anemia, ataxia, numbness, irritability | Numbness, decreased muscle coordination, irritability, confusion |
| **Vitamin C (ascorbic acid)** | Increases wound healing, decreases cholesterol and heart disease, boosts immune system, makes healthy bones and teeth, nourishes the sex organs, alleviates male infertility, decreases cancer, improves vision, acts as an antihistamine and antioxidant | Fragility of capillaries, poor wound healing, degenerative bone disease | Diarrhea, stomach pain |

GI, gastrointestinal; PMS, premenstrual syndrome.

B$_6$ (pyridoxine), B$_7$ (biotin), B$_9$ (folic acid), and B$_{12}$ (cobalamin). These B vitamins work to support the immune and nervous systems, as well as improve metabolism and maintain healthy skin and muscles. They also help with stress, depression, and cardiac disease. Vitamin C (ascorbic acid) is needed for the production and maintenance of connective tissue, bones, and teeth.

Minerals are **inorganic** (lack carbon) chemical elements that are necessary to the health and maintenance of the body's many biological processes. Minerals are required for almost every single function in the body. They act as catalysts for many essential vitamins. One example is magnesium, which allows calcium and vitamin C to be metabolized and helps to convert blood sugar into energy. Without magnesium, these nutrients would be excreted from the body without ever being used. Another example is iron. Iron is one key to hemoglobin production, which is necessary to transport oxygen throughout the body. Minerals can be major or trace. Major minerals are those that the body needs in large amounts such as calcium, magnesium, phosphorus, potassium, sodium, and chloride, and trace minerals are those the body needs in minute amounts. Trace minerals include chromium, cobalt, copper, iron, iodine, manganese, molybdenum, selenium, silica, and zinc. Table 21.3 lists both major and trace minerals and their functions.

## TABLE 21.3  Minerals

| Mineral | Function | Deficiency | Excess and Side Effects |
|---|---|---|---|
| **Major Minerals** | | | |
| Calcium | Decreases osteoporosis, cancer, heart disease, and high blood pressure; alleviates arthritis; keeps skin healthy; decreases leg cramps; encourages healthy heart rhythms; helps metabolize iron; decreases insomnia | Bone deformities and fractures, leg cramps, tetany, heart dysrhythmias | Constipation, irritation of tissue if IV infiltrates |
| Magnesium | Produces energy, replicates cell materials, transmits nerve impulses, prevents kidney stones and gallstones, repairs body cells, is required for hormonal activity | Kidney stones and gallstones, endocrine disorders, nerve numbness | None noted |
| Phosphorus | Forms bones and teeth, cofactor for many enzymes, activates B-complex vitamins, produces energy, increases endurance, fights fatigue, forms RNA and DNA | Malformed bones and teeth, poor growth and healing, fatigue, malabsorption | None noted |
| Potassium | Stabilizes the internal structure of cells, activates enzymes that control energy production, decreases blood pressure and stroke, improves athletic performance, acts with sodium to conduct nerve impulses | Confusion, muscular weakness, paralysis, arrhythmias, lethargy, fatigue | Hypotension, listlessness, paralysis, confusion, arrhythmias |
| Sodium and chloride | Found in every cell of body, necessary to maintain fluid balance, muscle relaxation, nerve signal transmission, and blood pressure | Nausea, vomiting, dizziness, headache, muscle cramps | Hypertension, malfunction in cells |
| **Trace Minerals** | | | |
| Chromium | Improves the production of insulin, metabolizes carbohydrates and fats, improves cholesterol levels, improves synthesis of proteins in the body, increases resistance to infection, decreases hunger | Rare: Diabetes mellitus symptoms: impairs ability to use glucose for energy | None known |
| Cobalt | Decreases pernicious anemia, increases the production of red blood cells, helps the synthesis of DNA and choline, decreases blood pressure; aids the nervous system and the formation of myelin | Blood abnormalities, neurological disorders | Toxic cardiomyopathy, polycythemia, goiter |
| Copper | Decreases cancer and CV disorders, improves arthritis, boosts the immune system, acts as an antioxidant | Infection, CV disease | Anxiety, insomnia, poor concentration, depression, tinnitus, headaches, rash |

*Continued*

## TABLE 21.3 Minerals—cont'd

| Mineral | Function | Deficiency | Excess and Side Effects |
|---|---|---|---|
| **Trace Minerals** | | | |
| **Fluoride** | Decreases dental caries and osteoporosis, improves heart functioning, decreases calcium buildup in organs | Dental caries, kidney stones | Mottling of teeth, possible brain under-development in children |
| **Iron (ferrous)** | Increases energy and physical performance, decreases cancer and learning disabilities, boosts the immune system, decreases iron-deficiency anemia, encourages sleep | Fatigue, anemia, pallor, pica (craving to eat nonfoods such as clay and laundry starch), lethargy, weakness, vertigo, air hunger, confusion, irregular heartbeat, learning disabilities in children, insomnia | Constipation, GI bleeding |
| **Iodine** | Aids metabolism, reduces fibrocystic breast disease, protects against toxic effects of exposure to radioactive materials, prevents goiter and thyroid disorders, loosens respiratory tract mucus, acts as an antiseptic | Goiters, thyroid disease | Thyroid underactivity |
| **Manganese** | Aids the nervous system, necessary for synthesis of structural proteins and normal bone structure, helps female sex hormones, metabolizes glucose, needed for formation of thyroxine in the thyroid gland, improves brain function, decreases nervous disorders | Hearing loss, dizziness, ataxia, fainting, weakness in joints; linked to myasthenia gravis, impaired glucose metabolism, reduced insulin production | Decreased iron absorption leading to iron-deficiency anemia |
| **Molybdenum** | Necessary for the utilization of iron, carbohydrates, and fats; excretes uric acid; decreases impotence and cancer; prevents dental caries; alleviates anemia | Cavities, anemia, impotence, gout, malabsorption | Weight loss, stunted growth, anemia, diarrhea, swollen joints |
| **Selenium** | Improves vision, skin, and hair; boosts the immune system; decreases cancer, improves liver function; decreases CV disease; detoxifies alcohol and other drugs; increases male potency and sex drive; decreases hot flashes and menopausal symptoms; alleviates dandruff | Immune, CV, liver, and sexual disorders | Nausea, vomiting, diarrhea, hair loss, rash, brittle nails, fatigue, nerve damage, garlic odor to breath |
| **Silica** | Decreases CV disease and osteoporosis; prevents hair from falling out; helps bones, skin, and fingernails grow | Hair, skin, CV, and bone disorders | None noted |
| **Zinc** | Boosts the immune system; prevents cancer; improves senses of sight, taste, and smell; decreases hair loss and acne; alleviates rheumatoid arthritis | Alcohol tolerance, anemia, poor wound healing, decreased taste, hair loss, dermatitis, immune deficiency, growth retardation | Nausea and vomiting, diarrhea, headaches |

CV, cardiovascular; GI, gastrointestinal.

Amino acids are compounds that contain an amino group and have an acidic function. They are considered the building blocks of protein. The eight "essential" amino acids include alanine, valine, tryptophan, isoleucine, methionine, lysine, threonine and leucine (Table 21.4). They are called essential because the body can only obtain them through diet and does not store them for future use. In addition, there are 12 "nonessential" amino acids; nonessential means that they can usually be made from other substances in the body if needed.

Lipids (fats) are necessary for life in that they store energy, insulate body tissues from heat and cold, and cushion and protect our internal organs. Saturated fats are obtained from animals and are solid at room temperature. Unsaturated fats originate from plant sources and are liquid at room temperature. Cholesterol is used to synthesize hormones, vitamin D, and bile. It also serves to stabilize cell membranes throughout the body. Fatty acids found in fish are available as fish oil and are considered helpful in patients with high triglycerides or familial history of heart disease, and they may also lower blood pressure. An IV form of lipids (Intralipid 20%) is available for administration to those patients who are receiving all their nutrients through IV therapy, to provide essential fatty acids and calories. Lipids are available as supplements (Table 21.5). They are used to prevent wrinkles, unclog arteries, and decrease cholesterol and heart disease.

### CRITICAL THINKING

If an athlete takes excessive amounts of vitamins and complains that his urine has changed color and has a strong odor, what is the likely cause?

## Virtual Field Trip

Using your preferred search engine, find information to help you make a brochure on safe herbal medication use for patients.

## TABLE 21.4 Key Amino Acids

| Amino Acid | Purpose |
| --- | --- |
| Alanine | Kills pain, acts as an antidepressant |
| Glycine | Increases pituitary function, decreases spasms, increases blood glucose |
| Arginine | Boosts immunity, decreases tremors, increases muscle tone, burns fat, promotes wound healing, protects the liver from toxins |
| Aspartic acid | Disposes of ammonia, decreases fatigue, may improve stamina and endurance |
| Cysteine | Protects against copper toxicity, decreases damage from free radicals (molecules that cause many kinds of chemical reactions in the body), may reverse damage done by smoking and alcohol abuse, protects against x-rays and radiation exposure damage |
| Glutamine | Decreases craving for alcohol, heals peptic ulcers, acts as an antidepressant, energizes the brain, heals colitis |
| Histidine | Increases suppressor T cells, decreases arthritis |
| Lysine | Prevents or treats herpes, builds muscle mass, improves concentration, increases fertility |
| Methionine | Eliminates fatty substances, decreases the risk of heart attack, regulates the nervous system, decreases tumors, is necessary for biosynthesis of taurine and cysteine |
| Phenylalanine | Acts as an antidepressant, controls addictive behavior, increases alertness and sexual arousal, decreases hunger |
| Tryptophan | Decreases pain sensitivity and craving for alcohol, acts as an antidepressant, acts as a sleep aid |
| Tyrosine | Acts as an antidepressant, decreases stress and premenstrual syndrome, decreases addiction and withdrawal symptoms |

**TABLE 21.5 Examples of Lipid Supplements**

| Supplement | Purpose |
|---|---|
| Fish oils | Reduce kidney disease, decrease cancer, slow arthritis progression, decrease blood pressure, have cardiovascular effects, decrease psoriasis signs and symptoms |
| Inositol | Dissolves fat, decreases anxiety, grows hair and nails, decreases cholesterol, improves sleep |
| Lecithin | Decreases cardiovascular illness and memory loss, balances mood in bipolar disorder, acts as an antiviral, decreases gallstones, is palliative for viral hepatitis |

● ● ● SUMMARY

This chapter discusses herbs, vitamins, minerals, amino acids, and fats and their role in a person's diet to maintain health. Herbs are often used to supplement health or medications and are considered CAM. Herbs and vitamin and mineral supplements are not regulated by the government, so an awareness of their effects and interactions with other herbs or medications is important. Always ask your patients about the type, if any, of CAM therapies they may be using, so you can be aware of any potential interactions with prescribed medications.

# Activities

To make sure that you have learned the key points covered in this chapter, complete the following activities.

## True or False

Write true if the statement is true. Beside the false statements, write false, and correct the statement to make it true.

Vitamin B is a water-soluble vitamin. _____

Vitamin A is stored in the liver. _____

Chamomile tea helps to keep someone alert. _____

Lipids are the building blocks of protein. _____

Niacin is a form of vitamin B. _____

Vitamins and minerals are regulated by the FDA as medications. _____

St. John's wort should not be taken by transplant recipients. _____

Herbs are available as a root that may be chewed. _____

Insurance companies routinely pay for CAM and herbal remedies. _____

CAM therapies are rooted in Eastern philosophy. _____

## Multiple Choice

Choose the best answer for each question.

**1. CAM therapies include all of the following EXCEPT ____.**
   A. Acupuncture
   B. Acupressure
   C. Reflexology
   D. Oncology
   E. Aromatherapy

**2. Which of the following is a substance closely regulated by the FDA?**
   A. Antibiotics
   B. Herbs
   C. Vitamins
   D. Minerals

**3. Which vitamin is important to blood clotting?**
   A. A
   B. D
   C. E
   D. K

**4. Herbal medicine forms include which of the following?**

A. Tablets

B. Teas

C. Roots

D. Topical preparations

E. All of the above

**5. The basis for Eastern philosophy is _____.**

A. The body's ability to heal itself

B. Medications to target specific problems

C. Disease is caused by physiological disorders

D. None of the above.

**6. Western philosophy focuses on _____.**

A. The body's ability to heal itself

B. Medications to target specific problems

C. Disease is caused by physiological disorders

D. None of the above

**7. B vitamins include which of the following?**

A. Niacin

B. Riboflavin

C. Folic acid

D. All of the above

**8. Which of the following vitamins must be taken on a daily basis?**

A. A

B. C

C. D

D. K

**9. Amino acids are the building blocks of what substance?**

A. Protein

B. Carbohydrate

C. Fat

D. None of the above

**10. RDA stands for _____.**

A. Ratio of daily allowance

B. Required daily allowance

C. Recommended daily allowance

D. None of the above

**Application Exercises**

Respond to the following situations on a separate sheet.

1. Patrick tells you that he is treating his depression with phenylalanine but still has very little energy and has no interest in his children's activities. What do you reply?

2. Ryan is undergoing chemotherapy for lung cancer. He is losing weight and has a very poor appetite. How will this affect his health? What would you suggest?

# Essentials Review

For further study and practice with drug classifications learned in this chapter, complete the following table to the best of your ability. Use resources such as the *PDR,* the Internet, or printed drug guides for help.

| Classification | Purpose | Side Effects | Contraindications and Precautions | Examples | Patient Eduction |
|---|---|---|---|---|---|
| Vitamin A | | | | | |
| Vitamin B | | | | | |
| B₁ | | | | | |
| B₂ | | | | | |
| B₃ | | | | | |
| B₅ | | | | | |
| B₆ | | | | | |
| B₇ | | | | | |
| B₉ | | | | | |
| B₁₂ | | | | | |
| Vitamin C | | | | | |
| Vitamin D | | | | | |
| Vitamin E | | | | | |
| Vitamin K | | | | | |
| Calcium | | | | | |
| Chromium | | | | | |
| Cobalt | | | | | |
| Copper | | | | | |

# Glossary

## A

Absorption—passage of a substance through some surface of the body into body fluids and tissues

a.c.—before meals

ACE inhibitor—drug that inhibits the action of angiotensin-converting enzyme

Acne—inflammatory disease of the sebaceous glands of the skin

Acromegaly—chronic syndrome of growth hormone excess, most often caused by a pituitary macroadenoma, and characterized by gradual coarsening and enlargement of bones and facial features

ACTH—adrenocorticotropic hormone

Active artificial immunity—immunity obtained through the administration of a vaccine that allows the patient to form antibodies to a virus, toxin, or bacterium

Active natural immunity—immunity obtained through a microorganism's entry into the body and the body's learning to fight it

Acupressure—traditional Chinese medicine's use of pressure on certain points on the body to promote healing

Acupuncture—traditional Chinese medicine's use of needles at certain points on the body to promote healing

a.d.—right ear

Addicting—a substance that encourages dependence on it

Addison's disease—gradual, progressive failure of the adrenal glands and insufficient production of steroid hormones

Addition—to combine two or more numbers together

Additive—effect that one drug or substance contributes to the action of another drug or substance

ADH—antidiuretic hormone

Adrenergic—relating to nerve fibers that release norepinephrine or epinephrine at the synapses

Adverse reaction—undesired side effects or toxicity caused by a treatment

Aerobic—taking place in the presence of oxygen

Agonist—drug that binds to the receptor and stimulates the receptor's function

Al-Hawi—large 20-volume Arabian medical book written by a single author Al-Razi and having a significant influence on medicine in Medieval Europe

Alimentary canal—another name for the gastrointestinal tract

Alopecia—absence or loss of hair

Alternative medicine—the practice of using natural healing in conjunction with mainstream medicine. Some examples are acupuncture, massage therapy, and aromatherapy

Alveoli—plural of alveolus; an air sac in the lungs

Ampule—small glass container that can be sealed and its contents sterilized

Anaerobic—taking place in the absence of oxygen

Analgesic—medication that relieves pain

Anaphylaxis—hypersensitivity reaction between an allergenic antigen and immunoglobulin E bound to mast cells; stimulates the sudden release of immunologic mediators locally or throughout the body

Androgen—substance producing or stimulating the development of male characteristics, such as the hormones testosterone and androsterone

Angina pectoris—oppressive pain or pressure in the chest caused by inadequate blood flow and oxygenation to heart muscle

Anoxia—absence of oxygen

Antagonist—that which counteracts the action of something else, such as a muscle or drug

Antibody—substance produced by lymphocytes in response to a unique antigen to fight against it

Antigen—any substance capable of eliciting an immune response (foreign invader)

Antihistamine—drug that opposes the action of histamine

Antihypertensive—drug used to treat hypertension

Antineoplastic—drug used to destroy neoplasms

Antispasmodic—drug that prevents or relieves spasm

Antitussive—drug that prevents or relieves coughing

Anxiolytic—medication that reduces anxiety

Apnea—cessation of breathing

Apothecary—druggist or pharmacist

Aqueous humor—thin watery fluid contained in the anterior chamber of the eye

Aromatherapy—use of fragrant oils in baths, as inhalants, or during massage to relieve stress and to treat skin conditions

a.s.—left eye

Atherosclerosis—the most common form of arteriosclerosis, marked by cholesterol-lipid-calcium deposits in the walls of the arteries

Attenuate—to render weak or make less virulent

a.u.—both ears

Aura—subjective, but recognizable sensation that precedes and signals the onset of a convulsion or migraine headache

Automatic stop order—an order that discontinues a medication at a certain time

Autoimmune disorder—condition in which the immune system attacks tissue normally present in the body (attacks itself)

Autonomic—self-controlling, functioning independently

Available dose—amount of medication on hand to administer to a patient

Avoirdupois—system of weighing or measuring articles in which 7,000 grains equal 1 pound

## B

Bactericidal—capable of killing bacteria

Bacteriostatic—inhibits the growth of bacteria

Barrel—part of the syringe through which the plunger passes

Benign—not recurrent or progressive, not malignant

Beta-adrenergic agent—synthetic or natural drug that stimulates beta receptors

bid—two times per day

Biotransformation—chemical alteration that a substance undergoes in the body

Bisphosphonates—any of a class of medications that inhibit the resorption of bones by osteoclasts

Blister pack—method of delivering medications; usually contains one dose in each small sac

Blood-borne pathogens—microorganisms capable of producing disease, transmitted by body fluids

Blood-brain barrier—densely packed cells that allow nutrients and certain other chemicals, but no others, to pass into the central nervous system

Blood-placental barrier—densely packed cells that allow nutrients and certain other chemicals, but not others, to pass through the placenta

Blood-testicular barrier—densely packed cells that allow nutrients and certain other chemicals, but not others, to pass into the testicles

Booster—additional dose of an immunizing agent to increase the protection afforded by the original series of injections

Bovine—refers to products produced from cows

BPH—benign prostatic hypertrophy

Brand name—drug name given by the drug manufacturer

Broad spectrum—in reference to antibiotics; ones that combat a wide variety of microorganisms

BSA—body surface area (computed using height and weight)

Buccal—route in which a medication is administered into the buccal pouch (cheek)

Buffered—treated in such a way to offset the reaction of an agent administered in conjunction with it

Bulk—mass; in reference to medication, a container holding multiple doses

BUN—blood urea nitrogen

## C

c̄—with

cc—unit of measure in which one cubic centimeter of space will hold 1 mL of fluid

C & S—culture and sensitivity

Calcitonin—hormone produced by the human thyroid gland that is important for maintaining a dense, strong bone matrix and regulating the blood calcium level

Calculus—stone commonly formed from calcium found in the gallbladder or kidneys

Calibrated—determined as accurate

CAM—complementary and alternative medicine

Cannula—tube used to deliver oxygen or through which a trocar is withdrawn after insertion

Cap.—abbreviation for capsule

Caplet—delivery mode for medication that is similar to both capsules and tablets

Capsule—delivery mode for medication that holds a measured drug inside a substance that dissolves

Carcinogen—any substance or agent that produces cancer or increases the risk of developing cancer in humans or animals

Cathartic—purging the body quickly; example, cleaning the bowels of stool

Centi—prefix used in the metric system to denote one-hundredth (1/100)

Cerumen—earwax; secreted by the glands at the outer third of the ear canal

Chemotherapy—also known as antineoplastic medications; those used to fight cancer cells or neoplasms

Chemical name—drug name that reflects the chemical makeup of the drug

CHF—congestive heart failure

Cholinergic—agent that produces the effect of acetylcholine

Chyme—mixture of food and stomach acid passing into the small intestine

Clinical trials—scientific tests that research the efficacy and safety of a medication

CNS—central nervous system

$CO_2$—carbon dioxide

Comedo—small skin lesion of acne vulgaris and seborrheic dermatitis

Compassionate use—the use of an investigational new drug (IND) in patients who are suffering greatly and may die without the drug

Compound—mix

Condyloma—wart, found on the genitals or near the anus, with a textured surface that may resemble coral, cauliflower, or cobblestone

Constipation—stool with lowered liquid content and less frequent

Contractility—having the ability to contract or shorten

Contraindications—symptoms or circumstances that make treatment with a drug or device unsafe or inappropriate

Control group—group of people in clinical trials who receive the placebo or usual treatment, in contrast to the group given the treatment or medication being studied

Controlled substances—substances monitored under the Comprehensive Drug Abuse Prevention and Control Act, a law enacted in 1971 to control the distribution and use of all depressant and stimulant drugs and other drugs of abuse or potential abuse as may be designated by the Drug Enforcement Administration of the Department of Justice

Conversion factor—number used to change a mathematical number from one condition to another

COPD—chronic obstructive pulmonary disease

CPAP—continuous positive airway pressure

Cream—semisolid delivery system for medications

Cretinism—congenital condition caused by a lack of thyroid hormones and characterized by arrested physical and mental development, myxedema, dystrophy of the bones and soft tissues, and lowered basal metabolism

Crystalloid—substance capable of crystallization, which in solution can be diffused through animal membranes

CSF—cerebrospinal fluid

Cumulation—increasing in effect by successive additions

Curative—having healing or remedial properties

Cushing's disease—caused by excessive production of adrenocorticotropic hormone (ACTH) in the body

CVA—cerebrovascular accident

Cyanosis—blue, gray, slate, or dark purple discoloration of the skin or mucous membranes caused by deoxygenated or reduced hemoglobin in the blood

# D

d/c—discontinue(d)

DEA—Drug Enforcement Agency of the Department of Justice

Débride—to perform the action of débridement, the removal of foreign material and dead or damaged tissue, especially in a wound

Deci—prefix used in the metric system to denote one-tenth (1/10)

Decimal—numeric system using numbers from 0 to 9

Decongestant—agent that reduces congestion, especially nasal

Delayed action—action occurring a considerable time after a stimulus

Deltoid—triangular muscle on the upper arm

Delusion—false belief brought about without appropriate external stimulation and inconsistent with the individual's own knowledge and experience

Dementia—progressive, irreversible decline in mental function, marked by memory impairment and, often, deficits in reasoning, judgment, abstract thought, registration, comprehension, learning, task execution, and use of language

Denominator—number on lower part of a fraction; used to divide into the numerator

Dependent—supported by, nurtured by, or relying on another person or variable

Depression—mood disorder marked by loss of interest or pleasure in living

Desired dose—dose of medication ordered by the prescriber (also known as ordered dose)

Destructive—causing injury or death

Dextrose—glucose, sugar

Diabetes insipidus—excessive urination caused by inadequate amounts of antidiuretic hormone (ADH) in the body or by failure of the kidney to respond to ADH

Diabetes mellitus—chronic metabolic disorder marked by hyperglycemia

Diagnostic—pertaining to the disease or syndrome a person has or is believed to have

Dialysis—passage of a solute through a membrane

Diarrhea—increased frequency of stool and higher fluid content

Digestion—the process of converting food into chemical substances that can be used in the body

Diluent—fluid used to reconstitute a powdered medication

Dimensional analysis—calculating dosages using the measurement, such as milligrams or milliliters, to set up the calculation

Distribution—dividing and spreading of a medication to a target organ

Dividend—number being divided in a division problem

Division—to separate into smaller parts

Divisor—number doing the division in a division problem

DMARD—disease-modifying antirheumatic drug

Dorsogluteal—injection site in the gluteus maximus on the dorsal (back) side

Double-blind—neither the patient nor the researcher in the clinical trial knows who has the placebo and who has the drug being tested

Drip chamber—part of an intravenous line where the medication drips into the chamber at a regulated rate

Droog—Dutch word meaning dry, as in dried herbs used for healing; source of the word drug

Drug—substance that can change a function in a living being

Drug cycle—absorption, distribution in the body, metabolism, and excretion of medications

Drug holiday—period in which a patient with Parkinson's disease stops taking medications for a period of time to allow the medications to be resumed at much lower doses while still obtaining desired benefits

DVT—deep vein thrombosis

Dwarfism—condition of being abnormally small

Dyspnea—difficult breathing

Dysrhythmias—abnormal heart rhythms

Dystonia—prolonged involuntary muscular contractions that may cause twisting of body parts, repetitive movements, and increased muscular tone

## E

Ebers Papyrus—preserved medical document listing some 700 recipes to remedy a wide range of illnesses; written in approximately 1550 BC in Egypt

Eczema—general term for an itchy red rash that initially weeps or oozes serum and may become crusted, thickened, and scaly

EEG—electroencephalogram

Effervescent—bubbling, rising in little bubbles of gas

Efficacy—ability to produce a desired effect

Electrolytes—substances that, in solution, conduct an electric current and are decomposed by its passage

Elix.—abbreviation for elixir

Elixir—sweetened, aromatic, hydroalcoholic liquid used when compounding oral medication

Embolus—mass of undissolved matter present in a blood or lymphatic vessel and brought there by the blood or lymph

Emesis—evacuation of stomach contents

Emulsions—mixtures of two liquids not mutually soluble

Endogenous—produced or originating from within a cell or organism

Enema—introduction of a solution into the rectum and colon to stimulate bowel activity and cause emptying of the lower intestine for feeding or therapeutic purposes; sometimes used to give anesthesia or to aid in radiographic studies

Enteric-coated—coated with a substance so the drug is dissolved and absorbed only in the small intestine

Enuresis—bedwetting

Equivalent—equal in power or force or value

ERT—estrogen replacement therapy

Estrogen—any natural or artificial substance that induces estrus and the development of female sex characteristics; more specifically, an estrogenic hormone produced by the ovaries

EtOH—ethyl alcohol

Excretion—elimination of waste products from the body

Expectorant—agent, such as guaifenesin, that promotes clearance of mucus from the respiratory tract

Expiration—death or end of usefulness; relaxation of lungs causing the exhalation of waste in the form of $CO_2$

Extremes—numbers on the far ends (front and back) of a ratio and proportion problem

## F

FDA—Food and Drug Administration

Fight or flight—body's natural response to prepare to flee or defend itself from attack

Filter—to pass a liquid through any porous substance that prevents particles larger than a certain size from passing through

Fissure—cracks in the anus

Flatulence—air in the gastrointestinal system

Flow regulator—piece of equipment on the intravenous line that regulates the rate of passage of fluid; can be used to stop or start the flow

Formula—rule prescribing how to calculate a dosage; for example, $D/H \times Q$ = answer

Fraction—ratio of a numerator to a denominator

FSH—follicle-stimulating hormone

## G

GABA—gamma-aminobutyric acid

Gauge—measurement representing the circumference of the inner opening of an object such as a needle

Gel—semisolid condition of a precipitated or coagulated colloid, jelly, or jelly-like colloid

Generic name—official name of the drug; nonproprietary

GERD—gastroesophageal reflux disease; acid regurgitates from the stomach up into the esophagus and causes irritation and erosion

Geriatrics—branch of health care concerned with care of the aged

GH—growth hormone

Gigantism—excessive development of a body or body part

Glucocorticoids—general classification of adrenal cortical hormones primarily active in protecting against stress and affecting protein and carbohydrate metabolism

g—abbreviation for gram

Goiter—enlarged thyroid

Gout—form of arthritis marked by the deposition of monosodium urate crystals in joints and other tissues

gr—abbreviation for grain

Gram negative—bacterial microorganism that is unable to retain the color applied in a Gram stain test

Gram positive—bacterial microorganism that is able to retain the color applied in a Gram stain test

Graves' disease—distinct type of hyperthyroidism caused by an autoimmune attack on the thyroid gland

gtt—abbreviation for drop

## H

Habituated—process of becoming accustomed to a stimulus

Halitosis—bad breath

Half-life—the length of time required for the concentration of a drug to decrease by one-half in the plasma

Hallucination—false perception having no relation to reality and not accounted for by any exterior stimulus

HCl—hydrochloric acid

HDL—high-density lipoprotein

Heartburn—pain in the area of the heart caused by irritation of refluxed acid into the esophagus

Hemorrhoid—varicose veins found in the anus

Hemostasis—arrest of bleeding or of circulation

HIPAA—Health Insurance Portability and Accountability Act

HMO—health maintenance organization

Homeopathy—school of American healing, founded by Dr. Samuel Hahnemann, based on the idea that very dilute doses of medicines that produce symptoms of a disease in healthy people can cure that disease in affected patients

Host—human, animal, or thing that harbors a potentially infectious microorganism

Household—measuring system used by lay persons, not apothecaries, in their home

*H. pylori*—bacterium responsible for the majority of ulcers

HPV—human papillomavirus

HRT—hormone replacement therapy

HTN—hypertension

Hub—part of the needle where syringe attaches

Hydantoins—colorless bases; glycolyl urea; derived from urea and allantoin

Hyperglycemia—abnormally high blood glucose levels, as are found in people with diabetes mellitus or people treated with some drugs

Hyperlipidemia—abnormally high lipids in the blood

Hypocalcemia—abnormally low calcium in the blood

Hypodermic—under or inserted under the skin

Hypoglycemia—abnormally low glucose levels in the blood

Hypoxia—oxygen deficiency in body tissues

## I

ICSH—interstitial cell–stimulating hormone

ID—intradermal

IDDM—insulin-dependent diabetes mellitus

Idiosyncratic—relating to idiosyncrasy; how a person differs from another

IM—intramuscular

Impaired provider—professional caregiver who is under the influence of a drug or disease and thus is not as competent

Impetigo—a bacterial infection of the skin

Implanted device—object inserted into the body

Improper—referring to a fraction, one in which the numerator is larger than the denominator

IND—investigational new drug

Induration—area of hardened tissue

Inert—having little or no tendency or ability to react with other chemicals; not active

Infarction—area of tissue in an organ or part that undergoes necrosis following cessation of blood supply

Infiltration—deposition and accumulation of an external substance in a cell, tissue, or organ, such as fat deposition in a damaged liver

Infusion—any liquid substance (other than blood) introduced into the body for therapeutic purposes

Inhalation—introduction of dry or moist air or vapor into the lungs for therapeutic purposes, such as by metered-dose bronchodilators in the treatment of asthma

Inhaler—device for administering medications by inhalation

Inorganic—not containing carbon; not derived from animal or vegetable matter

Inscription—body of the prescription, which gives the names of the drug prescribed and the dosage

Insert—implanting something inside something else

Insomnia—inability to sleep

Inspiration—inhalation, breathing in

Intradermal—within the dermis, intracutaneous

Intramuscular—within a muscle

Invert—to turn inside out or upside down

IOP—intraocular pressure

Ischemia—temporary deficiency of blood flow to an organ or tissue

IUD—intrauterine device, usually for contraception

IV—intravenous

IV push (IVP)—inject quickly, not drip, a small amount of medication into an intravenous line

## J
Jelly—thick, semisolid, gelatinous mass

## K
Keratinization—process of keratin formation that takes place in keratocytes as they progress upward through the layers of the epidermis of skin to the stratum corneum

Ketoacidosis—faulty fat metabolism

Kilo—prefix used in the metric system to denote 1,000

## L
Lactated Ringer's—intravenous medication containing fluid, dextrose, and electrolytes in a healthy combination, developed by Sydney Ringer

Latent TB—harboring of the tuberculosis tubercle, but without active infection

Lavage—irrigation of a cavity

LDL—low-density lipoprotein

LH—luteinizing hormone

Liniment—liquid vehicle (usually water, oil, or alcohol) containing a medication to be rubbed on or applied to the skin

Lipid—fat

Lotion—liquid medicinal preparation for local application to, or bathing, a part

Lowest common denominator—number on the bottom of a fraction that is common to the multiples of another number but is the least denominator those numbers have in common

Lozenge—small, dry, medicinal solid to be held in the mouth until it dissolves

Lumen—space within a tube

Lymphatic—pertaining to the lymph system

## M
Magma—mass left after extraction of principal; salve or paste; suspension of finely divided material in a small amount of water

Malignant—growing worse; resisting treatment; said of cancerous growth; tending or threatening to produce death; harmful

Mania—mental disorder characterized by excessive excitement

MAO inhibitor—medication that affects the action of monoamine oxidase at the synapse; used to treat depression and Parkinson's disease

Mast cell stabilizer—stabilizes large tissue cells; resembles a basophil; essential for inflammatory reactions; does not circulate in the blood

mcg—microgram; one-millionth part of a gram

Means—numbers in the center of a ratio and proportion problem, not those at the ends

Megadosage—overly large dosage

Melanocyte—cell that forms melanin; found in the lower epidermis of the skin

Melatonin—peptide hormone produced by the pineal gland; influences sleep-wake cycles and other circadian rhythms

Meniscus—curved upper surface of a liquid in a container

mEq—milliequivalent; one-thousandth of a chemical equivalent

Metabolism—breaking down into its constituents

Metastasis—change in location of a disease

Metric—measurement system based on grams for weight, liters for liquid, and meters for distance

mg—milligram, one-thousandth of a gram

MI—myocardial infarction; heart attack

Micro—small

Migraine headache—familiar disorder marked by periodic, usually unilateral, pulsatile headaches that begin during childhood or early adult life and tend to recur with diminishing frequency in later life

Milli—prefix used in the metric system to denote one-thousandth (1/1,000)

Mixed—when referring to numbers, a fraction that contains a whole number and a fractional part

mL—milliliter, one-thousandth of a liter

Morbidly obese—weight 20% or more above the recommended ideal weight; usually associated with increased health risks

Mortar—vessel with a smooth interior in which crude drugs are crushed or ground with a pestle

Mucolytic—medication that breaks down mucus and improves breathing

Multiplication—adding repetitively

Myxedema—clinical and metabolic manifestations of hypothyroidism in adults, adolescents, and children

## N

Narcotic—strong painkiller, generally made from opium, or synthetically made; may be addictive both psychologically and physically

Nausea—feeling of impending vomiting

NDA—new drug application

Nebulizer—apparatus for producing a fine spray or mist

Negative feedback system—result of a process that reverses or shuts off a stimulus

Nephrotoxic—substance with the potential to damage the kidney

Neuroleptic—medication used to treat psychoses

Neurotransmitter—substance released when the axon terminal of a presynaptic neuron is excited and acts by inhibiting or exciting a target cell

Nevus (nevi)—congenital discoloration of a circumscribed area of the skin resulting from pigmentation; a mole

NIDDM—non–insulin-dependent diabetes mellitus

Nit—egg of a louse or any other parasitic insect

Nodule—a small node or cluster of cells

Normal flora—normally occurring microorganisms on the human body; nonpathogenic with normal immune system

Nosocomial—infection contracted in a health-care facility

NPO—nothing by mouth

NSS—normal saline solution; isotonic solution

Numerator—number on the top of a fraction

## O

$O_2$—oxygen

o.d.—right eye

Ointment—viscous, semisolid vehicle to apply medication to the skin

Ophthalmic—pertaining to the eye

Oral—concerning the mouth; taking medications by mouth

Ordered dose—dose ordered by the prescriber (also known as desired dose)

Organic—containing carbon; composed of animal or vegetable matter

o.s.—left eye

OSHA—Occupational Safety and Health Administration

Osmosis—passage of a solvent through a semipermeable membrane that separates solutions of different concentrations

Osteoarthritis—inflammation of bone and joints

Osteomalacia—softening of bone in (adult form of rickets)

Osteoporosis—loss of bone mass that occurs throughout the skeleton and predisposes patients to fractures

OTC—over-the-counter

Otic—pertaining to the ear

Ototoxicity—having a detrimental effect on the eighth nerve or organs of hearing

o.u.—both eyes

Oxytocin—pituitary hormone that stimulates the uterus to contract and thus induces parturition

oz—abbreviation for ounce

## P

Package insert—information included with the product and written by the manufacturer

Packed cells—red blood cells that have been separated from plasma; used in treating conditions that require red blood cells but not liquid components of whole blood

Palliative—relieving or alleviating without curing

Papules—small lump or pimple, typically larger than a grain of salt but smaller than a peppercorn, that rises above the surface of the neighboring skin

Paranoia—condition in which patients show persistent persecutory delusions or delusional jealousy

Parasympathetic—of or pertaining to the craniosacral division of the autonomic nervous system

Parasympathomimetic—medication that stimulates the parasympathetic nervous system

Parathormone—hormone produced by the parathyroid; increases blood calcium

Parenteral—denoting any medication route other than the alimentary canal, such as intravenous, subcutaneous, intramuscular, or mucosal

Particulate—made up of particles

Passive artificial immunity—immunity obtained when patient is given antibodies from a donor to provide immunity

Passive natural immunity—immunity passed from mother to the newborn that is temporary

Patch—drug delivery system that enhances uptake of a medicine through the skin

Patent medicine—remedy of questionable value that may harm the patient

Pathogenic—disease-causing microorganism

p.c.—after meals, on a full stomach

PCA—patient-controlled analgesia; delivery of pain medication that is controlled by the patient

PDR—Physician's Desk Reference

Pediatric—concerning the treatment of children

Percent—number divided by 100

Peripheral—located at, or pertaining to, the periphery; occurring away from the center

Peristalsis—movement of food and stool through the gastrointestinal tract

Pernicious anemia—chronic, macrocytic anemia; an autoimmune disease marked by a reduction in the mass of circulating red blood cells

Pestle—device for macerating drugs in a mortar

Pharmacodynamics—study of drugs and their actions in living organisms

Pharmacokinetics—study of metabolism and action of drugs with particular emphasis on the time required for absorption, duration of action, distribution in the body, and method of excretion

Pharmacology—study of drugs and their origin, nature, properties, and effects on living organisms

Pharmakon—the study of medicine; also means poison or remedy

Phlebitis—inflammation of the vein

PICC (catheter)—peripherally inserted central catheter; ends in a large vein close to the heart, but is inserted from a peripheral site such as the lower arm

Piggyback—when medication is hung above another intravenous line and delivered before the main line is allowed to drip in

Placebo—inactive substance given to satisfy a patient's demand for medicine; a drug or treatment used as a nonspecific or inactive control in a test of a therapy that is suspected of being useful for a particular disease or condition

Plasma—liquid part of blood or lymph

Plaster—topical preparation in which the constituents are formed into a tenacious mass of substance harder than an ointment and spread on muslin, linen, skin, or paper

Platelet—round or oval disk found in the blood of vertebrates; fragments of megakaryocytes that contribute to forming a clot

Plunger—part of a syringe that pushes the medication out of the syringe

PO—by mouth

Polymerized hemoglobin—hemoglobin that has been chemically changed; when added to solutions, polymerized hemoglobin gives concentrated hemoglobin; used only when other blood products are not available

Polypharmacy—concurrent use of a large number of drugs, a condition that increases the likelihood of unwanted side effects and adverse drug-drug interactions

Porcine—indicates substance is derived from pigs

Port—site of entry into the intravenous system of tubing allowing a health-care professional to insert medication

Potency—power

Potentiate—strengthen

Powder—an aggregation of fine particles of one or more substances that may be passed through fine meshes; a dose of such a powder, contained in a paper

PPD—purified protein derivative; substance used in an intradermal test for tuberculosis

Priming—removing air from an intravenous line by allowing fluid to flow through it

Productive cough—cough producing and expectorating mucus

prn—as needed

Progestin—corpus luteum hormone that prepares the endometrium for implantation of the fertilized ovum; a term used to cover a large group of synthetic drugs that have a progesterone-like effect on the uterus

Prolactin—hormone produced by the anterior pituitary gland; in humans, in association with estrogen and progesterone, stimulates breast development and the formation of milk during pregnancy

Proper—in mathematics, a fraction in which the numerator is smaller than the denominator

Prophylactic—pertaining to prevention

Proportion—in mathematics, a comparison or relationship of numbers

Proprietary name—name given to a medication by the pharmaceutical company that developed it; trade name

Prostaglandins—any of a large group of biologically active, carbon-20, unsaturated fatty acids produced by the metabolism of arachidonic acid through the cyclooxygenase pathway

Protective cap—top devised to maintain sterility or to prevent accidental injury

Psoriasis—chronic skin disorder in which red, scaly plaques with sharply defined borders appear on the body surface

Psychotropic—affecting the mind, emotions, or behaviors

## Q

qd—every day

qid—four times per day

Quotient—answer in a division problem

## R

Random—in research, a method used to assign subjects to experimental groups without introducing bias into a study

Ratio—relation in degree or number between two things

RDA—recommended daily allowance

Receipts—recipes for preparation and administration of a treatment

Reconstitute—return a substance previously altered for preservation or storage to its original state

Reflux—regurgitation of acid up into the esophagus from the stomach

Releasing factor—chemical that triggers the release of hormones

Remainder—in mathematics, the amount left after subtracting two numbers

Replacement—restoration of something depleted or missing

Respiration—interchange of gases ($CO_2$ and $O_2$)

Rheumatoid arthritis—acute and chronic conditions marked by inflammation, muscle soreness and stiffness, and pain in joints and associated structures

Rickets—disease of bone formation in children, most commonly the result of vitamin D deficiency and marked by inadequate mineralization of developing cartilage and newly formed bone; causes abnormalities in the shape, structure, and strength of the skeleton

Rosacea—chronic eruption, usually localized in the middle of the face, in which papules and pustules appear on a flushed or red background

RSV—respiratory syncytial virus

Rx—means take; prescription; therapy

## S

s̄—without

Saline—sodium chloride solution

Salve—ointment; viscous, semisolid vehicle for applying medications to the skin

SC—under the skin, subcutaneous

Schlemm canal—drainage tube in the eye that drains aqueous humor

Scored—marked with a line to facilitate taking a half of a tablet

Seborrhea—disease of the sebaceous glands marked by an increase in the amount; often an alteration of the quality of the fats secreted by the sebaceous glands

Shock—clinical syndrome marked by inadequate perfusion and oxygenation of cells, tissues, and organs; usually a result of marginal or markedly lowered blood pressure

SIADH—syndrome of inappropriate antidiuretic hormone

Side effect—any action or effect other than that intended

Signature—part of the prescription; giving instructions to the patient

Six Rights of medication administration—six rules to follow to administer medication safely

Smoking cessation—stopping smoking

Solution—liquid containing dissolved substances

Somatic—pertaining to the body

Somatotropin—human growth hormone

Spacer—attachment to inhalers that promotes easier hand-holding; saves the medication in a chamber for entry during the next inhalation

Spastic—afflicted with spasms

Spike—in relation to intravenous (IV) therapy, opening an IV bag with a sharp device (spike) to allow fluid to flow out of the bag

ss—half

SSRI—selective serotonin reuptake inhibitor; drug used to treat depression related to low amounts of the neurotransmitter serotonin

Standing orders—orders that a prescriber leaves to administer certain medications automatically, usually in the prescriber's absence

Stat orders—orders to be executed immediately

Status asthmaticus—persistent and intractable asthma

Status epilepticus—continuous seizure activity without a pause

STD—sexually transmitted disease

Stomatitis—inflammation of the mouth including the gums, lips, and tongue

Street name—slang name for a drug; drug name used on the "street"

Subcutaneous—under the skin

Sublingual—under the tongue

Subscription—the part of the prescription that contains directions for compounding ingredients

Substance abuse—misuse or improper use of medications

Subtraction—removing one amount from another

Succinimides—class of antiseizure drugs that delay calcium moving over the neurons

Sum—answer to an addition problem

Superinfection—new infection caused by an organism different from that which caused the initial infection

Superscription—beginning of the prescription, denoted by the symbol $R_x$, meaning take

Suppository—semisolid substance for introduction into the rectum, vagina, or urethra, where it dissolves

Suspension—state of a solid when its particles are mixed with, but not dissolved in, a fluid or another solid

Sympathetic—division of the autonomic nervous system that produces a general rather than a specific effect and prepares the body to cope with stressful circumstances

Sympathomimetic—medication that stimulates the sympathetic nervous system

Synapse—space at the junction of two neurons

Synergism—action of two or more agents or organs working with each other

Synthetic—related to or made by synthesis; artificially prepared

Syrup—concentrated solution of sugar in water to which specific medicinal substances are usually added

Systemic—concerning a system or organized according to a system, pertaining to the whole body rather than one of its parts

# T

t—teaspoon

T—tablespoon

$T_3$—triiodothyronine, a thyroid hormone

$T_4$—thyroxine, a thyroid hormone

Tab.—abbreviation for tablet

Tablet—a small, disklike mass of medicinal powder

Telephone orders—orders received from a prescriber over the telephone

Tension headache—head pain that feels like pressure on the skull

Teratogenic—literally, creating a monster; anything that adversely affects normal cellular development in the embryo or fetus

Therapeutic dose—dose that causes the medication to promote wellness

Therapeutic level—blood value showing amount of medication in the system to be in the range that is desired

Therapeutic range—the range of blood levels from low to high in which the medication will work as desired

Therapeutic touch—the use of hand movements to stimulate circulation and healing

Thrombolytic—substance that breaks apart clots

Thrombus—blood clot that adheres to the wall of a blood vessel or organ

Thrush—candidal (yeast) infection of the mouth where white patches are noted

Thyroid storm—life-threatening situation resulting from untreated hyperthyroidism and characterized by hyperthermia, tachycardia, chest pain, sweating, weakness, heart failure, anxiety, shortness of breath, and disorientation

tid—three times daily

Timed-release—medication that is released over a period of time to allow continuous treatment

Tinnitus—subjective ringing, buzzing, tinkling, or hissing sound in the ear

Tip—part of the syringe where the needle is attached

Titer—level of a specific item in the blood

TNF—tumor necrosis factor

Tocolytic—capable of relieving uterine contraction by reducing the excitability of myometrial muscle

Tolerance—capability to endure a large amount of a substance without an adverse effect and show decreased sensitivity to subsequent doses of the same substance

Tonometer—instrument for measuring tension or pressure

Topical—pertaining to a definite surface area; local

Toxic—pertaining to, resembling, or caused by poison

Toxin—poisonous substance

TPN—total parenteral nutrition; the patient receives nutrition only through this parenteral route; also known as hyperalimentation

Trade name—name given to a drug by the pharmaceutical company that developed it; brand name

Transdermal—method of delivering medicine by placing it in a special gel-like matrix that is applied to the skin

Troche—solid, discoid, or cylindrical mass consisting of chiefly medicinal powder, sugar, and mucilage

TSH—thyroid-stimulating hormone

Tuberculin—solution of purified protein derivative of tuberculosis that is injected intradermally to determine the presence of a tuberculosis infection

## U

Ulcer—lesion of the skin or mucous membranes

Unit—a determined amount; insulin, vitamins, and some antibiotics are usually measured in units

Urticaria—multiple swollen raised areas on the skin that are intensely itchy and last up to 24 hours

USP/NF—the official source of information for drugs approved by the Food and Drug Administration

USP/DI—published by the United States Pharmacopeial Convention, Inc., in Rockville, Maryland; the first of this two-volume set is *Drug Information for Health Providers* and is written primarily for prescribers; the other volume, *Advice for the Patient*, is written in language that is easy for patients to understand, with tips for proper use of drugs and a pronunciation key

USP/NF—United States Pharmacopeia/National Formulary

## V

Vasopressin—causes contraction of smooth muscle, including blood vessels

Vastus lateralis—muscle on the side of the thigh; usual site for injecting medication in infants

Ventrogluteal—site for injecting medication wherein the patient is lying on the side and the gluteus maximus muscle is accessed

Verbal orders—orders given by a prescriber that are not written

Verruca(e)—wart(s)

Vertigo—sensation of moving around in space or having objects move about the person

Vial—small glass or plastic bottle for medicine or chemicals

Viscous—sticky, gummy, gelatinous

Vitamin—accessory, but vital, nutrient that serves as a coenzyme or cofactor in an essential metabolic process

Vitreous humor—thick liquid found in the posterior chamber of the eye

VLDL—very low-density lipoprotein

## W

Wheal—more or less round, temporary elevation of the skin, white in the center with a pale red periphery, accompanied by itching

Whole blood—all blood components, including plasma

Whole numbers—numbers that have no fractional component, except to be placed over 1

Withdrawal—cessation of administration of a drug, especially a narcotic; cessation of ingesting alcohol to which the individual has become either physiologically or psychologically addicted

## Z

Z-track—intramuscular injection route that displaces the skin before entry to decrease skin staining

# Drug Classifications

Drugs are classified according to what they do in the body. They may be used to treat specific illness or symptoms and to diagnose diseases. It is important to understand the general effects of drugs in these classifications. You can then learn about drugs more easily because those in the same class share many of the same purposes and effects.

## A

**Analgesics**—reduce pain. Non-narcotic analgesics are used for mild pain. Narcotic analgesics are used to treat moderate to severe pain.

**Anti-Alzheimer's agents**—work to manage the dementia that occurs with Alzheimer's disease. They attempt to prevent further deterioration of the reasoning and memory. They are not curative.

**Antianemics**—prevent and treat anemias, which are most commonly caused by low iron levels in the blood.

**Antianginals**—treat and prevent angina, or chest pain.

**Antianxiety medications**—used to treat anxiety, such as generalized anxiety disorder (GAD) or post-traumatic stress disorder (PTSD).

**Antiarrhythmics**—suppress cardiac arrhythmias, or irregular heart beats.

**Antiasthmatics**—manage both acute and chronic attacks of bronchospasm or asthma.

**Anticholinergics**—have many uses, including slowing a fast heart rate and relieving spasms of the respiratory system and nasal discharge. They may also be used to treat nausea and vomiting, motion sickness, and dizziness; some decrease gastric secretions and increase esophageal sphincter muscle tone. Finally, anticholinergics can be used for treating eye and urinary tract disorders, as well as neurological disorders.

**Anticoagulants**—prevent blood from clotting. They can cause a prolonged bleeding time (a laboratory test).

**Anticonvulsants**—decrease the incidence and severity of seizures. Sometimes they are used for immediate relief of symptoms (usually given intramuscularly, intravenously, or via endotracheal tube for this purpose). Blood levels may be measured to evaluate the effectiveness of the therapy.

**Antidepressants**—treat depression and elevate mood, usually in conjunction with psychotherapy. They are also used for the following: to treat anxiety, bedwetting, and chronic pain syndromes; for smoking cessation and eating disorders; and for obsessive-compulsive and generalized anxiety disorders.

**Antidiabetics**—manage diabetes mellitus. In some cases, injecting insulin is necessary. In others, tablets can be given to stimulate the body to release its own insulin.

**Antidiarrheals**—control and give symptomatic relief for both acute and chronic diarrhea.

**Antiemetics**—manage nausea, vomiting, and motion sickness.

**Antifungal agents**—treat fungal infections. Usually, they are rubbed on the skin or mucosa. Severe cases may require systemic treatment with an oral or intravenous form.

**Antihistamines**—relieve symptoms associated with allergies, including nose inflammation, itching, and vessel swelling. They are used to treat anaphylaxis.

**Antihypertensives**—decrease blood pressure. They are usually taken orally to reduce chronic hypertension, although some may be given intravenously in an emergency.

**Anti-infectives**—treat bacterial infections. They may be used for a current infection or to prevent infection (prophylaxis). For example, frequently anti-infectives can be given before surgery to prevent infections that could result from opening the patient's body during surgery.

**Anti-inflammatories**—decrease swelling.

**Antineoplastics**—fight new growths caused by cancer. They are also used against autoimmune diseases, such as rheumatoid arthritis.

**Antiparkinsonian agents**—treat Parkinson's disease, a neurological disorder caused by low levels of dopamine, a chemical substance that transmits nerve impulse in the body.

**Antiplatelet agents**—prevent thromboembolic (clots that move) events, such as a stroke (cerebrovascular accident [CVA]) or heart attack. They are frequently used after cardiac surgery and can be combined with anticoagulants and thrombolytic (clot-busting) drugs.

**Antipsychotic drugs**—treat both acute and chronic psychoses, such as schizophrenia. They are also used to suppress tics that originate in the brain, such as in Tourette's syndrome.

**Antipyretics**—lower fevers resulting from infection, inflammation, or cancer.

**Antiretrovirals**—manage human immunodeficiency virus (HIV) infections. They increase the CD4 cell count and decrease the viral load.

**Antirheumatics**—manage symptoms of rheumatoid arthritis (pain and swelling), slow joint destruction, and preserve joint function.

**Antituberculars**—prevent and treat tuberculosis. They are also used to prevent meningitis and influenza.

**Antiulcer agents**—prevent or treat stomach ulcers. They are also used in the management of gastroesophageal reflux disease (GERD).

**Antiviral medications**—manage viral infections, such as herpes, chickenpox, influenza A, and cytomegalovirus (CMV) infection.

## B

**Beta blockers**—help to manage blood pressure, chest pain, fast heart rates, vessel narrowing, migraine headaches, glaucoma, and heart failure. They can also prevent heart attacks and manage symptoms of low thyroid function.

**Bone resorption inhibitors**—primarily used to treat and prevent osteoporosis in postmenopausal women. They are also used to manage high blood calcium and Paget's disease of bone.

**Bronchodilators**—treat reversible airway obstruction resulting from asthma or chronic obstructive pulmonary disease (COPD).

## C

**Calcium channel blockers**—treat high blood pressure, chest pain, and coronary artery spasm. They act to control the rhythm of the heart and to prevent neurological damage.

**Central nervous system stimulants**—treat narcolepsy, attention deficit disorder (ADD), and attention deficit hyperactivity disorder (ADHD).

**Corticosteroids**—correct adrenocortical insufficiency. In large dosages, corticosteroids are used for anti-inflammatory, immunosuppressive, and antineoplastic activity. They can be used to reduce blood calcium and to treat autoimmune diseases. Topically, they are used to decrease inflammation and allergic conditions. Inhaled corticosteroids are used for asthma and vasoconstriction. They are also used for eye disorders.

## D

**Diuretics**—used alone or in combination to reduce high blood pressure and swelling resulting from congestive heart failure (CHF) and other disorders. Potassium-sparing diuretics conserve potassium while decreasing fluid.

## H

**Hormones**—used to treat deficiencies in disorders such as diabetes and thyroid disease.

## I

**Immunosuppressants**—prevent transplant rejection. However, they also suppress the body's own immune system. For this reason, they may be used to treat some autoimmune disorders.

## L

**Laxatives**—treat and prevent constipation. They are also used to cleanse the bowel in preparation for radiological or endoscopic procedures.

**Lipid-lowering agents**—used in conjunction with diet and exercise to lower blood lipid levels in an effort to decrease the morbidity associated with cardiovascular disease.

## M

**Minerals/electrolytes/pH modifiers**—treat deficiencies or excesses of electrolytes to maintain correct acid-base balance.

## N

**Natural/herbal products**—used for a wide variety of disorders. As discussed in the text, the Food and Drug Administration (FDA) does not regulate herbal remedies, so the quality and effectiveness of herbal remedies can vary. Herbs are used extensively to treat menopausal symptoms, improve mood, reduce nausea, prevent motion sickness, boost the immune system, strengthen muscles, and improve gastric and urinary functioning.

**Nonsteroidal anti-inflammatory drugs (NSAIDs)**—control mild to moderate pain, fever, and inflammatory symptoms resulting from conditions such as rheumatoid arthritis and osteoarthritis. Ophthalmic NSAIDs decrease inflammation after eye surgery.

## S

**Sedative-hypnotics**—provide sedation. They are frequently given before procedures or to induce sleep.

**Skeletal muscle relaxants**—reduce spasticity associated with neurological disorders or for symptomatic relief of musculoskeletal conditions.

## T

**Thrombolytic agents**—dissolve clots and prevent heart attacks. As their name suggests, they are "clot-busters."

## V

**Vaccines/immunizing agents**—prevent infectious diseases by promoting the body's own production of antibodies against diseases.

**Vascular headache suppressants**—change vascular tension to decrease pain.

**Vitamins**—prevent and treat vitamin deficiencies. They are also used as supplements in metabolic disorders.

## W

**Weight control agents**—used in the management of obesity. This therapy should be combined with a reduced-calorie diet and exercise.

# Drug Classification Index by Generic Name

| Generic Name | Trade Names | Classification |
|---|---|---|
| acetaminophen | Acephen, Aceta, Aminofen, Apacet, APAP, Aspirin Free Anacin, Aspirin Free Pain Relief, Children's Pain Reliever, Dapacin, FeverAll, Extra Strength Dynafed (Billups, P.J.), Extra Strength Dynafed E.X., Genapap, Genebs, Halenol, Infant's Pain Reliever, Liquiprin, Mapap, Maranox, Meda, Neopap, Oraphen-PD, Panadol, paracetamol, Redutemp, Ridenol, Silapap, Tapanol, Tempra, Tylenol, Uni-Ace | Antipyretics, nonopioid analgesics |
| acyclovir | Zovirax | Antivirals |
| adenosine | Adenocard, Adenoscan | Antiarrhythmics |
| albuterol | Accuneb, ProAir HFA, Proventil HFA, Ventolin HFA, VoSpire ER | Bronchodilators |
| alendronate | Fosamax | Bone resorption inhibitors |
| allopurinol | Alloprim, Lopurin, Zyloprim | Antigout agents, antihyperuricemics |
| alprazolam | Niravam, Xanax, Xanax XR | Antianxiety agents |
| aluminum hydroxide | AlternaGel, Alu-Cap, Aluminet, Alu-Tab, Amphojel, Basalgel, Dialume | Antiulcer agents, hypophosphatemics |
| alteplase | Activase, Cathflo Activase, tissue plasminogen activator | Thrombolytics |
| aminocaproic acid | Amicar, epsilon-aminocaproic acid | Hemostatic agents |
| amiodarone | Cordarone, Nexterone, Pacerone | Antiarrhythmics (class III) |
| amitriptyline | Elavil | Antidepressants |
| amlodipine | Norvasc | Antihypertensives |
| amoxicillin | Amoxil, DisperMox, Moxatag, Trimox, | Anti-infectives, antiulcer agents |
| amoxicillin/clavulanate | Amoclan, Augmentin, Augmentin ES, Augmentin XR | Anti-infectives |
| amphetamine mixtures | Adderall, Adderall XR, Amphetamine Salt | Central nervous system stimulants |
| amphotericin B liposome | AmBisome | Antifungals |
| ampicillin | Marcillin, Omnipen, Penbritin, Polycillin, Principen, Totacillin | Anti-infectives |
| asparaginase | Elspar | Antineoplastics |
| atazanavir | Reyataz | Antiretrovirals |
| atenolol | Tenormin | Antianginals, antihypertensives |
| atorvastatin | Lipitor | Lipid-lowering agents |
| atropine | AtroPen | Antiarrhythmics |
| azacitidine | Vidaza | Antineoplastics |
| azathioprine | Azasan, Imuran | Immunosuppressants |

*Continued*

| Generic Name | Trade Names | Classification |
|---|---|---|
| desmopressin | DDAVP, DDAVP Rhinal Tube, DDAVP Rhinyle Drops, Stimate | Hormones |
| desvenlafaxine | Pristiq | Antidepressants |
| dexlansoprazole | Dexilant | Antiulcer agents |
| dexmedetomidine | Precedex | Sedative-hypnotics |
| dexmethylphenidate | Focalin, Focalin XR | Central nervous system stimulants |
| dextroamphetamine | Dexedrine | Central nervous system stimulants |
| dextromethorphan | Benylin Adult, Benylin Pediatric, Children's Hold, Creo-Terpin, Delsym, DexAlone, Drixoral Liquid Cough Caps, ElixSure Children's Cough Syrup, Hold, Little Colds Cough Formula Drops, Mediquell, PediaCare, Infant's Long Acting Cough Drops, Pertussin Cough Suppressant, Pertussin CS, Pertussin ES, Robitussin Cough Calmers, Robitussin CoughGels, Robitussin Maximum Strength Cough Suppressant, Robitussin Pediatric, Simply Cough, Sucrets Cough Control Formula, Theraflu Thin Strips Long Acting Cough, Triaminic Thin Strips Long Acting Cough, Vicks 44 Cough Relief, Vicks Formula 44 Pediatric Formula | Allergy, cold, and cough remedies, antitussives |
| diazepam | Diastat, Valium | Antianxiety agents, anticonvulsants, sedative-hypnotics, skeletal muscle relaxants (centrally acting) |
| diclofenac sodium | Voltaren, Voltaren XR | Nonopioid analgesics, nonsteroidal anti-inflammatory agents |
| dicyclomine | Bentyl | Antispasmodics |
| digoxin | Lanoxicaps, Lanoxin | Antiarrhythmics, inotropics |
| diltiazem | Cardizem, Cardizem CD, Cardizem LA, Cardizem SR, Cartia XT, Dilacor XR, Diltia XT, Nu-Diltiaz, Tiamate, Taztia XT, Tiazac | Antianginals, antiarrhythmics (class IV), antihypertensives |
| dinoprostone | Cervidil Vaginal Insert, Prepidil Endocervical Gel, Prostin E Vaginal Suppository | Cervical ripening agent |
| diphenhydramine (oral, parenteral) | Allergy Medication, AllerMax, Banophen, Benadryl, Benadryl Allergy, Benadryl Dye-Free Allergy, Compoz, Compoz Nighttime Sleep Aid, Diphen AF, Diphen Cough, Diphenhist, Dormin, Genahist, 40 Winks, Hyrexin-50, Maximum Strength Nytol, Maximum Strength Sleepinal, Midol PM, Miles Nervine, Nighttime Sleep Aid, Nytol, Scot-Tussin Allergy DM, Siladryl, Silphen, Sleep-Eze 3, Sleepwell 2-night, Snooze Fast, Sominex, Tusstat, Twilite, Unisom Nighttime Sleep-Aid | Allergy, cold, and cough remedies; antihistamines; antitussives |
| diphenoxylate-atropine | Logen, Lomate, Lomotil, Lonox | Antidiarrheals |
| dipyridamole | Dipridacot, Persantine, Persantine IV | Antiplatelet agents, diagnostic agents (coronary vasodilators) |
| dobutamine | Dobutrex | Inotropics |
| docetaxel | Taxotere | Antineoplastics |
| docosanol | Abreva | Antivirals |
| docusate sodium | Colace, Correctol Stool Softener Soft Gels, Diocto, Docu, Docusoft S, DOK, DOS Softgels, DOS, DOSS, DSS, Dulcolax Stool Softener, Ex-Lax Stool Softener, Fleet Sof-Lax, Modane Soft, Phillips Liqui-Gels, Regulax-SS, Silace, Soflax, Stool Softener, Therevac SB | Laxatives |
| dofetilide | Tikosyn | Antiarrhythmics |
| dolasetron | Anzemet | Antiemetics |
| donepezil | Aricept, Aricept ODT | Anti-Alzheimer's agents |

| Generic Name | Trade Names | Classification |
|---|---|---|
| dopamine | Intropin | Inotropics, vasopressors |
| doripenem | Doribax | Anti-infectives |
| doxazosin | Cardura, Cardura XL | Antihypertensives |
| doxepin | Sinequan, Zonalon | Antianxiety agents, antidepressants, antihistamines (topical) |
| doxorubicin hydrochloride | Adriamycin PFS, Adriamycin RDF, Rubex | Antineoplastics |
| dronedarone | Multaq | Antiarrhythmics |
| droperidol | Inapsine | Sedative-hypnotics |
| drotrecogin | Xigris | Anti-infectives |
| duloxetine | Cymbalta | Antidepressants |
| dutasteride | Avodart | Benign prostatic hyperplasia (BPH) agents |
| efavirenz | Sustiva | Antiretrovirals |
| eletriptan | Relpax | Vascular headache suppressants |
| emtricitabine | Emtriva | Antiretrovirals |
| enalapril, enalaprilat | Vasotec, Vasotec IV | Antihypertensives |
| enoxaparin | Lovenox | Anticoagulants |
| entacapone | Comtan | Antiparkinsonian agents |
| entecavir | Baraclude | Antivirals |
| epinephrine | Adrenalin, Ana-Guard, AsthmaHaler Mist, AsthmaNefrin (racepinephrine), EpiPen, micro-Nefrin, Nephron, Primatene, S-2, Sus-Phrine | Antiasthmatics, bronchodilators, vasopressors |
| epirubicin | Ellence | Antineoplastics |
| eplerenone | Inspra | Antihypertensives |
| epoetin | EPO, Epogen, erythropoietin, Procrit | Antianemics |
| eprosartan | Teveten | Antihypertensives |
| eptifibatide | Integrilin | Antiplatelet agents |
| ergotamine | Ergomar | Vascular headache suppressants |
| erlotinib | Tarceva | Antineoplastics |
| ertapenem | Invanz | Anti-infectives |
| erythromycin base | E-Mycin, Eryc, Ery-Tab | Anti-infectives |
| erythromycin (topical) | Akne-Mycin, Erygel | Anti-infectives |
| escitalopram | Lexapro | Antidepressants |
| esmolol | Brevibloc | Antiarrhythmics (class II) |
| esomeprazole | Nexium | Antiulcer agents |
| eszopiclone | Lunesta | Sedative-hypnotics |
| etanercept | Enbrel | Antirheumatics |
| ethambutol | Myambutol | Antituberculars |
| etidronate | Didronel | Bone resorption inhibitors |
| etodolac | Lodine, Lodine XL | Antirheumatics, nonopioid analgesics |
| etoposide | VePesid, VP-16 | Antineoplastics |
| etravirine | Intelence | Antiretrovirals |
| exenatide | Byetta | Antidiabetics |
| ezetimibe | Zetia | Lipid-lowering agents |
| famciclovir | Famvir | Antivirals |
| famotidine | Pepcid, Pepcid AC | Antiulcer agents |
| febuxostat | Uloric | Antigout agents |
| fenofibrate | Antara, Fenoglide, Lipofen, Lofibra, Tricor, Triglide | Lipid-lowering agents |
| fenofibric acid | Trilipix | Lipid-lowering agents |
| fenoldopam | Corlopam | Antihypertensives |
| fentanyl (parenteral) | Sublimaze | Opioid analgesics |
| fentanyl (transdermal) | Duragesic | Opioid analgesics, analgesic adjuncts |
| ferumoxytol | Feraheme | Antianemics |
| fesoterodine | Toviaz | Urinary tract antispasmodics |
| fexofenadine | Allegra | Allergy, cold, and cough remedies; antihistamines |

*Continued*

| Generic Name | Trade Names | Classification |
|---|---|---|
| filgrastim | G-CSF, granulocyte colony-stimulating factor, Neupogen | Colony-stimulating factors |
| finasteride | Propecia, Proscar | Hair regrowth stimulants |
| flecainide | Tambocor | Antiarrhythmics |
| fluconazole | Diflucan | Antifungals (systemic) |
| fludarabine | Fludara, Oforta | Antineoplastics |
| flumazenil | Romazicon | Antidotes (for sedative-hypnotics) |
| flunisolide | AeroBid, AeroBid-M, Aerospan | Antiasthmatics, anti-inflammatories (steroidal) |
| fluorouracil | Carac, Efudex, Fluoroplex, 5-FU | Antineoplastics |
| fluoxetine | Prozac, Prozac Weekly, Sarafem | Antidepressants |
| fluphenazine | Prolixin, Prolixin Decanoate | Antipsychotics |
| flurazepam | Dalmane | Sedative-hypnotics |
| fluticasone (inhaled) | Flovent Diskus, Flovent HFA | Antiasthmatics, anti-inflammatories (steroidal) |
| fluticasone (nasal) | Flonase, Veramyst | Anti-inflammatories (steroidal) |
| fluvastatin | Lescol, Lescol XL | Lipid-lowering agents |
| folic acid | folate, Folvite, vitamin B | Antianemics, vitamins |
| fondaparinux | Arixtra | Anticoagulants |
| formoterol | Foradil, Perforomist | Bronchodilators |
| fosamprenavir | Lexiva | Antiretrovirals |
| foscarnet | None listed | Antivirals |
| fosinopril | Monopril | Antihypertensives |
| fosphenytoin | Cerebyx | Anticonvulsants |
| frovatriptan | Frova | Vascular headache suppressants |
| furosemide | Lasix | Diuretics |
| gabapentin | Neurontin | Analgesic adjuncts, therapeutic; anticonvulsants; mood stabilizers |
| galantamine | Razadyne, Razadyne ER | Anti-Alzheimer's agents |
| ganciclovir | Cytovene, Vitrasert | Antivirals |
| gatifloxacin | Zymar | Anti-infectives |
| gefitinib | Iressa | Antineoplastics |
| gemcitabine | Gemzar | Antineoplastics |
| gemfibrozil | Lopid | Lipid-lowering agents |
| gemifloxacin | Factive | Anti-infectives |
| gemtuzumab ozogamicin | Mylotarg | Antineoplastics |
| gentamicin | Garamycin, G-Mycin, Jenamicin | Anti-infectives |
| glimepiride | Amaryl | Antidiabetics |
| glipizide | Glucotrol, Glucotrol XL | Antidiabetics |
| glucagon | GlucaGen | Hormones |
| glyburide | DiaBeta, Glynase PresTab | Antidiabetics |
| glycopyrrolate | Robinul, Robinul-Forte | Antispasmodics |
| golimumab | Simponi | Antirheumatics |
| goserelin | Zoladex | Antineoplastics, hormones |
| granisetron | Kytril | Antiemetics |
| guaifenesin | Alfen Jr, Altarussin, Breonesin, Diabetic Tussin, Ganidin NR, Guiatuss, Hytuss, Hytuss-2X, Mucinex, Naldecon Senior EX, Organidin NR, Robitussin, Scot-tussin Expectorant, Siltussin DAS, Siltussin SA | Allergy, cold, and cough remedies; expectorants |
| haloperidol | Haldol, Haldol Decanoate | Antipsychotics |
| heparin | Hep-Lock, Hep-Lock U/P | Anticoagulants |
| human papillomavirus quadrivalent (types 6, 11, 16, and 18) | Gardasil | Vaccines/immunizing agents |
| hydralazine | Apresoline | Antihypertensives |
| hydrocodone | Hycodan, Tussigon (U.S. antitussive formulations contain homatropine) | Allergy, cold, and cough remedies (antitussive); nonopioid analgesics; opioid analgesics |

| Generic Name | Trade Names | Classification |
|---|---|---|
| hydromorphone | Dilaudid, Dilaudid-HP, Hydrostat IR, PMS Hydromorphone | Allergy, cold, and cough remedies (antitussives); opioid analgesics |
| hydroxychloroquine | Plaquenil | Antimalarials, antirheumatics (DMARDs) |
| hydroxyzine | Atarax, Hyzine-50, Vistaril | Antianxiety agents, antihistamines, sedative-hypnotics |
| hyoscyamine | Anaspaz, A-Spas S/L, Cystospaz, Cystospaz-M, Donnamar, ED-SPAZ, Gastrosed, Levbid, Levsin, Levsinex, L-hyoscyamine, NuLev | Antispasmodics |
| ibandronate | Boniva | Bone resorption inhibitors |
| ibuprofen, oral | Advil, Advil Migraine Liqui-Gels, Children's Advil, Children's Motrin, Excedrin IB, Genpril, Haltran, Junior Strength Advil, Medipren, Menadol, Midol Maximum Strength Cramp Formula, Motrin, Motrin Drops, Motrin IB, Motrin Junior Strength, Motrin Migraine Pain, Nu-Ibuprofen, Nuprin, PediaCare Children's Fever | Antipyretics, antirheumatics, nonopioid analgesics, nonsteroidal anti-inflammatory agents |
| ibutilide | Corvert | Antiarrhythmics (class III) |
| idarubicin | Idamycin | Antineoplastics |
| ifosfamide | Ifex | Antineoplastics |
| iloperidone | Fanapt | Antipsychotics |
| imatinib | Gleevec | Antineoplastics |
| imipenem/cilastatin | Primaxin | Anti-infectives |
| imipramine | Norfranil, Tipramine, Tofranil, Tofranil PM | Antidepressants |
| imiquimod | Aldara | Antivirals, immune modifiers |
| indomethacin | Indocin, Indocin I.V., Indocin SR | Antirheumatics, ductus arteriosus patency adjuncts (IV only), nonsteroidal anti-inflammatory agents |
| infliximab | Remicade | Antirheumatics (DMARDs), gastrointestinal anti-inflammatories |
| insulin, regular (injection, concentrated) | Humulin R, Humulin R Regular U-500 (Concentrated), Novolin R | Antidiabetics, hormones |
| ipratropium | Atrovent, Atrovent HFA | Allergy, cold, and cough remedies; bronchodilators |
| irbesartan | Avapro | Antihypertensives |
| irinotecan | Camptosar | Antineoplastics |
| isoniazid | INH | Antituberculars |
| isosorbide | Dilatrate-SR, Isordil | Antianginals |
| isotretinoin | Amnesteem, Claravis, Sotret | Antiacne agents |
| isradipine | DynaCirc, DynaCirc CR | Antianginals |
| itraconazole | Sporanox | Antifungals (systemic) |
| ixabepilone | Ixempra | Antineoplastics |
| ketoconazole (systemic) | Nizoral | Antifungals (systemic) |
| ketorolac | Toradol | Nonsteroidal anti-inflammatory agents, nonopioid analgesics |
| labetalol | Trandate | Antianginals, antihypertensives |
| lactulose | Cholac, Constilac, Constulose, Enulose, Generlac, Kristalose | Laxatives |
| lamivudine | Epivir, Epivir-HBV, 3TC | Antiretrovirals, antivirals |
| lamotrigine | Lamictal | Anticonvulsants |
| lansoprazole | Prevacid, Prevacid 24 HR | Antiulcer agents |
| lapatinib | Tykerb | Antineoplastics |
| leflunomide | Arava | Antirheumatics |
| lepirudin (rDNA) | Refludan | Anticoagulants |
| letrozole | Femara | Antineoplastics |
| leucovorin | Folinic acid | Antidotes (for methotrexate), vitamins |
| leuprolide | Eligard, Lupron, Lupron Depot, Lupron Depot-Ped, Lupron Depot-3 Month, Lupron Depot-4 Month | Antineoplastics |

*Continued*

| Generic Name | Trade Names | Classification |
|---|---|---|
| nisoldipine | Sular | Antihypertensives |
| nitrofurantoin | Furadantin, Macrobid, Macrodantin | Anti-infectives |
| nitroglycerin | Capsules: Nitro-Time<br>IV: Nitro-Bid IV, Tridil<br>Translingual spray: Nitrolingual, NitroMist<br>Ointment: Nitro-Bid<br>Sublingual: Nitrostat, NitroQuick<br>Transdermal: Minitran, Nitrek, Nitro-Dur | Antianginals |
| nitroprusside | Nitropress | Antihypertensives |
| nizatidine | Axid, Axid AR | Antiulcer agents |
| norfloxacin | Noroxin | Anti-infectives |
| norepinephrine | Levophed | Vasopressors |
| nortriptyline | Aventyl, Pamelor | Antidepressants |
| NPH insulin (isophane insulin suspension) | Humulin N, Novolin N, NPH Iletin II | Antidiabetics, hormones |
| nystatin | Mycostatin, Nilstat | Antifungals (topical/local) |
| octreotide | Sandostatin, Sandostatin LAR | Antidiarrheals, hormones |
| ofloxacin | Floxin | Anti-infectives |
| olanzapine | Zyprexa, Zyprexa Zydis | Antipsychotics, mood stabilizers |
| olmesartan | Benicar | Antihypertensives |
| olopatadine (nasal spray) | Patanase | Allergy, cold, and cough remedies |
| olsalazine | Dipentum | Gastrointestinal anti-inflammatories |
| omalizumab | Xolair | Antiasthmatics |
| omega-3 acid ethyl esters | Lovaza | Lipid-lowering agents |
| omeprazole | Prilosec, Prilosec OTC | Antiulcer agents |
| ondansetron | Zofran, Zofran ODT | Antiemetics |
| oprelvekin | Neumega | Colony-stimulating factors |
| orlistat | Alli, Xenical | Weight control agents |
| oxaliplatin | Eloxatin | Antineoplastics |
| oxaprozin | Daypro | Antirheumatics, nonsteroidal anti-inflammatory agents |
| oxazepam | Serax | Antianxiety agents, sedative-hypnotics |
| oxcarbazepine | Trileptal | Anticonvulsants |
| oxybutynin (oral) | Ditropan, Ditropan XL | Urinary tract antispasmodics |
| oxybutynin (transdermal) | Oxytrol | Urinary tract antispasmodics |
| oxycodone | Endocodone, M-Oxy, OxyContin, Oxy-FAST, OxyIR, Percolone, Roxicodone | Opioid analgesics |
| oxymorphone | Opana, Opana ER | Opioid analgesics |
| oxytocin | Pitocin | Hormones |
| paclitaxel | Onxol, Taxol | Antineoplastics |
| palifermin | Kepivance | Cytoprotective agents |
| palonosetron | Aloxi | Antiemetics |
| pamidronate | Aredia | Bone resorption inhibitors |
| pancrelipase | Creon, Enzymase-16, Pancrease MT 4, Pancrease MT 10, Pancrease MT 16, Pancrease MT 20, Pancrecarb MS08, Ultrase MT 12, Ultrase MT 20, Viokase, Zenpep | Digestive agent |
| pancuronium | None listed | Neuromuscular blocking agents |
| panitumumab | Vectibix | Antineoplastics |
| pantoprazole | Protonix, Protonix IV | Antiulcer agents |
| paroxetine hydrochloride | Paxil, Paxil CR | Antianxiety agents, antidepressants |
| pazopanib | Votrient | Antineoplastics |
| pegaspargase | Oncaspar, PEG-L-asparaginase | Antineoplastics |
| pegfilgrastim | Neulasta | Colony-stimulating factors |
| pemetrexed | Alimta | Antineoplastics |
| penciclovir | Denavir | Antivirals |

| Generic Name | Trade Names | Classification |
|---|---|---|
| penicillin G | Pfizerpen | Anti-infectives |
| pentamidine | NebuPent, Pentam 300 | Antiprotozoals |
| pentazocine | Talvin, Talwin NX | Opioid analgesics |
| perindopril | Aceon | Antihypertensives |
| permethrin | Acticin, Elimite, Nix | Pediculicides |
| phenazopyridine | Azo-Standard, Baridium, Prodium, Pyridium, Pyridium Plus, UTI Relief | Nonopioid analgesics |
| phenobarbital | Luminal, Solfoton | Anticonvulsants, sedative-hypnotics |
| phentermine | Adipex-P, Banobese, Fastin, Ionamin, Obi-Nix, OBY-CAP, Phentercot, Phentride, T-Diet, Teramine, Zantryl | Weight control agents |
| phentolamine | Oraverse, Regitine | Agents for pheochromocytoma |
| phenytoin | Dilantin, Phenytek | Antiarrhythmics, anticonvulsants |
| phosphate-biphosphate | Fleet Enema, OsmoPrep, Visicol | Laxatives |
| phytonadione | Mephyton, vitamin K | Antidotes, vitamins |
| pimecrolimus | Elidel | Immunosuppressants (topical) |
| pioglitazone | Actos | Antidiabetics (oral) |
| piperacillin-tazobactam | Zosyn | Anti-infectives |
| piroxicam | Feldene | Antirheumatics, nonsteroidal anti-inflammatory agents |
| polyethylene glycol | GlycoLax, MiraLax | Laxatives |
| polyethylene glycol-electrolyte | Colyte, GoLYTELY, MoviPrep, NuLYTELY, TriLyte | Laxatives |
| posaconazole | Noxafil | Antifungals |
| potassium chloride | Cena-K, Gen-K, K+ Care, K+ 10, Kaochlor, Kaochlor S-0F, Kaon-Cl, Kay Ciel, KCL, K-Dur, K-Lease, K-Lor, Klor-Con, Klorvess Liquid, Klotrix, K-Lyte/Cl Powder, K-Med, K-Norm, K-Sol, K-Tab, Micro-K, Micro-K Extencaps, Micro-LS, Potasalan, Roychlor, Rum-K, Slow-K, Ten-K | Mineral and electrolyte replacements/supplements |
| pramipexole | Mirapex | Antiparkinsonian agents |
| pramlintide | Symlin | Antidiabetics |
| prasugrel | Effient | Antiplatelet agents |
| pravastatin | Pravachol | Lipid-lowering agents |
| prazosin | Minipress | Antihypertensives |
| prednisolone | Orapred, Orapred ODT, Pediapred, Prelone | Antiasthmatics, corticosteroids |
| prednisone | Sterapred | Antiasthmatics, corticosteroids |
| pregabalin | Lyrica | Analgesics, anticonvulsants |
| procainamide | None listed | Antiarrhythmics (class IA) |
| procarbazine | Matulane | Antineoplastics |
| prochlorperazine | Compo | Antiemetics, antipsychotics |
| progesterone | Crinone, Endometrin, Prochieve, Prometrium | Hormones |
| promethazine | Promethacon | Antiemetics, antihistamines, sedative-hypnotics |
| propafenone | Rythmol, Rythmol SR | Antiarrhythmics (class IC) |
| propofol | Diprivan | General anesthetics |
| propoxyphene napsylate | Darvon N | Opioid analgesics |
| propranolol | Inderal, Inderal LA, InnoPran XL | Antianginals, antiarrhythmics (Class II), antihypertensives, vascular headache suppressants |
| propylthiouracil | PTU | Antithyroid agents |
| protamine sulfate | None given | Antidotes (heparin) |
| pseudoephedrine | Cenafed, Congestaid, Decofed, Dimetapp Maximum Strength 12-Hour Non-Drowsy Extentabs, Dimetapp Decongestant Pediatric, Drixoral 12 Hour Non-Drowsy Formula, Efidac 24, Genafed, Halofed, Kid Kare, Medi-First Sinus | Allergy, cold, and cough remedies; nasal drying agents/decongestants |

*Continued*

| Generic Name | Trade Names | Classification |
|---|---|---|
| | Decongestant, PediaCare Infants' Decongestant Drops, Pediatric Nasal Decongestant, Simply Stuff, Sinustop, Silfedrine, Sudafed, Sudafed Children's Non-Drowsy Maximum Strength, Sudodrin, Triaminic Allergy Congestion Softchews, Unifed | |
| psyllium | Alramucil, Cillium, Effer-Syllium, Fiberall, Fibrepur, Hydrocil, Konsyl, Metamucil, Modane Bulk, Mylanta Natural Fiber Supplement, Naturacil Caramels, Perdiem, Pro-Lax, Reguloid Natural, Serutan, Siblin, Syllact, Vitalax, V-Lax | Laxatives |
| pyridostigmine | Mestinon, Mestinon Timespan, Regonol | Antimyasthenics |
| pyridoxine | Beesix, Doxine, Nestrex, Pyri, Rodex, Vitabee 6, vitamin B$_6$ | Vitamins |
| pyrimethamine | Daraprim | Antimalarials, antiprotozoals |
| quetiapine | Seroquel | Antipsychotics, mood stabilizers |
| quinapril | Accupril | Antihypertensives |
| quinine | Qualaquin | Antimalarials |
| rabeprazole | Aciphex | Antiulcer agents |
| raloxifene | Evista | Bone resorption inhibitors |
| raltegravir | Isentress | Antiretrovirals |
| ramelteon | Rozerem | Sedatives-hypnotics |
| ramipril | Altace | Antihypertensives |
| ranitidine | Zantac, Zantac EFFERdose, Zantac 75, Zantac 150 | Antiulcer agents |
| ranolazine | Ranexa | Antianginals |
| rasagiline | Azilect | Antiparkinsonian agents |
| rasburicase | Elitek | Antigout agents, antihyperuricemics |
| repaglinide | Prandin | Antidiabetics |
| reteplase | Retavase | Thrombolytics |
| ribavirin | Copegus, Rebetol, Virazole | Antivirals |
| rifabutin | Mycobutin | Agents for atypical mycobacterium |
| rifampin | Rifadin, Rimactane | Antituberculars |
| rifaximin | Xifaxan | Anti-infectives |
| risedronate | Actonel | Bone resorption inhibitors |
| risperidone | Risperdal, Risperdal Consta, Risperdal M-TAB | Antipsychotics, mood stabilizers |
| ritonavir | Norvir | Antiretrovirals |
| rituximab | Rituxan | Antineoplastics |
| rivastigmine | Exelon | Anti-Alzheimer's agents |
| rizatriptan | Maxalt, Maxalt-MLT | Vascular headache suppressants |
| ropinirole | Requip, Requip XL | Antiparkinsonian agents |
| rosiglitazone | Avandia | Antidiabetics |
| salmeterol | Serevent Diskus | Bronchodilators |
| sargramostim | Leukine, rHu GM-CSF (recombinant human granulocyte-macrophage colony-stimulating factor) | Colony-stimulating factors |
| saxagliptin | Onglyza | Antidiabetics |
| scopolamine | Scopace, Transderm-Scop | Antiemetics |
| selegiline | Apo-Selegiline, Carbex, Eldepryl, Gen-Selegiline, Nu-Selegiline | Antiparkinsonian agents |
| selegiline transdermal | Emsam | Antidepressants |
| sennosides | Black-Draught, Ex-Lax, Ex-Lax Chocolated, Fletchers' Castoria, Maximum Relief Ex-Lax, Senna-Gen, Senexon, Senokot, SenokotXTRA | Laxatives |
| sertaconazole | Ertaczo | Antifungals |
| sertraline | Zoloft | Antidepressants |
| sevelamer | Renagel, Renvela | Electrolyte modifiers |
| sibutramine | Meridia | Weight control agents |
| sildenafil | Revatio, Viagra | Erectile dysfunction agents |
| silodosin | Rapaflo | Benign prostatic hyperplasia (BPH) agents |

| Generic Name | Trade Names | Classification |
|---|---|---|
| simethicone | Degas, Extra Strength Gas-X, Flatulex, Gas-X, Genasyme, Maximum Strength Mylanta Gas, Mylanta Gas, Mylicon, Phazyme | Antiflatulents |
| simvastatin | Zocor | Lipid-lowering agents |
| sirolimus | Rapamune | Immunosuppressants |
| sitagliptin | Januvia | Antidiabetics |
| sodium bicarbonate | Baking soda, Bell-Ans, Citrocarbonate, Neut, Soda Mint | Antiulcer agents |
| sodium chloride (IV, oral) | Slo-Salt | Mineral and electrolyte replacements/ supplements |
| sodium citrate and citric acid | Bicitra, Oracit, Shohl's Solution modified | Antiurolithics, mineral and electrolyte replacements/ supplements |
| sodium polystyrene sulfonate | Kalexate, Kayexalate, Kionex, SPS | Hypokalemic, electrolyte modifiers |
| solifenacin | Vesicare | Urinary tract antispasmodics |
| sotalol | Betapace, Betapace AF, Sorine | Antiarrhythmics (classes II and III) |
| spironolactone | Aldactone | Diuretic |
| stavudine | d4T, Zerit, Zerit XR | Antiretrovirals |
| streptokinase | Streptase | Thrombolytics |
| streptomycin | None listed | Anti-infectives |
| sucralfate | Carafate | Antiulcer agents |
| sulfasalazine | Azulfidine, Azulfidine EN-tabs | Antirheumatics (DMARDs), gastrointestinal anti-inflammatories |
| sulindac | Clinoril | Antirheumatics, nonsteroidal anti-inflammatory agents |
| sumatriptan | Imitrex, Imitrex STATdose, Sumavel DosePro | Vascular headache suppressants |
| sunitinib | Sutent | Antineoplastics |
| tacrine | Cognex | Anti-Alzheimer's agents |
| tadalafil | Adcirca, Cialis | Erectile dysfunction agents, vasodilators |
| tamoxifen | None listed | Antineoplastics |
| tamsulosin | Flomax | None assigned |
| tapentadol | Nucynta | Analgesic (centrally acting), opioid analgesics |
| telmisartan | Micardis | Antihypertensives |
| temazepam | Restoril | Sedative-hypnotics |
| tenecteplase | TNKase | Thrombolytics |
| tenofovir | Viread | Antiretrovirals |
| terazosin | Hytrin | Antihypertensives |
| terbinafine | Lamisil | Antifungals (systemic) |
| terbutaline | None listed | Bronchodilators |
| teriparatide | Forteo | Hormones |
| tetracycline | Sumycin | Anti-infectives |
| thalidomide | Thalomid | Immunosuppressants |
| theophylline | Quibron-T, Theochron, Theo-24, Uniphyl | Bronchodilators |
| thiamine | Biamine, vitamin $B_1$ | Vitamins |
| thioridazine | None listed | Antipsychotics |
| thyroid | Armour thyroid, Westhroid | Hormones |
| tiagabine | Gabitril | Anticonvulsants |
| ticarcillin-clavulanate | Timentin | Anti-infectives |
| ticlopidine | None listed | Antiplatelet agents |
| tigecycline | Tygacil | Anti-infectives |
| timolol | None listed | Antihypertensives, vascular headache suppressants |
| tinidazole | Tindamax | Antiprotozoals |
| tiotropium | Spiriva | Bronchodilators |
| tirofiban | Aggrastat | Antiplatelet agents |
| tizanidine | Zanaflex | Antispasticity agents (centrally acting) |

*Continued*

| Generic Name | Trade Names | Classification |
|---|---|---|
| tolcapone | Tasmar | Antiparkinsonian agents |
| tolterodine | Detrol, Detrol LA | Urinary tract antispasmodics |
| tolvaptan | Samsca | Electrolyte modifiers |
| topiramate | Topamax | Anticonvulsants, mood stabilizers |
| topotecan | Hycamtin | Antineoplastics |
| torsemide | Demadex | Antihypertensives |
| tramadol | Ultram, Ultram ER | Analgesics (centrally acting) |
| trandolapril | Mavik | Antihypertensives |
| tranylcypromine | Parnate | Antidepressants |
| trastuzumab | Herceptin | Antineoplastics |
| trazodone | None listed | Antidepressants |
| triazolam | Halcion | Sedative-hypnotics |
| trimethoprim-sulfamethoxazole | Bactrim, Bactrim DS, Septra, Septra DS, SMZ/TMP, Sulfatrim, TMP/SMX, TMP/SMZ | Anti-infectives, antiprotozoals |
| trospium | Sanctura, Sanctura XR | Urinary tract antispasmodics |
| valacyclovir | Valtrex | Antivirals |
| valganciclovir | Valcyte | Antivirals |
| valproate sodium | Depacon | Anticonvulsants, vascular headache suppressants |
| valproic acid | Depakene, Stavzor | Anticonvulsants, vascular headache suppressants |
| valsartan | Diovan | Antihypertensives |
| vancomycin | Vancocin | Anti-infectives |
| vardenafil | Levitra | Erectile dysfunction agents |
| varenicline | Chantix | Smoking deterrents |
| vasopressin | Pressyn | Hormones |
| venlafaxine | Effexor, Effexor XR | Antidepressants, antianxiety agents |
| verapamil | Calan, Calan SR, Covera-HS, Isoptin, Verelan, Verelan PM | Antianginals, antiarrhythmics (class IV), antihypertensives, vascular headache suppressants |
| vinblastine | None listed | Antineoplastics |
| vincristine | Vincasar PFS | Antineoplastics |
| vinorelbine | Navelbine | Antineoplastics |
| vitamin E | alpha-tocopherol, Amino-Opti-E, Aquasol E, E-200, E-400, #-1000, E-Complex-600, E-Vitamin, Liqui-E, Pheryl-E, Vita Plus E | Vitamins |
| voriconazole | VFEND | Antifungals |
| warfarin | Coumadin, Jantoven | Anticoagulants |
| zafirlukast | Accolate | Antiasthmatics, bronchodilators |
| zaleplon | Sonata | Sedative-hypnotics |
| zanamivir | Relenza | Antivirals |
| ziconotide | Prialt | Analgesics |
| zidovudine | azidothymidine, AZT, Retrovir | Antiretrovirals |
| zinc sulfate | Orazinc, Verazinc, Zinc 220, Zincate, Zinkaps | Mineral and electrolyte replacements/supplements |
| ziprasidone | Geodon | Antipsychotics, mood stabilizers |
| zoledronic acid | Reclast, Zometa | Bone resorption inhibitors, electrolyte modifiers, hypocalcemics |
| zolmitriptan | Zomig, Zomig-ZMT | Vascular headache suppressants |
| zolpidem | Ambien, Ambien CR, Edluar, Zolpimist | Sedative-hypnotics |
| zonisamide | Zonegran | Anticonvulsants |

DMARD, disease-modifying antirheumatic drug

# Pregnancy Drug Categories and Controlled Substances Schedules

## ■ PREGNANCY DRUG CATEGORIES

### Category A
Adequate, well-controlled studies in pregnant women have not shown an increased risk of fetal abnormalities.

### Category B
Animal studies have revealed no evidence of harm to the fetus; however, there are no adequate and well-controlled studies in pregnant women; **or** animal studies have shown an adverse effect, but adequate and well-controlled studies in pregnant women have failed to demonstrate a risk to the fetus.

### Category C
Animal studies have shown an adverse effect, and there are no adequate and well-controlled studies in pregnant women; **or** no animal studies have been conducted, and there are no adequate and well-controlled studies in pregnant women.

### Category D
Studies—adequate and well-controlled or observational—in pregnant women have demonstrated a risk to the fetus. However, the benefits of therapy may outweigh the potential risk.

### Category X
Studies—adequate and well-controlled or observational—in animals or pregnant women have demonstrated positive evidence of fetal abnormalities. Use of the product is contraindicated in women who are or may become pregnant.

## ■ CONTROLLED SUBSTANCES SCHEDULES

Classes or schedules are determined by the Drug Enforcement Agency (DEA), an arm of the United States Department of Justice, and are based on the potential for abuse and dependence liability (physical and psychological) of the medication. Some states have stricter prescription regulations. Physicians, dentists, podiatrists, and veterinarians may prescribe controlled substances. Nurse practitioners and physician's assistants may prescribe controlled substances with certain limitations.

### Schedule I (C-I)
The potential for abuse is so high as to be unacceptable. These substances may be used for research with appropriate limitations, but otherwise have no acceptable medical use. Examples are LSD and heroin.

### Schedule II (C-II)

These substances have high potential for abuse and extreme liability for physical and psychological dependence (amphetamines, opioid analgesics, dronabinol, certain barbiturates). Outpatient prescriptions must be in writing. In emergencies, telephone orders may be acceptable if a written prescription is provided within 72 hours. No refills are allowed.

The following are examples of Schedule II drugs included in *Davis's Drug Guide for Nurses:*

- Amphetamine
- Codeine (single entity; solid dosage form or injectable)
- Fentanyl
- Hydromorphone
- Methylphenidate
- Morphine

### Schedule III (C-III)

These substances have intermediate potential for abuse (less than C-II) and intermediate liability for physical and psychological dependence (certain nonbarbiturate sedatives, certain nonamphetamine central nervous system stimulants, limited dosages of certain opioid analgesics). Outpatient prescriptions can be refilled five times within 6 months from the date of issue if authorized by the prescriber. Telephone orders are acceptable.

The following are examples of Schedule III drugs included in *Davis's Drug Guide for Nurses:*

- Codeine (in combination with nonopioid analgesics: solid oral dosage forms)
- Hydrocodone (in combination with nonopioid analgesics)
- Nandrolone decanoate

### Schedule IV (C-IV)

These substances have less abuse potential than Schedule III, with minimal liability for physical or psychological dependence (certain sedative-hypnotics, certain antianxiety agents, some barbiturates, benzodiazepines, chloral hydrate, pentazocaine, propoxyphen). Outpatient prescriptions can be refilled six times within 6 months from the date of issue if authorized by the prescriber. Telephone orders are acceptable.

The following Schedule IV drugs are included in *Davis's Drug Guide for Nurses:*

- Alprazolam
- Codeine (elixir or oral suspension with acetaminophen)
- Diazepam
- Pentazocaine
- Phenobarbital
- Zolpidem

### Schedule V (C-V)

These substances have minimal abuse potential. The number of outpatient refills is determined by the prescriber. Some products (cough suppressants with small amounts of codeine, antidiarrheals containing paregoric) may be available without a prescription to patients more than18 years of age.

The following Schedule IV drugs are included in *Davis's Drug Guide for Nurses:*

- Buprenorphine
- Diphenoxylate/atropine

# Routine Pediatric and Adult Immunizations

Immunization recommendations change frequently: For the latest recommendations, see www.cdc.gov.

## Routine Pediatric Immunizations (0–18 Years)

| Generic Name (Brand Names) | Route and Dosage | Contraindications and Precautions | Adverse Reactions and Side Effects | Notes |
|---|---|---|---|---|
| Hepatitis B vaccine (HepB, Engerix-B, Recombivax HB) | 0.5 mL IM at 0, 1–2, and 6–18 mo; dose is same for patients age 0–19 yr. *Infants born to HBsAg-positive mothers:* Administer 0.5 mL hepatitis B immune globulin IM and first dose of hepatitis B vaccine; give second and third doses of hepatitis B vaccine at 1 mo and 6 mo, respectively. | Hypersensitivity to yeast | Local soreness | A two-dose series (separated by ≥4 mo) of the adult formulation (Recombivax HB) can be used in children 11–15 yr |
| Rotavirus vaccine (RV, Rotarix [RV1], RotaTeq [RV5]) | *Rotarix:* 1 mL PO at 2 and 4 mo. *RotaTeq:* 2 mL PO at 2, 4, and 6 mo; first dose of either product may be given as early as age 6 wk; final dose should be given no later than age 8 mo. | History of uncorrected congenital malformation of the GI tract (Rotarix) | Fever, irritability, diarrhea, vomiting | Series should not be started in infants older than 15 wk |
| Diphtheria toxoid, tetanus toxoid, and acellular pertussis vaccine (DTaP, Daptacel, Infanrix, Tripedia) | 0.5 mL IM at 2, 4, 6, 15–18 mo and 4–6 yr (first dose may be given as early as age 6 wk; fourth dose may be given at 12 mo). | Acute infection, previous CNS damage, convulsions | Redness, tenderness, induration at site; fever; malaise; myalgia; urticaria; hypotension; neurological reactions; allergic reactions all less than with DTwP) | Individual components may be given as separate injections if unusual reactions occur |
| *Haemophilus* b conjugate vaccine (Hib, PedvaxHIB, ActHIB, Hiberix) | *ActHIB:* 0.5 mL IM at 2, 4, 6 mo, with a booster dose at 12–15 mo. *Hiberix:* can be used only for the booster dose (any of the products can be used for the booster dose). | If coadministered with other immunizations, consider contraindications of all products | Induration, erythema, tenderness at injection site; fever | |

*Continued*

## Routine Pediatric Immunizations (0–18 Years)—cont'd

| Generic Name (Brand Names) | Route and Dosage | Contraindications and Precautions | Adverse Reactions and Side Effects | Notes |
|---|---|---|---|---|
| Pneumococcal conjugate vaccine (7-valent) (PCV, Prevnar) | 0.5 mL IM at 2, 4, 6, and 12–15 mo | Hypersensitivity to all components including diphtheria toxoid, moderate to severe febrile illness | Erythema induration, tenderness, nodule formation at injection site; fever | One dose may also be given to previously unvaccinated healthy children age 24–59 mo and for high-risk children (e.g., sickle cell disease; anatomic or functional asplenia; chronic cardiac, pulmonary, or renal disease; diabetes; HIV; immunosuppression; cochlear implant), age 24–59 mo; give two doses (≥8 wk apart) if previously received more than three doses or one dose if previously received three doses) |
| Polio vaccine, inactivated (IPV, IPOL, Poliovax) | 0.5 mL IM or subcutaneously at 2, 4, and 6–18 mo and at 4–6 yr (first dose may be given as early as age 6 wk) | Hypersensitivity to neomycin, streptomycin, or polymyxin B; acute febrile illness; pregnancy | Erythema, induration, pain at injection site; fever | Oral polio vaccine (OPV) no longer recommended for use in the United States |
| Influenza vaccine *injection (trivalent inactivated):* (Afluria, Fluarix, FluLaval, Fluvirin, Fluzone); *intranasal (live attenuated):* (FluMist) | Injection: *age 6–35 mo:* two doses of 0.25 mL IM given 4 wk apart for initial season, then one dose annually; *age 3–8 yr:* two doses of 0.5 mL IM given 4 wk apart for initial season, then one dose annually; *age ≥9 yr:* 0.5 mL IM single dose annually. Intranasal: *age 2–8 yr:* if not previously vaccinated with influenza vaccine, two doses of 0.2 mL (given as 0.1 mL in each nostril) 4 wk apart, then one dose annually; if previously vaccinated with influenza vaccine, one dose of 0.2 mL (given as 0.1 mL in each nostril) annually; *age ≥9 yr:* one dose of 0.2 mL (given as 0.1 mL in each nostril) annually. | Hypersensitivity to eggs or egg products; hypersensitivity to thimerosal (injection only); avoid use in patients with acute neurological compromise; Fluvirin should only be used in children ≥4 yr; Fluarix should only be used in children age ≥3 yr; FluMist should be avoided in pregnancy; chronic pulmonary (including asthma), cardiovascular (not hypertension), renal, hepatic, | Injection: local soreness, fever, myalgia, possible neurological toxicity  Intranasal: upper respiratory congestion, malaise | Immunosuppression may decrease antibody response to injection and increase the risk of viral transmission with intranasal route |

## Routine Pediatric Immunizations (0–18 Years)—cont'd

| Generic Name (Brand Names) | Route and Dosage | Contraindications and Precautions | Adverse Reactions and Side Effects | Notes |
|---|---|---|---|---|
| | | neurological, hematological, or metabolic (including diabetes) disorders; immunosuppression (including HIV); chronic salicylate therapy (children 6 mo–18 yr) | | |
| Measles, mumps, and rubella vaccines (MMR II) | 0.5 mL subcutaneously at 12–15 mo and at 4–6 yr | Allergy to egg, gelatin, or neomycin; active infection; severe immunosuppression (in the absence of severe immunosuppression, HIV is not a contraindication); pregnancy | Burning, stinging, pain at injection site; arthritis or arthralgia; fever; encephalitis; allergic reactions | If unusual reactions occur, individual components may be given as separate injections; immunosuppression may decrease antibody response to injection and increase the risk of viral transmission |
| Varicella vaccine (Var, Varivax) | 0.5 mL subcutaneously at 12–15 mo and at 4–6 yr (second dose may be given earlier if ≥3 mo have elapsed since the first dose); for persons 7–18 yr who have not been vaccinated or without a history of chickenpox, two doses should be given (≥3 mo apart if 7–12 yr or ≥28 days apart if ≥13 yr). | Allergy to gelatin or neomycin; active infection; immunosuppression (including HIV); pregnancy | Local soreness, fever | Given to children and adolescents who do not have evidence of immunity; immunosuppression may decrease antibody response to injection and increase the risk of viral transmission |
| Hepatitis A vaccine (HepA, Havrix, Vaqta) | Should be given to all children age 12–23 mo; give a total of two doses of pediatric formulation (each 0.5 mL) IM at least 6 mo apart | Acute febrile illness | Local reactions, headache | Also recommended in children ≥2 yr old who live in areas with high rates of hepatitis A or in other high-risk groups (e.g., chronic liver disease, clotting factor disorders, illicit drug users) |
| Meningococcal conjugate vaccine (MCV4, Menactra) | 0.5 mL IM single dose at 11–12 yr or at age 13–18 yr if not previously vaccinated | Hypersensitivity to any component | Fatigue, malaise, anorexia, pain at injection site | Routine vaccination with meningococcal vaccine also recommended for college freshmen living in dormitories who are previously unvaccinated and for children ≥2 yr |

*Continued*

## Routine Pediatric Immunizations (0–18 Years)—cont'd

| Generic Name (Brand Names) | Route and Dosage | Contraindications and Precautions | Adverse Reactions and Side Effects | Notes |
|---|---|---|---|---|
| | | | | old who are at high risk (anatomic or functional asplenia, persistent complement component deficiency, travel or residence in areas in which meningococcal disease is hyperendemic or epidemic) |
| Human papillomavirus vaccine (HPV, Gardasil) | ≥9 yr, 0.5 mL IM, repeat at 2 and 6 mo after initial dose | Hypersensitivity to yeast: pregnancy | Headache, dizziness, fever, nausea, diarrhea, syncope, local soreness | All previously unvaccinated women through age 26 yr; also recommended for boys and men through age 26 yr for prevention of genital warts caused by HPV types 6 and 11 |

CNS, central nervous system; DTwP, diphtheria toxoid, tetanus toxoid, and whole cell pertussis vaccine; GI, gastrointestinal; HBsAg, hepatitis B surface antigen; IM, intramuscularly; PO, orally.

# NURSING IMPLICATIONS

## Assessment

Assess the previous immunization history and history of hypersensitivity.

Assess the patient for a history of asthma or reactive airway disease. Patients with a positive history should not receive FluMist.

Assess for a history of latex allergy. Some prefilled syringes may use latex components and should be avoided in patients with hypersensitivity.

Potential Nursing Diagnoses

Infection, risk for (indications)

Knowledge, deficient, related to medication regimen (patient/family teaching)

## Implementation

The following may be given concomitantly: measles, mumps, and rubella (MMR) vaccine; trivalent oral poliovirus vaccine; and diphtheria toxoid, tetanus toxoid, and pertussis vaccine.

Do not administer FluMist concurrently with other vaccines or in patients who have received a live virus vaccine within 1 month or an inactivated vaccine within 2 weeks or vaccination.

Administer each immunization by the appropriate route:

- Oral: Rotavirus vaccine
- Subcutaneous: MMR; Varicella vaccine
- Intramuscular: Hepatitis B, Diphtheria toxoid; tetanus toxoid, and acellular pertussis; *Haemophilus* b; Pneumococcal; Polio vaccine; Influenza vaccine; Hepatitis A; Meningococcal and Human papillomavirus
- Intranasal: FluMist

## Patient and family teaching

Inform the parent of potential and reportable side effects of immunization. The physician should be notified if the patient develops the following: a fever higher than 39.4°C (103°F); difficulty breathing; hives; itching; swelling of the eyes, face, or inside of the nose; sudden, severe tiredness or weakness; convulsions.

Review the next scheduled immunization with the parent.

## Evaluation

Effectiveness of therapy can be demonstrated by prevention of diseases through active immunity.

## Routine Adult Immunizations

| Generic Name (Brand Names) | Indications | Dosage and Route | Contraindications | Adverse Reactions and Side Effects |
|---|---|---|---|---|
| Tetanus toxoid, reduced diphtheria toxoid and acellular pertussis vaccine absorbed (Tdap, Adacell, Boostrix) | Single dose should be given instead of Td in adults (19–64 yr) if they received their last dose of Td≥10 yr ago (and did not previously receive a dose of Tdap) | 0.5 mL IM to replace one dose of DTaP | Previous reactions to DTaP, progressive neurological disease, recent (within 7 days) CNS disease | Fatigue, headache, gastrointestinal symptoms, pain at injection site |
| Tetanus-diphtheria (Td, Decavac) | All adults who lack written documentation of a primary series of tetanus-and diphtheria-toxoid–containing vaccine; booster dose should be given to all adults every 10 yr (see foregoing information on use of Tdap to replace one dose of Td in booster series) | Unimmunized: two doses 0.5 mL IM 1–2 mo apart, then a third dose 6–12 mo later. Immunized: 0.5 mL IM booster every 10 yr. | Neurological or severe hypersensitivity reaction to prior dose | Local pain and swelling |
| Human papillomavirus vaccine (HPV, Gardasil) | All previously unvaccinated women through age 26 yr; also recommended for boys and men through age 26 yr for prevention of genital warts caused by HPV types 6 and 11 | 0.5 mL IM, repeat at 2 and 6 mo after initial dose | Hypersensitivity to yeast: pregnancy | Headache, dizziness, fever, nausea, diarrhea, syncope, local soreness |
| Varicella vaccine (Var, Varivax) | Any adult without a history of chickenpox or herpes zoster (shingles), a history of receiving two doses of varicella vaccine, or laboratory evidence of immunity. Health-care workers and pregnant women born in United States before 1980 who do not meet the foregoing criteria should be tested for immunity. | 0.5 mL subcutaneously; repeated 4–8 wk later | Allergy to gelatin or neomycin, active infection, immunosuppression (including HIV), pregnancy (also avoid becoming pregnant for 4 wk after immunization) | Local soreness, fever Immunosuppression may decrease antibody response to injection and increase the risk of viral transmission |
| Zoster vaccine (Zos, Zostavax) | All adults ≥60 yr (regardless of previous history of chickenpox or herpes zoster). | 0.65-mL subcutaneous single dose | Allergy to gelatin or neomycin, active infection, immunosuppression (including HIV), pregnancy | Local soreness, fever Immunosuppression may decrease antibody response to injection and increase the risk of viral transmission |

*Continued*

## Routine Adult Immunizations—cont'd

| Generic Name (Brand Names) | Indications | Dosage and Route | Contraindications | Adverse Reactions and Side Effects |
|---|---|---|---|---|
| Measles, mumps, and rubella vaccine (MMR II) | Adults born in 1957 or later with unreliable history of MMR illness or immunization, high-risk groups (e.g., health-care workers, college students, international travelers), women of childbearing age (with no evidence of rubella immunity or immunization) | 0.5 mL subcutaneously, one or two doses in adults born in 1957 or later with unreliable history; high-risk groups should receive a total of two doses given 1 mo apart | Allergy to egg, gelatin, or neomycin; active infection; severe immunosuppression (in the absence of severe immunosuppression, HIV is not a contraindication); pregnancy (also avoid becoming pregnant for 4 wk after immunization) | Burning, stinging pain at injection site; arthritis or arthralgia; fever; encephalitis; allergic reactions; immunosuppression may decrease antibody response to injection and increase the risk of viral transmission |
| Influenza vaccine *injection (trivalent inactivated):* (Afluria, Fluarix, FluLaval, Fluvirin, Fluzone;) *intranasal (live attenuated):* (FluMist) | All adults | Injection: 0.5 mL IM annually Intranasal (for adults <50 yr): single dose of 0.2 mL (given as 0.1 mL in each nostril) annually | Hypersensitivity to eggs or egg products; hypersensitivity to thimerosal (injection only); avoid use in patients with acute neurological compromise; FluMist should be avoided in pregnancy; chronic pulmonary (including asthma), cardiovascular (not hypertension), renal, hepatic, neurological, hematological, or metabolic (including diabetes) disorders; immunosuppression (including HIV); age ≥50 yr | Injection: local soreness, fever, myalgia, possible neurological toxicity; intranasal: upper respiratory congestion, malaise; immunosuppression may decrease antibody response to injection and increase the risk of viral transmission |
| Pneumococcal polysaccharide vaccine (PPSV, Pneumovax 23) | All adults ≥65 yr; high-risk patients (e.g., chronic cardiac or pulmonary disease [including asthma], chronic liver disease, alcoholism, diabetes, cigarette smoker, anatomic or functional asplenia, sickle cell disease; immunosuppression [including HIV], cochlear implants) | 0.5 mL IM or subcutaneously; one-time revaccination should also be given ≥5 yr after first dose to those ≥65 yr (if first dose was given before age 65) and to high-risk patients | Hypersensitivity to all components including diphtheria toxoid | Erythema induration, tenderness, nodule formation at injection site, fever |
| Hepatitis A vaccine (HepA, Havrix, Vaqta) | High-risk groups (e.g., chronic liver disease, clotting factor disorders, illicit drug users, men who have sex with men, some health-care workers, food handlers), travel to endemic areas, recent (<2 wk) exposure to HepA (if less than 40 yr old) | 1 mL IM, followed by 1 mL IM 6–18 mo later (adult dose form) | Hypersensitivity to aluminum or 2-phenoxy-ethanol | Local reactions, headache |

## Routine Adult Immunizations—cont'd

| Generic Name (Brand Names) | Indications | Dosage and Route | Contraindications | Adverse Reactions and Side Effects |
|---|---|---|---|---|
| Hepatitis B vaccine (HepB, Engerix-B, Recombivax HB) | High-risk patients (e.g., household contacts or sex partners of HBsAg-positive persons, IV drug users, sexually active persons not in a monogamous relationship, men who have sex with men, HIV, STDs, hemodialysis, health-care workers, inmates), chronic liver disease, all unvaccinated adolescents | Three doses of 1 mL IM, given at 0, 1–2, and 4–6 mo | Anaphylactic allergy to yeast | Local soreness |
| Meningococcal conjugate vaccine (MCV4, Menactra) | College freshmen living in dormitories who are previously unvaccinated, anatomic or functional asplenia, persistent complement component deficiency, travel or residence in areas in which meningococcal disease is hyperendemic or epidemic | 0.5-mL IM single dose; revaccination with MCV4 indicated in patients previously vaccinated with MCV4 or meningococcal polysaccharide vaccine (MPSV4) and who also remain at increased risk for infection (revaccinate after 5 yr of previous dose) | Hypersensitivity to any components | Fatigue, malaise, anorexia, pain at injection site |

CNS, central nervous system; DTaP, diphtheria toxoid, tetanus toxoid, and acellular pertussis vaccine; HBsAg, hepatitis B surface antigen; IM, intramuscularly; STDs, sexually transmitted diseases.

Source: Adapted from the recommendations of the National Immunization Program: http://www.cdc.gov. Davis's Drug Guide for Nurses, ed 12. Philadelphia: FA Davis; 2010.

# Administering Medications to Children

## GENERAL GUIDELINES

Medication administration to a pediatric patient can be challenging. Prescribers should order dosage forms that are age appropriate for their patients, but they do not always specify beyond the route desired. If a child is unable to take a particular dosage form, ask the pharmacist whether another form is available. If no other form is available, you may need to crush a tablet and mix it with a small amount of food. Always verify that the ordered medication can be crushed.

## ORAL LIQUIDS

Pediatric liquid medicines may be given with plastic medicine cups, oral syringes, oral droppers, or cylindrical dosing spoons. Parents should be taught to use these calibrated devices, rather than household utensils, because household teaspoons, tablespoons, and cups have a variety of sizes. For young children, it is best to use an oral syringe to squirt a small amount of the dose at a time into the side of the cheek, away from the bitter taste buds at the back of the tongue. This approach also prevents choking and aspiration because you are not squirting the liquid directly toward the back of the throat.

## EYE DROPS AND OINTMENTS

Tilt the child's head back, gently press the skin under the lower eyelid, and pull the lower lid away slightly until a small pouch is visible. Insert the ointment or drop (one drop at a time), and close the eye for a few minutes to keep the medicine in place.

## EAR DROPS

Shake the otic suspensions well before administration. For children younger than 3 years of age, pull the outer ear outward and downward before you instill the drops. For children 3 years old and older, pull the outer ear outward and upward. Keep the child on his or her side for 2 minutes, and place a cotton plug in the ear.

## NOSE DROPS

First, clear the child's nose of secretions with a nasal aspirator (bulb syringe), or a cotton swab may be used in infants and young children. Ask older children to blow their nose. Then tilt the child's head back over a pillow, and squeeze the dropper without touching the nostril. Keep the child's head back for 2 minutes.

# SUPPOSITORIES

Keep suppositories refrigerated for easier administration. While wearing gloves, moisten the rounded end of the suppository with water or petroleum jelly before insertion. Using your pinky finger for children younger than 3 years of age and your index finger for those 3 years and older, insert the suppository into the rectum about 1/2 to 1 inch beyond the sphincter. If the suppository slides out, insert it a little farther than before. Hold the child's buttocks together for a few minutes, and have the child hold the position for about 20 minutes, if possible.

# TOPICALS

Clean the affected area and dry it well before topical application. Apply a thin layer of medication to the skin, and rub it in gently. Children absorb medication more rapidly through their skin than do adults, so it is important to keep the layer thin unless otherwise ordered. Do not apply a covering over the area unless instructed to do so by prescriber.

# METERED-DOSE INHALERS

Generally, the same principles apply to children as to adults, except the use of spacers is recommended for young children.

Source: Davis's Drug Guide for Nurses, ed 12. Philadelphia: F. A. Davis; 2010.

# Pediatric Dosage Calculations

Most drugs in children are dosed according to body weight (mg/kg) or body surface are (BSA) (mg/m$^2$). Care must be taken to convert body weight from pounds to kilograms (1 kg = 2.2 lb) before calculating doses based on body weight. Doses are often expressed as mg/kg/day or mg/kg/dose; therefore, orders written "mg/kg/d," which is confusing, require clarification from the prescriber.

Because of the caustic nature of these drugs, chemotherapy is commonly dosed according to the BSA, which requires an extra verification step (BSA) calculation before dosing. These calculations are done by the physician and pharmacist. The allied health professionals' role is obtaining extremely accurate height and weight measurements of the patient. It is a good idea to understand how these calculations are done, to assist in recognizing errors in calculations. Medications are available in multiple concentrations; therefore, orders written in "mL" rather than "mg" are not acceptable and require clarification.

Dosing also varies by indication; therefore, diagnostic information is helpful when calculating doses. The following examples are typically encountered when dosing medication in children.

## ■ EXAMPLE 1

Calculate the dose of amoxicillin suspension in milliliters for otitis media for a 1-year-old child weighing 22 lb. The dose required is 40 mg/kg/day divided twice daily (bid), and the suspension comes in a concentration of 400 mg/5 mL.

| | |
|---|---|
| Step 1: Convert pounds to kilograms: | 22 lb × 1 kg/2.2 lb = 10 kg |
| Step 2: Calculate the dose in milligrams: | 40 mg × 10 kg = 400 mg/day |
| Step 3: Divide the dose by the frequency: | 400 mg/day ÷ 2 (bid) = 200 mg/dose bid |
| Step 4: Convert the milligrams dose to milliliters: | 200 mg/dose ÷ 400 mg/5 mL = 2.5 mL bid |

## ■ EXAMPLE 2

Calculate the dose of ceftriaxone in milliliters for meningitis for a 5-year-old child weighing 20 kg. The dose required is 100 mg/kg/day given IV once daily, and the drug comes prediluted in a concentration of 500 mg/mL.

| | |
|---|---|
| Step 1: Calculate the dose in milligrams: | 100 mg × 20 kg = 2000 mg/day |
| Step 2: Divide the dose by the frequency: | 2000 mg/day ÷ 1 (daily) = 2000 mg/dose |
| Step 3: Convert the milligram dose to milliliters: | 2000 mg/dose ÷ 500 mg/mL = 4 mL once daily |

# ■ EXAMPLE 3

Calculate the dose of vincristine in milliliters for a 4-year-old child with leukemia who weighs 37 lb and is 97 cm tall. The dose required is 2 mg/m², and the drug comes in 1 mg/mL concentration.

| | |
|---|---|
| Step 1: Convert pounds to kilograms: | 37 lb × 1 kg/2.2 lb = 16.8 kg |
| Step 2: Calculate the BSA: | $\sqrt{}$ 16.8 kg × 97 cm/3600 = 0.67 m² |
| Step 3: Calculate the dose in milligrams: | 2 mg × 0.67 m² = 1.34 mg |
| Step 4: Calculate the dose in milliliters: | 1.34 mg ÷ 1 mg/mL = 1.34 mL |

Source: Davis's Drug Guide for Nurses, ed 12. Philadelphia: F. A. Davis; 2010.

# G

# Examples of Herbs, Vitamins, Minerals, Amino Acids, and Lipids Used in Illness

| Herb | Illnesses Patient May be Taking For |
|------|-------------------------------------|
| Alfalfa | • Anemia<br>• Diabetes mellitus |
| Aloe vera | • Eczema<br>• Sunburn<br>• Thrush |
| Aniseed (anise) | • Asthma<br>• Bronchitis<br>• Cough |
| Angelica | • Allergies<br>• Anemia<br>• Anorexia<br>• Motion sickness<br>• Neuralgia<br>• Thyroid disease |
| Barberry | • Heartburn<br>• Hepatitis<br>• Jaundice<br>• Thrush |
| Bayberry | • Colds<br>• Diarrhea<br>• Hemorrhoids |
| Bladderwrack | • Arthritis<br>• Obesity<br>• Thyroid disease |
| Broom | • Hypotension<br>• Palpitations |
| Bugleweed | • Thyroid disease |

*Continued*

| Herb | Illnesses Patient May be Taking For |
|------|-------------------------------------|
| Burdock | • Acne<br>• Chickenpox<br>• Seborrhea<br>• Sprains and strains<br>• Syphilis |
| Butternut | • Anal fissure<br>• Constipation<br>• Seborrhea |
| Cascara | • Anal fissure<br>• Constipation |
| Catnip | • Encephalitis<br>• Fever<br>• Insomnia<br>• Migraine |
| Cayenne | • Reynaud's disease<br>• Toothache |
| Cayenne pepper | • Worms |
| Chamomile | • Allergies<br>• Cirrhosis<br>• Eczema<br>• Encephalitis<br>• Hay fever<br>• Insomnia<br>• Irritable bowel syndrome<br>• Motion sickness<br>• Neuralgia<br>• Obsessions and compulsions<br>• Restless legs syndrome<br>• Sprains and strains<br>• Stress<br>• Tonsillitis<br>• Urticaria |
| Chickweed | • Asthma<br>• Constipation<br>• Eczema<br>• Urticaria |
| Comfrey | • Bunion<br>• Chickenpox<br>• Fractures<br>• Gingivitis<br>• Osteoporosis<br>• Peptic ulcers<br>• Pertussis (whopping cough)<br>• Tooth abscess |
| Comfrey root | • Gastroenteritis<br>• Pleurisy<br>• Tracheitis |

| Herb | Illnesses Patient May be Taking For |
|---|---|
| Dandelion | • Anal fissure<br>• Anemia<br>• Arthritis<br>• Edema<br>• Hemorrhoids<br>• Hepatitis<br>• Indigestion<br>• Jaundice<br>• Osteoporosis<br>• Warts |
| Dandelion leaves | • Gallstones |
| Dietary fiber | • Angina<br>• Atherosclerosis<br>• Constipation<br>• Hypertension |
| Dill | • Flatulence<br>• Indigestion |
| Echinacea | • Abscess<br>• AIDS<br>• Allergies<br>• Athlete's foot<br>• Boils<br>• Cold<br>• Encephalitis<br>• Enlarged spleen<br>• Guillain-Barré syndrome<br>• Laryngitis<br>• Tonsillitis<br>• Tuberculosis |
| Elderberry | • Chronic fatigue<br>• Influenza<br>• Sciatica<br>• Tonsillitis |
| Elderflower | • Allergies<br>• Measles<br>• Rubella<br>• Sinusitis |
| Eucalyptus | • Fever<br>• Hay fever |
| Fennel | • Motion sickness |
| Fenugreek | • Constipation<br>• Diabetes mellitus<br>• Flu (influenza) |
| Feverfew | • Arthritis<br>• Migraines<br>• Rheumatoid arthritis |

*Continued*

| Herb | Illnesses Patient May be Taking For |
|------|-------------------------------------|
| Garlic | • AIDS<br>• Allergies<br>• Aneurysm<br>• Angina<br>• Bronchitis<br>• Corns and calluses<br>• Diabetes mellitus<br>• Encephalitis<br>• Enlarged spleen<br>• Measles<br>• Pneumonia<br>• Sore throat<br>• Thyroid disease<br>• Tonsillitis<br>• Tooth abscess<br>• Tuberculosis |
| Ginger | • Alopecia (hair loss)<br>• Cold<br>• Hypotension<br>• Irritable bowel syndrome<br>• Motion sickness<br>• Nausea<br>• Reynaud's disease<br>• Sprains and strains<br>• Syncope (fainting) |
| Ginkgo biloba | • Stroke |
| Ginseng | • AIDS<br>• Allergies<br>• Bronchitis<br>• Bursitis<br>• Cold<br>• Enlarged spleen<br>• Flu (influenza<br>• Grinding teeth<br>• Guillain-Barré syndrome<br>• Memory loss<br>• Pneumonia<br>• Stress<br>• Tuberculosis |
| Golden seal | • Cough<br>• Diaper rash<br>• Gingivitis<br>• Hepatitis<br>• Jaundice<br>• Sinusitis<br>• Sore throat |
| Grapefruit | • Cirrhosis |
| Grapefruit seed | • Yeast infections |
| Green tea | • Cancer |
| Hawthorn | • Angina<br>• Atherosclerosis<br>• Hypertension |

| Herb | Illnesses Patient May be Taking For |
|---|---|
| Hops | • Attention deficit hyperactivity disorder (ADHD)<br>• Crohn's disease<br>• Insomnia<br>• Obsessions and compulsions |
| Horsetail | • Edema<br>• Fractures<br>• Incontinence<br>• Osteoporosis |
| Hyssop | • AIDS<br>• Asthma<br>• Pertussis (whopping cough) |
| Juniper | • Cirrhosis<br>• Sciatica |
| Lady's slipper | • Anxiety<br>• Hyperventilation |
| Lavender | • Atherosclerosis<br>• Dandruff<br>• Epistaxis (nosebleed)<br>• Hay fever<br>• Insomnia<br>• Perspiration<br>• Stress |
| Lemon | • Cirrhosis<br>• Pertussis (whopping cough) |
| Lemon balm | • Depression<br>• Irritable bowel syndrome<br>• Migraines<br>• Stress<br>• Urticaria |
| Lemon juice | • Corns and calluses |
| Licorice | • AIDS<br>• Anal fissure<br>• Constipation<br>• Cough<br>• Enlarged spleen<br>• Flu (influenza)<br>• Pancreatitis<br>• Peptic ulcers<br>• Tuberculosis |
| Lime blossom | • Anxiety |
| Lime flowers | • Hypertension<br>• Insomnia |
| Marigold | • Diaper rash<br>• Eczema<br>• Perspiration<br>• Varicose veins |

*Continued*

| Herb | Illnesses Patient May be Taking For |
|------|-------------------------------------|
| Marshmallow | • Bunion |
| Meadowsweet | |
| Melatonin | • Insomnia |
| Mint | • Halitosis |
| Mistletoe | • Palpitations |
| Motherwort | • Angina<br>• Asthma<br>• Palpitations |
| Mustard | • Cough |
| Myrrh | • Diarrhea<br>• Gingivitis<br>• Mouth ulcers<br>• Tonsillitis<br>• Tooth abscess |
| Nettles | • Alopecia (hair loss)<br>• Anemia<br>• Gout<br>• Obesity<br>• Osteoporosis<br>• Psoriasis |
| Oats | • Addictions<br>• Anxiety<br>• Depression<br>• Eczema<br>• Guillain-Barré syndrome<br>• Shingles<br>• Stress |
| Onions | • Diabetes mellitus<br>• Thyroid disease |
| Orange | • Cirrhosis |
| Parsley | • Halitosis |
| Passiflora | • Obsessions and compulsions<br>• Stress |
| Peppermint | • Bronchitis<br>• Chickenpox<br>• Cold<br>• Crohn's disease<br>• Indigestion<br>• Irritable bowel syndrome<br>• Motion sickness<br>• Neuralgia<br>• Rubella<br>• Emphysema<br>• Syncope (fainting) |

| Herb | Illnesses Patient May be Taking For |
|---|---|
| **Rosemary** | • Alopecia (hair loss)<br>• Atherosclerosis<br>• Dandruff<br>• Depression<br>• Halitosis<br>• Hypotension<br>• Memory loss<br>• Migraines<br>• Stroke<br>• Syncope (fainting) |
| **Red clover** | • Abscess<br>• Allergies |
| **Rhubarb** | • Constipation |
| **Sage** | • Laryngitis<br>• Pleurisy |
| **Sandalwood** | • Prickly heat |
| **Saw palmetto** | • Asthma<br>• Benign prostatic hypertrophy<br>• Sinusitis |
| **Senna** | • Constipation |
| **Skullcap** | • Anxiety<br>• Encephalitis<br>• Guillain-Barré syndrome<br>• Hyperventilation<br>• Migraines<br>• Shingles |
| **Slippery elm** | • Bunion<br>• Bursitis<br>• Irritable bowel syndrome<br>• Peptic ulcers<br>• Rheumatoid arthritis |
| **Slippery elm bark** | • Emphysema |
| **St. John's Wort** | • Cold sores<br>• Shingles |
| **Tarragon** | • Halitosis |
| **Thyme** | • Abscess<br>• Athlete's foot<br>• Cough<br>• Dermatitis<br>• Halitosis |
| **Tumeric** | • Asthma |
| **Valerian** | • Epilepsy<br>• Obsessions and compulsions<br>• Phobias<br>• Restless legs syndrome |

*Continued*

| Herb | Illnesses Patient May be Taking For |
|------|-------------------------------------|
| Valerian root | • Guillain-Barré syndrome |
| Verbena | • Dermatitis<br>• Hepatitis<br>• Jaundice |
| Vervain | • Depression<br>• Epilepsy<br>• Guillain-Barré syndrome |
| Watercress | • Anemia<br>• Cough<br>• Halitosis |
| White willow | • Arthritis<br>• Osteoporosis<br>• Rheumatoid arthritis |
| Wild indigo | • Tonsillitis |
| Wild yam | • Allergies<br>• Hepatitis<br>• Osteoporosis |
| Witch hazel | • Bruising<br>• Hemorrhoids |
| Wormwood tea | • Worms |
| Yams | • Jaundice |
| Yarrow | • Edema<br>• Psoriasis<br>• Rubella<br>• Stroke<br>• Tonsillitis |
| Yellow dock | • Pancreatitis |

| Vitamin | Illnesses Patient May be Taking For |
|---------|-------------------------------------|
| Beta-carotene (vitamin A) | • Sprains and strains |
| Choline (very similar to vitamin B) | • Alopecia (hair loss)<br>• Dementia<br>• Liver disease |
| Folic acid (vitamin B-complex ) | • Insomnia<br>• Multiple sclerosis |
| Inositol (very similar to vitamin B) | • Alopecia (hair loss)<br>• Diabetic neuropathy |
| Vitamin A | • Arthritis<br>• Bronchitis<br>• Corns and calluses<br>• Crohn's disease<br>• Eczema |

| Vitamin | Illnesses Patient May be Taking For |
|---|---|
| | • Irritable bowel syndrome<br>• Mouth ulcers<br>• Psoriasis |
| **Vitamin B** | • Addictions<br>• Allergies<br>• Alopecia (hair loss)<br>• Anemia<br>• Anxiety<br>• Bronchitis<br>• Constipation<br>• Crohn's disease<br>• Dandruff<br>• Eczema<br>• Guillain-Barré syndrome<br>• Hyperventilation<br>• Insomnia<br>• Memory loss<br>• Parkinson's disease<br>• Phobias<br>• Stress<br>• Psoriasis |
| **Vitamin B$_1$** | • Diarrhea<br>• Neuralgia |
| **Vitamin B$_2$** | • Mouth ulcers<br>• Neuralgia |
| **Vitamin B$_3$** | • Diarrhea<br>• Multiple sclerosis |
| **Vitamin B$_5$** | • Epilepsy<br>• Migraines |
| **Vitamin B$_6$** | • Asthma<br>• Depression<br>• Epilepsy<br>• Irritable bowel syndrome<br>• Multiple sclerosis<br>• Nausea |
| **Vitamin B$_{12}$** | • Anemia<br>• Depression<br>• Multiple sclerosis |
| **Vitamin C** | • AIDS<br>• Allergies<br>• Anemia<br>• Aneurysm<br>• Arthritis<br>• Athlete's foot<br>• Bronchitis<br>• Bruising<br>• Cold<br>• Cold sores<br>• Dandruff<br>• Depression<br>• Eczema |

*Continued*

| Vitamin | Illnesses Patient May be Taking For |
|---|---|
| | • Encephalitis<br>• Flu (influenza)<br>• Gingivitis<br>• Hay fever<br>• Hepatitis<br>• Insomnia<br>• Laryngitis<br>• Measles<br>• Migraines<br>• Multiple sclerosis<br>• Parkinson's disease<br>• Phobias<br>• Pneumonia<br>• Prickly heat<br>• Psoriasis<br>• Shingles<br>• Sore throat<br>• Sprains and strains<br>• Stress<br>• Reynaud's disease<br>• Tonsillitis<br>• Tracheitis<br>• Varicose veins |
| **Vitamin D** | • Crohn's disease<br>• Epilepsy |
| **Vitamin E** | • Aneurysm<br>• Arthritis<br>• Corns and calluses<br>• Dandruff<br>• Guillain-Barré syndrome<br>• Measles<br>• Migraines<br>• Mouth ulcers<br>• Multiple sclerosis<br>• Palpitations<br>• Psoriasis<br>• Restless legs syndrome<br>• Rubella<br>• Shingles<br>• Stroke<br>• Sunburn<br>• Varicose veins |
| **Vitamin K** | • Diarrhea |

| Mineral | Illnesses Patient May be Taking For |
|---|---|
| **Calcium** | • Guillain-Barré syndrome<br>• Insomnia<br>• Alopecia (hair loss)<br>• Anemia<br>• Hypertension |

| Mineral | Illnesses Patient May be Taking For |
|---|---|
| Chromium | • Neuralgia<br>• Obesity |
| Copper | • Anemia<br>• Arthritis |
| Fluoride | • Osteoporosis |
| Iodine | • Thyroid disease |
| Iron | • Anemia |
| Magnesium | • Alopecia (hair loss)<br>• Fractures<br>• Guillain-Barré syndrome<br>• Hypertension<br>• Multiple sclerosis |
| Manganese | • Guillain-Barré syndrome |
| Phosphorus | • Fractures |
| Potassium | • Hypertension |
| Selenium | • Sprains and strains |
| Zinc | • AIDS<br>• Bruising<br>• Cold<br>• Cold sores<br>• Dandruff<br>• Diaper rash<br>• Encephalitis<br>• Guillain-Barré syndrome |

| Amino Acid | Illnesses Patient May be Taking For |
|---|---|
| L-Tyrosine | • Stress |

| Lipid | Illnesses Patient May be Taking For |
|---|---|
| Fish oil | • Angina<br>• Arthritis<br>• Stroke<br>• Tonsillitis |
| Lecithin | • High cholesterol<br>• Memory loss |
| Olive oil | • Tooth abscess |

There are many other supplements not listed here, as well as additional reasons that patients take these substances. This is just a sampling.

# Answers to Check Ups

## CHAPTER 5

### Check Up Answers

1. ā: Before
2. a.c.: Before meals
3. a.d.: Right ear
4. a.s.: Left ear
5. a.u.: Both ears
6. bid: Twice daily
7. c̄ With
8. cap: Capsule(s)
9. d/c: Discontinue(d)
10. elix: Elixir
11. g: Gram
12. gr: Grain
13. gtt: Drop
14. hs: At bedtime
15. ID: Intradermal
16. IM: Intramuscular
17. IV: Intravenous
18. mcg: Milligram
19. mEq: Milliequivalent
20. mg: Milligram
21. mL: Milliliter
22. NPO: Nothing by mouth
23. o.d.: Right eye
24. o.s.: Left eye
25. o.u.: Both eyes
26. oz: Ounce
27. p̄: After
28. pc: After meals
29. prn: As needed
30. s̄: Without

**31.** SC: Subcutaneously
**32.** STAT: Immediately
**33.** Tb: Tablespoon(s)
**34.** tid: Three times daily
**35.** tsp: Teaspoon

## ■ CHAPTER 6

### Check Up 6.1: addition

**1.** 400
**2.** 7
**3.** 1480
**4.** 31
**5.** 176

### Check Up 6.2: subtraction

**1.** 75
**2.** 200
**3.** 14
**4.** 27
**5.** 30

### Check Up 6.3: multiplication

**1.** 40
**2.** 180
**3.** 21
**4.** 210
**5.** 300

### Check Up 6.4: division

**1.** 2
**2.** 2
**3.** 3
**4.** 3
**5.** 9

### Check Up 6.5: fraction

**1.** Circled fraction: 10/25   Underlined fraction: 4/25
**2.** Circled fraction: 1/100   Underlined fraction 1/300
**3.** Circle fraction: 5/3   Underlined fraction 2/3
**4.** Circled fraction 1/75   Underlined fraction 1/125
**5.** Circled fraction 4/8   Underlined fraction 1/8
**6.** Circled fraction 1/10   Underlined fraction 1/6
**7.** Circled fraction 2/6   Underlined fraction 5/6
**8.** Circled fraction 1/75   Underlined fraction 1/25
**9.** Circled fraction 1/16   Underlined fraction 4/16
**10.** Circled fraction 1/12   Underlined fraction 6/12

## Check Up 6.6: proper fractions

**1.** 1/4

**2.** 1/2

**3.** 2/6

**4.** 2/3

**5.** 3/8

**6.** 5/6

## Check Up 6.7: improper fractions

**1.** 16/5

**2.** 8/4

**3.** 13/5

**4.** 5/3

**5.** 3/2

**6.** 15/6

## Check Up 6.8: least common denominator

**1.** 4/45

**2.** 17/24

**3.** 31 /60

**4.** 9/20

**5.** 13/24

**6.** 73/60

**7.** 43/30

**8.** 21/38

**9.** 13/75

**10.** 7/16

## Check Up 6.9: equivalent

**1.** 4

**2.** 1/4

**3.** 3

**4.** 3

**5.** 4

## Check Up 6.10: mixed numbers to improper fraction

**1.** 10/3

**2.** 19/2

**3.** 25/4

**4.** 52/5

**5.** 7/6

## Check Up 6.11: improper fraction to mixed numbers

**1.** 5 3/5

**2.** 8 2/5

**3.** 4 2/7

**4.** 5 2/10

**5.** 1 1/6

## Check Up 6.12: reducing fractions to their lowest terms

**1.** 1/3
**2.** 4/5
**3.** 1/3
**4.** 1/2
**5.** 1/4
**6.** 3/10
**7.** 3/1
**8.** 7/9
**9.** 3/5
**10.** 1/3

## Check Up 6.13: fraction addition

**1.** 5/6
**2.** 5/10 or 1/2
**3.** 59/56 or 1 and 3/56
**4.** 5/12
**5.** 7/9

## Check Up 6.14: fraction subtraction

**1.** 1/3
**2.** 5/12
**3.** 200/500 or 2/5
**4.** 6/6 or 1
**5.** 15/2 or 7 and 1/2

## Check Up 6.15: multiplying and dividing fractions

**1.** 4/18 or 2/9
**2.** 5/80 or 1/16
**3.** 16/27
**4.** 5/36
**5.** 25/75 or 1/3
**6.** 8/6 or 1 and 1/3
**7.** 15/150 or 1/10
**8.** 4/9 or 2/3
**9.** 24/6 or 4
**10.** 16/18 or 8/9

## Check Up 6.16: rounding

**1.** 1
**2.** 1.5
**3.** 1
**4.** 2
**5.** 2.5
**6.** 1
**7.** 2
**8.** 2

**9.** 2

**10.** 3

## Check Up 6.17: larger/smaller

**1.** 0.52

**2.** 0.355

**3.** 0.322

**4.** 0.5

**5.** Equal

## Check Up 6.18: adding decimals

**1.** 0.37

**2.** 233.82

**3.** 28.17

**4.** 66.10

**5.** 9.034

## Check Up 6.19: subtracting decimals

**1.** 6.38

**2.** 1.123

**3.** 18.97

**4.** 62.101

**5.** 21.5

## Check Up 6.20: multiplying decimals

**1.** 96.8

**2.** 1002

**3.** 1002

**4.** 21.692

**5.** 170.3047

## Check Up 6.21: decimal division

**1.** 15.909

**2.** 285.714

**3.** 80

**4.** 800

**5.** 250

## Check Up 6.22: converting fractions to decimal

**1.** 0.4

**2.** 0.06

**3.** 0.71

**4.** 0.192

**5.** 0.020

**6.** 0.3

**7.** 0.43

**8.** 0.005

**9.** 0.417

**10.** 0.055

## Check Up 6.23: converting fractions to percentage

**1.** 20%

**2.** 2%

**3.** 20%

**4.** 20%

**5.** 2%

## Check Up 6.24: ratio

**1.** 40

**2.** 10

**3.** 8

**4.** 10

**5.** 1

## Check Up 6.25: converting ratios to decimal

**1.** 0.125

**2.** 0.2

**3.** 0.1

**4.** 0.01

**5.** 0.001

## Check Up 6.26: converting decimals to ratios

**1.** 125:1000

**2.** 12:100

**3.** 1:10

**4.** 2:10

**5.** 22:100

## Check Up 6.27: converting ratios to percentages

**1.** 67%

**2.** 50%

**3.** 50%

**4.** 10%

**5.** 33%

## Check Up 6.28: converting percentages to ratios

**1.** 5:10 or 1:2

**2.** 1:10

**3.** 75:100 or 3:4

**4.** 67:100 or 2:3

**5.** 33:100 or 1:3

## Check Up 6.29: ratios (proportional)

**1.** False

**2.** True

3. False

4. True

5. False

### Check Up 6.30: ratios (equal)

1. False

2. True

3. True

4. False

5. True

### Check Up 6.31: solve for the unknown

1. 1

2. 200

3. 3

4. 1

5. 2

## ■ CHAPTER 7

### Check Up 7.1

1. 88.6 kg

2. 25 kg

3. 18.2 kg

4. 136.4 kg

5. 56.8 kg

6. 1.02 kg

7. 3.27 kg

8. 2.05 kg

9. 3.07 kg

10. 5.63 kg

11. 187 lb

12. 22 lb

13. 264 lb

14. 440 lb

15. 46.2 lb

### Check Up 7.2

1. Juice glass = 4 oz

2. Teacup = 6 oz

3. Glass = 8 oz

4. 1 T = 1/2 oz

5. 1 oz = 6 t

6. 1 cup = 8 oz

7. 1 pint = 2 cups

8. 1 quart = 2 pints

**9.** 1 gallon = 4 quarts

**10.** 1 cup = 1/2 pint

## Check Up 7.3

**1.** 8

**2.** 2

**3.** 60

**4.** 2

**5.** 10

**6.** 4

**7.** 16

**8.** 2

**9.** 1/2

**10.** 4

**11.** 1

**12.** 360-480

**13.** 360-480

## Check Up 7.4

Microgram, milligram, centigram, decigram, gram, kilogram

## Check Up 7.5

1.5 mL

3 mL

2.25 mL

## Check Up 7.6

**1.** Multiply

**2.** Divide

    **3.** Divide

    **4.** Divide

    **5.** Multiply

    **6.** 350 mg

    **7.** 500 mg

    **8.** 125 mg

### Check Up 7.7

    **1.** 1000

    **2.** 1000

    **3.** 15

    **4.** 15

    **5.** 60

    **6.** 60

    **7.** 1/15

    **8.** 1/15

    **9.** 1/1000

    **10.** 1/1000

    **11.** 1/60

    **12.** 1/60

## ■ CHAPTER 8

### Check Up 8.1: ratio and proportion

    **1.** 0.5 mL

    **2.** 3 mL

    **3.** 1 mL

    **4.** 3 mL

    **5.** 2 tablets

    **6.** 0.5 mL

    **7.** 3 mL

    **8.** 1 mL

    **9.** 3 mL

    **10.** 2 tablets

### Check Up 8.2: formulation method

    **1.** 2 mL

    **2.** 1/2 tablet

    **3.** 1 capsule

    **4.** 2 oz

    **5.** 45.5 kg

    **6.** 1 mL

    **7.** 0.5 or 1/2 tablet

    **8.** 1 mL

**9.** 2 tablets

**10.** 2 bottles

## Check Up 8.3: dimensional analysis

**1.** 1 mL

**2.** 2 mL

**3.** 0.5 mL

**4.** 3 mL

**5.** 2.5 mL

## Check Up 8.4: dimensional analysis

$$15 \text{ mL} \times \frac{1 \text{ teaspoon}}{\textbf{5 mL}} = 3 \text{ teaspoons}$$

## Check Up 8.5: fraction method

**1.** 0.5 mL

**2.** 2 tablets

**3.** 0.5 oz

**4.** 2 capsules

**5.** 0.5 bottle

## Check Up 8.6: fraction method to verify results

**1.** False

**2.** True

**3.** True

**4.** False

**5.** True

## Check Up 8.7: pediatric dosages

**1.** 91 mg/day

**2.** 30 mg per dose

**3.** 182 mg/day

**4.** 45.5 mg/dose

**5.** Two

**6.** 227 mg/dose

**7.** 681 mg/day

**8.** 455 mg/dose

**9.** 1820 mg/day

## Check Up 8.8: body surface area (BSA)

**1.** 0.18 $m^2$

**2.** 0.6 $m^2$

**3.** 0.42 $m^2$

**4.** 0.165 $m^2$

**5.** 0.32 $m^2$

### Check Up 8.9: reconstitution of powdered medications

**1.** 4 mL

**2.** 250 mg/5 mL

**3.** 1.7 mL

**4.** 250 mg/1mL

**5.** 33 mL

**6.** 500,000 units/mL

**7.** 19 mL

**8.** 10 mg/mL

### Check Up 8.10: IV electronic milligrams per hour

**1.** 333 mL/hour

**2.** 250 mL/hour

**3.** 250 mL/hour

**4.** 250 mL/hour

**5.** 50 mL/hour

### Check Up 8.11: manual IV rate calculations

**1.** 10 gtt/min

**2.** 14 gtt/min

**3.** 50 gtt/min

**4.** 23 gtt/min

**5.** 17 gtt/min

### Check Up 8.12: intake calculations

**1.** John exceeded his fluid restriction by 80 mL:

$$
\begin{aligned}
10 \times 30 \text{ mL} &= 300 \text{ mL} \\
10 \times 30 \text{ mL} &= 300 \text{ mL} \\
8 \times 30 \text{ mL} &= 240 \text{ mL} \\
8 \times 30 \text{ mL} &= \underline{240 \text{ mL}} \\
& \quad\; 1080 \text{ mL}
\end{aligned}
$$

**2.** Kathy met her goal of 1200 mL:

$$
\begin{aligned}
12 \times 30 \text{ mL} &= 360 \text{ mL} \\
12 \times 30 \text{ mL} &= 360 \text{ mL} \\
8 \times 30 \text{ mL} &= 240 \text{ mL} \\
8 \times 30 \text{ mL} &= \underline{240 \text{ mL}} \\
& \quad\; 1200 \text{ mL}
\end{aligned}
$$

# INDEX

## A